FOOD ALLERGY

Food Allergy

Editors

Dietrich Reinhardt   Eberhard Schmidt

Department of Pediatrics
University of Düsseldorf
Düsseldorf, Federal Republic of Germany

Nestlé Nutrition
Workshop Series
Volume 17

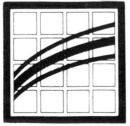

NESTLÉ NUTRITION

RAVEN PRESS ■ NEW YORK

Nestec Ltd., Avenue Nestlé, 1800 Vevey, Switzerland
Raven Press, Ltd., 1185 Avenue of the Americas, New York,
New York 10036

Made in the United States of America

Library of Congress Cataloging-in-Publication Data

Food allergy.
   (Nestlé Nutrition workshop series ; v. 17)
   Includes bibliographical references and index.
   1. Food allergy.   I. Schmidt, Eberhardt.   II. Nestlé Nutrition
S.A.   III. Series
RC596.F654   1988   616.97′5   88-42557
ISBN 0-88167-438-9 (Raven Press)

The material contained in this volume was submitted as previously
unpublished material, except in the instances in which credit has been given to
the source from which some of the illustrative material was derived.

Great care has been taken to maintain the accuracy of the information
contained in the volume. However, neither Nestec nor Raven Press can be held
responsible for errors or for any consequences arising from the use of the
information contained herein.

9 8 7 6 5 4 3 2 1

Preface

Pediatric allergology has experienced increasing importance within pediatric subspecialties, whether it be the cause or the consequence of increasing incidence of allergic diseases in childhood. In this context, several efforts have been undertaken to elucidate the role of nutrition in infancy in causing or preventing atopic disease, mainly in infants with a high genetic risk.

The contributions of this workshop attempt to pinpoint the scientific background of early atopic disease, focusing especially on the possibilities of nutritional interventions. The concept of reduction of allergen content in special formulas, hitherto only applied in dietetic therapy, is an interesting prospect in regard to dietetic prophylaxes. Solutions in this direction will be a first step toward opening the possibility for clinical trials on dietetic prophylaxes of atopic disease in early infancy and in determining the possible role of these dietetic prophylaxes in long-term prevention.

E. SCHMIDT
D. REINHARDT

Foreword

The importance of giving the right type of food to atopic babies was recognized many decades ago; however, for a long time, pediatric allergologists and gastroenterologists were not particularly interested in the early diagnosis of atopic predisposition, since there had been no simple method of preventing food allergy manifestations. This situation was mainly due to the general consensus that soya protein was as allergenic as cow's milk protein and to the confusing number of publications reporting that breast-feeding did not give protection.

The recent confirmation that foreign protein could pass unchanged into mother's milk, that the level of secretory IgA was low in the atopic mother's milk, and that the exclusion of foreign protein should be prolonged and total helped explain many failures of prophylaxis of atopic manifestations by breast-feeding. The conditions under which breast-feeding can be protective are now better defined and, together with the recent development of "hypoallergenic starter formula" with an acceptable taste and a competitive price, an interest has been regenerated in early diagnosis of atopic children. In addition, new studies are being undertaken in the field of food allergy.

We believe that the findings of this Nestlé Nutrition Workshop on food allergy, summarizing the knowledge on this topic, will be used for many years to come as a basis for measuring the progress made in this now fast-moving subject.

PIERRE R. GUESRY, M.D.
Vice President
Nestlé Products Technical Assistance Co. Ltd.

Contents

Contributors

Kjell Aas
Rikshospitalet Universitetsklinik
Boks 50, Voksenkollen
0326 Oslo 3, Norway

Joseph A. Bellanti
Departments of Pediatrics and
*   Microbiology*
Georgetown University
School of Medicine
Washington, D.C. 20007

A. Blanco Quiros
Hospital Clinico Universitario
Valladolid, Spain

D. Blum
Pediatric Sleep Laboratory and
*   Department of Immunology*
Free University of Brussels
1090 Brussels, Belgium

J.L. Bresson
Department of Pediatrics
Hôpital des Enfants Malades
75015 Paris, France

Jonathan Brostoff
The Middlesex Hospital
London, W1N 8AA, England

Andrew J. Cant
Department of Paediatrics
Guy's Hospital Medical School
St. Thomas Street
London SE1 9RT, England

G. Casimir
Pediatric Sleep Laboratory and
*   Department of Immunology*
Free University of Brussels
1090 Brussels, Belgium

Michel Deneyer
Academic Children's Hospital
Free University of Brussels
1090 Brussels, Belgium

Alain L. de Weck
Institute for Clinical Immunology
Inselspital Bern
3010 Bern, Switzerland

J. Duchateau
Pediatric Sleep Laboratory and
*   Department of Immunology*
Free University of Brussels
1090 Brussels, Belgium

Paolo Durand
Istituto Giannina Gaslini
Via V Maggio 39
16147 Genoa, Italy

J. Egger
Universitätskinderklinik
Lindwurmstr. 4
8000 Munich 2, West Germany

Ahmed El-Rafei
International Center for Interdisciplinary
*   Studies of Immunology*
Georgetown University
School of Medicine
Washington, D.C. 20007

M. Eran
Pediatric Research Laboratories
Shaare Zedek Medical Center
Jerusalem 91-000, Israel

S. Freier
Pediatric Research Laboratories
Shaare Zedek Medical Center
P.O. Box 293
Jerusalem 91-000, Israel

Oscar L. Frick
University of California
San Francisco, California

R. Gerke
Department of Pediatrics
University of Düsseldorf
4000 Düsseldorf 1, West Germany

D. Granato
Nestlé Research Department
Nestec Ltd.
1000 Lausanne 26, Switzerland

Nick Harris
Departments of Pediatrics and
Microbiology
Georgetown University
School of Medicine
Washington, D.C. 20007

I. Jakobsson
Malmö General Hospital
21401 Malmö, Sweden

R. Jost
Nestlé Research Department
Nestec Ltd.
Vers-chez-les-Blanc
1000 Lausanne 26, Switzerland

A. Kahn
Hôpital Universitaire des Enfants
AV. JJ Crocq 15
1020 Bruxelles, Belgium

D. Kaiserlian
Pavillon P
Hôpital Edouard Herriot
69374 Lyon Cedex 08, France

M.D. Kemeny
Department of Internal Medicine
Guy's Hospital Medical School
London SE1 9RT, England

N.-I. Max Kjellman
Department of Pediatrics
Linköping University Hospital
58185 Linköping, Sweden

S. Lafont
Pavillon P
Hôpital Edouard Herriot
69374 Lyon Cedex 08, France

Helmuth Loeb
Academic Children's Hospital
Free University of Brussels
1090 Brussels, Belgium

F. Lorenz
University Children's Hospital
4000 Düsseldorf 1, West Germany

M.J. Mozin
Pediatric Sleep Laboratory and
Department of Immunology
Free University of Brussels
1090 Brussels, Belgium

J.J. Pahud
Nestlé Research Department
Nestec Ltd.
Vers-chez-les-Blanc
1000 Lausanne 26, Switzerland

Stephen M. Peters
Departments of Pediatrics and
Microbiology
Georgetown University
School of Medicine
Washington, D.C. 20007

E. Rebuffat
Pediatric Sleep Laboratory and
Department of Immunology
Free University of Brussels
1090 Brussels, Belgium

D. Reinhardt
Department of Pediatrics
University of Düsseldorf
Moorenstrasse 5
4000 Düsseldorf 1, West Germany

J.P. Revillard
Pavillon P
Hôpital Edouard Herriot
69374 Lyon Cedex 08, France

Johannes Ring
*Dermatologische Klinik und Poliklinik
der Ludwig-Maximilians-Universität
8000 Munich 2, Federal Republic of
Germany*

Liliane Sacre
*Academic Children's Hospital
Free University of Brussels
1090 Brussels, Belgium*

E. Sanchez Villares
*Hospital Clinico Universitario
Valladolid, Spain*

Glenis K. Scadding
*The Middlesex Hospital
Mortimer Street
London W1N 8AA, England*

E. Schmidt
*Department of Pediatrics
University of Düsseldorf
4000 Düsseldorf 1, West Germany*

J. Schmitz
*Department of Pediatrics
Hôpital des Enfants Malades
149 rue de Sèvres
75015 Paris, France*

K. Schwarz
*Nestlé Research Department
Nestec Ltd.
1000 Lausanne 26, Switzerland*

M. Seid
*University Children's Hospital
4000 Düsseldorf 1, West Germany*

Stephan Strobel
*Institute of Child Health
University of London
30 Guiford Street
London WC1N 1EH, U.K.*

Y. Suranyi
*Pediatric Research Laboratories
Shaare Zedek Medical Center
Jerusalem 91-000, Israel*

R. Tangermann
*University Children's Hospital
4000 Düsseldorf 1, West Germany*

R. Urbanek
*Universität-Kinderklinik Freiburg
Mathildenstr. 1
7800 Freiburg, West Germany*

Yvan Vandenplas
*Academic Children's Hospital
Free University of Brussels
Laarbecklaan 101
1090 Brussels, Belgium*

J.K. Visakorpi
*Department of Clinical Sciences
University of Tampere
33101 Tampere 10, Finland*

U. Wahn
*Children's Hospital
Free University of Berlin
Fachbereich 3
Heubnerweg 6
1000 Berlin 19, West Germany*

V. Wahn
*University Children's Hospital
Moorenstrasse 5
4000 Düsseldorf 1, Federal Republic of
Germany*

W. Allan Walker
*Department of Pediatrics
Harvard Medical School
Boston, Massachusetts 02115; and
Chief, Combined Program in Pediatric
Gastroenterology and Nutrition
Children's Hospital and Massachusetts
General Hospital
Boston, Massachusetts 02181*

Invited Attendees

T. Abdeslam/*Tanger, Morocco*
F. Argüelles Martín/*Sevilla, Spain*
M. Atmodjo/*Indonesia*
K. Baerlocher/*St. Gallen, Switzerland*
A.F. Bakken/*Oslo, Norway*
C.P. Bauer/*Munich, West Germany*
N. Benincori/*Italy*
H. Berger/*Innsbruck, Austria*
C. Billeaud/*Bordeaux, France*
M. Bowie/*South Africa*
P.B. Calderón/*Valladolid, Spain*
G. Casimir/*Brussels, Belgium*
P. Chairuddin/*Indonesia*
D.N. Challacombe/*Taunton, Great Britain*
G. Couillaud/*Dijon, France*
J.P. Chouraqui/*Grenoble, France*
J. Cousin/*Lille, France*
B. Descos/*Lyon, France*
E. Eggermont/*Leuven, Belgium*
M.M. Esteban/*Madrid, Spain*
M. Fall/*Dakar, Senegal*
F. Fernàndez de las Heras/*Valladolid, Spain*
H. Gaze/*Neuchâtel, Switzerland*
A.A. Gerung/*Indonesia*
J. Ghisolfi/*Toulouse, France*
J. Glatzl/*Innsbruck, Austria*
M. Goetz/*Vienna, Austria*
F. Haschke/*Vienna, Austria*
G. Hendrickx/*Lommel, Belgium*
I. Jakobsson/*Malmö, Sweden*
A.S. Kemp/*Sydney, Australia*
J. Leclercq/*Liège, Belgium*
M. Lentze/*Bern, Switzerland*

J. Leroy/*Gent, Belgium*
H. Loeb/*Brussels, Belgium*
F. Macagno/*Italy*
A. Marini/*Milano, Italy*
C. Maurage/*Tours, France*
A. Miadonna/*Italy*
S.K. Mittal/*New Delhi, India*
A. Morali/*Nancy, France*
J.-C. Mouterde/*Rouen, France*
J. Navarro/*Paris, France*
D. Nusslé/*Geneva, Switzerland*
O. Østerballe/*Viborg, Denmark*
J.S. Partana/*Indonesia*
L. Partana/*Indonesia*
P. Reinert/*Paris, France*
J. Rey/*Paris, France*
M. Rieu/*Montpellier, France*
L. Ros Mar/*Zaragoza, Spain*
E. Rossipal/*Graz, Austria*
G. Salvioli/*Bologna, Italy*
E. Sànchez y Sànchez-Villares/*Valladolid, Spain*
P. Saye/*Liège, Belgium*
R. Seger/*Zürich, Switzerland*
D.H. Shmerling/*Zürich, Switzerland*
A. Signoretti/*Roma, Italy*
P. Solis Sanchez/*Valladolid, Spain*
A. Ugazio/*Brescia, Italy*
I.B. Umoh/*Calabar, Nigeria*
B.D. Van Caillie/*Antwerpe, Belgium*
J.-C. Vitoria Cormenzana/*Bilbao, Spain*
K. Widhalm/*Vienna, Austria*
M. Willems/*Brussels, Belgium*

Nestlé Participants

P.R. Guesry
Vice President
Nestec, Vevey, Switzerland

P. Goyens
Nestec
Vevey, Switzerland

M.-C. Secretin
Nestec
Vevey, Switzerland
U. Preysch
SPN Zürich, Switzerland
A. Reith
SPN Zürich, Switzerland
K. De Block
Nestlé Belgilux SA.
M.J. Mozin
Nestlé Belgilux SA.
C. De Prelle
Nestlé Belgilux SA.
M.O. Gailing
Dietina Courbevoie, France

L. Morhedec
Dietina Courbevoie, France
L. Franguelli
Nestlé Italiana SpA., Italy
A. Latronico
Nestlé Italiana SpA., Italy
C. Conill
Sociedad Nestlé A.E.P.A.
Barcelona, Spain
F.J. Dorca
Sociedad Nestlé A.E.P.A.
Barcelona, Spain
M. Romano
Sociedad Nestlé A.E.P.A.
Barcelona, Spain

Nestlé Nutrition Workshop Series

Food Allergy, edited by Eberhardt Schmidt.
Nestlé Nutrition Workshop Series, Vol. 17.
Nestec Ltd., Vevey/Raven Press, Ltd.,
New York © 1988.

The Biochemistry of Food Allergens: What Is Essential for Future Research?

Kjell Aas

*Voksentoppen Allergy and Asthma Institute, Rikshospitalet University Hospital,
0326 Oslo 3, Norway*

In this presentation the topic of food allergens is approached from an angle different from that of comprehensive reviews. A number of such reviews are available (1–5). Together with a recent book on food allergy (6) they compile almost everything about food allergens that is worth knowing—and some information that is not so valuable. The present discussion is concerned only with IgE-mediated allergy and natural allergens found in food. It does not take into consideration possible antigenicity of additives used for preservation, flavoring, or food cosmetic purposes.

DEFINITION OF TERMS USED

Scientific work and clinical work in the study of allergy must both satisfy strict criteria with regard to specificity and precision. Thus it appears appropriate to be specific and precise with respect to the terms and definitions used.

Allergy is used in the context of hypersensitivity reactions caused by immune reactions that are harmful to the tissues or disruptive of the physiology of the host. The immune reaction triggers complex biochemical and/or inflammatory responses that result in clinical symptoms. These responses are dependent on the degree of reactivity of the involved tissue receptors and of the effector cells.

Allergen indicates the antigenic molecule that takes part in the immune reaction resulting in allergy. *Food allergen* indicates allergens found in food.

Allergenic source indicates the material (or food) that contains allergens.

Immunogen indicates the molecule (or part of it) that is able to initiate proliferation of immunocompetent lymphocytes or trigger the synthesis of specific antibodies.

ISOLATED ALLERGENS

In recent years many allergen sources have been studied. A wide variety of allergens have been isolated and characterized. The list of isolated allergens has become too long to be given here. The time has come to bring order to a rather chaotic situation concerning allergen nomenclature. Those interested are referred to the nomenclature system advocated by the International Union of Immunological Societies (IUIS) presented in the Bulletin of the World Health Organization 1986 (7).

FOOD ALLERGENS ARE (MOSTLY) PROTEINS

All natural allergens that react with IgE antibodies have, so far, been shown to be proteins.

A protein is made up of a number of amino acids bound together in peptide linkages with or without additional carbohydrate residues in the primary structure. Each amino acid is characterized by its side chain. The side chains together represent chemically active sites and contribute to the final shape and the power field of the molecule. The chain or sequence of amino acids is twisted and is given its final shape through conformational changes resulting from the chemical forces between the side chains, which then fold the molecule into its tertiary structure. Chemical forces from outside also influence the final shape and the net chemical power of the molecule.

The amino acids can, in a way, be said to act as letters in a *chemical* alphabet containing 20 different letters. Different combinations of these chemical letters create a multitude of words (peptide fragments) and phrases (proteins) in the language of protein chemistry. Some of the words are made by the amino acid letters as found in the original sequence of the chain. These words are sequential denominators. Other words are made when amino acid "letters" that are remote in the primary sequence chain are brought close together by folding of the chain. These words are conformational denominators.

The complexity of proteins found in allergen sources and in extracts of allergenic foods is well demonstrated by a number of techniques: Sodium docedyl sulfate polyacrylamide gel electrophoresis (SDS-PAGE); isoelectrofocusing (IEF); and PAGE or starch gel electrophoresis with immunoprinting and crossed radioimmunoelectrophoresis (CRIE). A wide variety of modifications of these and similar methods have been used, and new methods are being invented. We can rightly speak about *immunoacrobatics* in this connection. Combined with each other and, for example, with immunosorbent techniques, as well as by means of selected patients' sera, monospecific antisera may be produced to almost any of the allergenic components in food. The monoclonal antibody technique adds further possibilities for research in the field (8). Progress in protein separation methods has been an important propagator. Many possibilities have been opened for those interested.

I am not saying that this is easy work! On the contrary, it is a demanding, tedious, and time-consuming process full of challenges, problems, and pitfalls. If we want to spent time and resources on it, we ought to consider our ultimate goals with this kind of work. An isolated and well-characterized allergen is not a goal in itself but only a tool of value for further research. Then we have to ask ourselves: What is essential for future research with regard to food allergy? Answers to this question should influence (a) what food allergens we select for study and (b) the research protocol in allergen purification and characterization.

MAJOR, INTERMEDIATE, AND MINOR ALLERGENS

Only one or very few of the several proteins found in a given allergen source act as essential allergens in the majority of allergic patients. The most important ones are called *major allergens*. Less important allergens, statistically speaking, are called *intermediate allergens* and *minor allergens*. It should be kept in mind that a so-called "minor allergen" may play a major role in rare individual patients.

CRIE can be used to define these terms more precisely in order to promote meaningful communication, provided that a CRIE reference system is included (9). A *major allergen* is then defined as one that binds IgE antibodies in 50% or more of sera from all the patients allergic to the matter, with strong binding in at least 25% of the sera. A *minor allergen* binds IgE antibodies in not more than 10% of the sera from the same patient population. Allergens with binding capacities between these two are called *intermediate allergens*. Most, if not all, allergen sources seem to contain several distinct allergens of major, intermediate, or minor importance. The egg white in hen's egg, for example, is a complex mixture of at least 20 distinct proteins, but only four or five of them are allergenic (10,11).

Blands et al. (12) demonstrated 40 antigens in wheat flour. Eighteen of them were able to bind IgE, and three were considered to be major allergens. Theobald et al. (13), in a study of the sera from patients with "bakers's asthma," concluded that IgE and IgG antibodies seemed to react with the same components in wheat. A clear-cut distinction between antigens and allergens was not obtained in their study. Baldo et al. (14) found a high degree of allergenic cross-reactivity between several cereals, particularly between wheat, rye, barley, and oats. All the studies were concerned with inhalant allergies to flour, and the results are not necessarily applicable to cereals in food. Some individuals allergic to wheat in food tolerate moderate amounts of gluten-free cereals, whereas others do not. This suggests that some, but not all, major or intermediate allergens in wheat are removed or inactivated by the processing of gluten-free cereals.

Cow's milk contains more than 25 distinct proteins that may act as antigens in humans, and a few more antigenic characteristics may arise during the intestinal passage. Absorption of antigenic molecules leads to antibody production. Increased absorption results in more prominent immune response and higher serum concentration of antibodies to milk components. Most of the antibodies do no harm; they are only innocent waste products and can, in a sense, be compared with sewage from the immunocompetent cell populations in the host.

The antigenicity differs from protein to protein and seems to depend on host factors as well as a combination of genetic, environmental, and adjuvant factors.

This applies also to allergens. The most important allergens are found in beta-lactoglobulin (60–80% of cow's milk allergic patients), casein (60%), lactalbumin (50%), and bovine serum albumin (50%) according to several investigators. Others claim that bovine serum albumin, casein, and bovine gammaglobulin rank the highest.

WHAT MAKES AN ALLERGEN AN ALLERGEN?

One may ask why some proteins act as strong allergens while others in the same food do not. Casein is by far the most prominent protein in cow's milk but is not as important in allergy as beta-lactoglobulin, which represents approximately 10% of the total protein. In hen's egg, one could get the idea that the proteins found in the highest concentrations may be the most important ones in allergy. Ovalbumin, which constitutes more than half of the total protein in the egg white, is the most important allergen. Lysozyme, however, is a very weak allergen even though it represents as much as 3.5% to 10% of the total protein.

It has not been possible to point out any physicochemical feature that is characteristic of major allergens reacting with IgE antibodies except for the fact that these allergens are proteins with a molecular weight usually between 10,000 and 100,000 daltons. Theoretically, there may be physicochemical traits that are important for the transport through living membranes, for passage of biochemical barriers, or for phagocyte handling without being directly related to antigenicity. Genetic host factors are probably as important as the molecular structure (4).

Those who study the classic scientific literature may easily become confused or be led astray. As evaluated today, some of the documentation has been confirmed, some has been shown to be only partially true, and some has been dismissed as being wrong. During one period (1960–1970) it was, for example, claimed that sugar moieties and N-glycosidic bonding elements were mandatory for allergenic activity. To study this, one has to work with completely pure allergen systems. The N-glycosidic bond theory was, however, a result of generalizations from studies with a restricted number of impure systems. These are pitfalls that many have fallen into. You may find many examples of this in the literature in question. Using a pure system we could show in 1971 that N-glycosidic bonds are not necessary for the allergic reaction as such.

DENATURATION AND DIGESTION

Identification of allergens in a given food starts with a crude extract of the matter. This involves the risk that some allergenic components are not represented in the original form or not at all in the extract. Some of them may be insoluble and lost in the sediment if the latter is not examined. Others may be present in an altered form. Denaturation and inactivation with respect to IgE binding may occur during the preparation of the extract. This occurs, for example, for some fruit allergens, as demonstrated by Bjørksten et al. (15).

Furthermore, the processes of fractionation and isolation of protein molecules imply great risks of inducing alterations in the conformation and charges of some of the molecules in question. The molecular folding and charge of proteins are influenced by forces exerted on them from the environmental electrolytes and other proteins. Dilution itself may induce marked changes. This may or may not affect the antigenicity of the molecule.

It is more likely than not that isolation and dilution will induce some changes in the allergenic molecules you try to purify. In fact, for a large number of allergens, you may find that a given fraction with all signs of immunologic homogeneity may be separated in an electrical field if you use the right kind of medium and buffer (or, in your opinion, the wrong kind). Such so-called *isoallergens* are antigenically identical molecules that migrate slightly differently in an electrical field. They may well represent molecules from the same origin which are slightly changed in conformation and charge during the separation manipulations, but the changes do not affect the antigenic sites.

Questions about the degree of resistance to denaturation and digestion are especially important for food allergens. Clinical observations indicate this. Thus many patients have fierce allergic reactions to fresh but not to cooked apples, carrots, and potatoes. A large number of bakers get allergic asthma or allergic rhinitis as occupational diseases from inhaling flour dust, but they tolerate the same cereals in the food.

Many of the allergens in question may be very susceptible to denaturation during preparation of the food. With regard to allergens in apples, for instance, inactivation may occur as soon as the apple is cut and crushed. The fruit contains phenolic compounds and enzymes that tend to denaturate the allergenic molecules quickly on manipulation. Apple allergens could, however, be extracted in active form with media containing agents which inhibit the phenol-protein reactions (15). Phenols combine with proteins by oxidation and hydrogen bonding. This results in denaturation with alterations of the antigenic properties of some molecules.

On the other hand, such foods as hen's eggs, peanuts, nuts, peas, fish, and seafood elicit allergic reactions almost irrespective of what you do to the food in question. They provoke allergic reactions even when found as steam droplets from the food being cooked or fried. New antigenic forms may be created during cooking and/or digestion and may be important in very rare cases. Küstner, in 1921, who delivered his serum for the first scientific demonstration of the presence of circulating reaginic antibodies associated with allergy, claimed that he reacted to fish only after it had been cooked. This suggests that allergenic sites not present in the original fish proteins were formed or made accessible only by denaturation. Küstner must have been quite unique in this respect. I myself have seen hundreds of fish-allergenic patients and all of them react both to raw and cooked fish proteins.

In other words, the antigenic determinants in question in some food allergens are affected and inactivated by denaturation and digestion. Others are not affected; they maintain the allergenic activity. Here we have arrived at something essential in the discussion of the biochemistry of food allergens.

EPITOPES (ANTIGENIC/ALLERGENIC DETERMINANTS)

The antibody (or immune receptor of an immunocompetent lymphocyte) binds specifically to a very limited part of the antigenic molecule. This binding site is called an *epitope or antigenic determinant*. In this review an *allergenic* determinant or epitope means an epitope in the IgE system. All proteins may be considered to be complex mosaics of epitopes—comparable, in a sense, to short or long words in the language of protein chemistry. Some feature may be decisive, others less so, as seen from the antibody viewpoint. Some components may act only as necessary spacing elements keeping the essential denominators at an optimal distance from each other, or they may take part through more or less essential binding forces. The factors that may determine the potency of the particular allergen, making it a major, intermediate, or minor allergen, are (a) the number of allergenic epitopes that are accessible for the specific antibodies and (b) the binding dynamics of these epitopes and antibodies.

CROSS-REACTIVITIES

A number of the proteins present in a given food may have some epitopes in common, as demonstrated for wheat flour by Theobald et al. (13) using monocolonal antibodies. This accounts for immunological cross-reactivities between different proteins within a given food as well as between different related food. Thus, patients allergic to the major allergen (Allergen M) in codfish therefore react also to haddock and carp white-muscle proteins. In fish allergy, some patients react to all fish species tested for, whereas other exhibit a marked species differentiation (16,17). Some patients who react to both codfish and salmon apparently have IgE antibodies reacting with identical allergenic epitopes on proteins found both in codfish and salmon. In other patients there are, however, quite distinct sensitizations to different allergens (epitopes) in the two species of fish.

Cross-reactivities are also found between eggs of different birds (11), between different seafoods (18), and between many other foods within the same order. Cross-reactivities are also found between certain pollen and vegetables/fruits (19).

CONFORMATIONAL AND SEQUENTIAL EPITOPES

Most epitopes are thought to be conformational. They result from the steric folding of the amino-acid–peptide chains. The folding of the molecule brings together important amino acids that are found quite remote in the amino acid sequence chain as such. Denaturation of the protein will usually alter the folding and break up this kind of epitope. Laboratory manipulation during protein fractionation may have similar effects, thus making it extremely difficult to identify essential epitopes. It is still more difficult to synthesize such epitopes.

A number of epitopes are sequential. They are organized from a number of amino acids (with or without sugar moieties) as found in the original linear sequence. They may be picked out directly from the amino acid sequence of the protein. This type of epitope often remains unchanged following denaturation of the protein and may be left untouched by enzymes not specific for amino acid bonds present within the epitope. Sequential epitopes lend themselves much more easily to identification and synthesization.

THE CODFISH ALLERGEN MODEL

The observation that the allergenic activity of hen's egg white, peas, and fish is unaffected by cooking and digestion in human intestines suggests that these foods contain major allergens with sequential epitopes. To begin with, it is wise to select such material for purification and characterization purposes. This is what I myself thought when I wanted to pick a model for molecular research in the immunology of allergic reactions.

An infant with severe atopic symptoms was admitted to my department. He had been solely breast-fed but suffered from atopic eczema, bronchial asthma, and bouts of severe angioedema and diarrhea. We could demonstrate that he was excessively sensitive to fish and that he got worse every time his mother had eaten fish herself.

The allergenic molecules in question had resisted cooking (denaturation) followed by digestion (proteolysis) in the mother's intestines, passage through several membranes (to the breast milk), and a second digestion in the infant's intestines. They were still active when reaching reaginic antibodies in various tissues in the infant. From these observations, the allergenic molecules in question had to be associated with sequential units of amino acids and could probably be found in rather short fragments. I wanted a model for investigation of what makes an allergen an allergen, and here the case history of the infant told me about a suitable model.

I selected codfish for this purpose and started a tedious protein fractionation and purification process including quite a number of trials and failures before succeeding. Codfish contains one major allergen (Allergen M) found in the white-muscle tissues. All the codfish-allergic patients I have seen react to this allergen. Codfish white muscle also contains other intermediate and minor allergens and so does the blood serum of the fish. In the most sensitive patient systems the purified allergen was extremely potent. It provoked marked local whealing reactions in passive transfer or so-called Prausnitz-Küstner tests (PK test) in concentrations corresponding to less than 10,000 molecules injected into the sensitized sites. Double-blind food challenges with microgram quantities given to the PK-test recipients provoked similar reactions. The latter experiments confirmed that the purified allergen was also absorbed in an active form through normal adult intestines. The major allergen is heat stable and quite resistant to proteolytic digestion and several denaturation procedures. This supported the idea that the allergenic activity is found in a linear sequence.

The purified allergen turned out to be a valuable tool for performing further work in basic study, as well as clinical study, within the immunology of allergy. Thus, it was shown that most of the IgG antibodies to codfish in patients' sera reacted with proteins other than the major allergen in question. Furthermore, some IgG antibodies (both human and rabbit) binding to the allergenic molecule reacted with the allergenic epitope as such, whereas others reacted with other epitopes on the same molecule. This is an important point in discussions about the role played by so-called *blocking antibodies*. It appears that only those blocking antibodies that react with the allergenic epitope as such are likely to affect the *in vivo* synthesis of the IgE antibodies in question. These antibodies could be referred to as *"allergenic epitope blocking antibodies"*.

AN ALLERGENIC EPITOPE

The amino acid sequence of the purified allergen was analyzed. This provided enough material to propose the hypothetical model for a sequential allergenic determinant (IgE-binding epitope) presented during the 1975 Nobel symposium in Stockholm (3). This hypothetical model has subsequently been substantiated and confirmed. It was based on the assumption that the epitope may be formed by a few critical amino acid side chains found in a sequence while one or several amino acids, acting only as rather indifferent spacers, keep the critical amino acids at the optimal distance from each other.

Furthermore, at that time it had become evident that the biological reaction in IgE-mediated allergy was brought about when the allergen bound two IgE antibody molecules on the surface of mast cells or basophils. To be allergenically active the allergen had to have at least two accessible allergenic determinants, probably of identical composition. Assuming this, the molecule in question could have six (or even more) allergenic determinants (IgE-binding epitopes) composed of two closely connected carboxylic side chains (ASP + GLU) kept at a critical distance from the basic residue (LYS). According to this the sequences (-ASP-GLU-LEU-LYS-), (-ASP-GLU-ASP-LYS-), and possibly (-ASP-ASP-LYS) stood out as particularly interesting candidates. The same constellations could possibly also occur as conformational units (Fig. 1). Short enzymatic cleavage products from the native Allergen M resulted in peptides containing ASP-GLU-LEU-LYS and ASP-GLU-ASP-LYS, which were allergenically active.

Preliminary efforts to synthesize such a tetrapeptide rendered a molecule that was only partially able to block PK-test reactions to the major allergen. At this

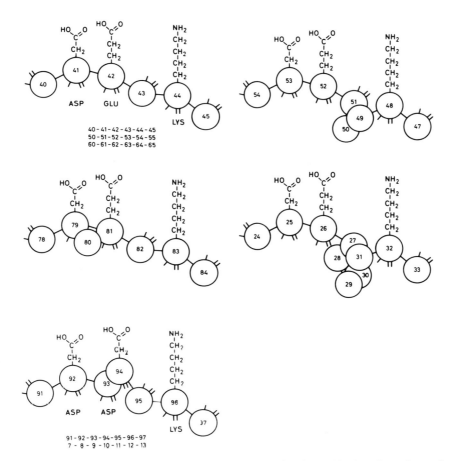

FIG. 1. Sequential and conformational combinations of amino acids thought to form allergenic epitopes in Allergen M of codfish.

point I had to abandon molecular and immunological research in order to devote most of my time to other tasks. The molecular research work was, however, carried on by my former collaborators.

The region composed of residues 41 through 64 of Allergen M encompassed three of the tetrapeptides described, kept apart by two segments of six variable amino acid residues. Elsayed and co-workers (20,21) produced synthetic peptides corresponding to the peptides in question. A peptide composed of 16 amino acids corresponding to residues 49 through 64 of Allergen M was produced by solid-phase synthesis (SPS). This hexadecapeptide bound IgE antibodies in the sera from cod-allergic patients. The peptide interfered also with rabbit antiserum IgC antibodies to Allergen M (20,21). The nature of the interspacing amino acids appeared to be without significance.

IMPLICATIONS FOR FUTURE RESEARCH

At least two of the epitopes in question are necessary for the binding to IgE antibodies in biological tests of allergy to codfish. Immunogenicity for IgE antibody synthesis in predisposed individuals probably demands only one epitope. Theoretically, a carrier substance may be provided by the host itself (i.e., as serum albumin or heparin). In any case, extremely small fragments containing one epitope would suffice for sensitization of a disposed individual. Then it is not likely that sensitization depends on the degree of permeability of the gut but rather on a combination of genetic and adjuvant factors in the host.

Peptides of the kind described could serve as valuable tools for molecular and cellular studies in this field. The availability of synthetic peptides that represent the allergenic determinants of natural allergens may open the field for studies involving variable fragments, the effects of amino acid substitution, the effects of conjugation to various carrier substances, and so on. This kind of information may serve as a useful key to some of the hidden mysteries of immune reactions in allergy. It may also prove valuable in efforts to unveil mechanisms of induction, as well as of suppression, of the immune responses in question.

There is, however, no room for generalization. The codfish allergen model functions only for certain limited aspects of our many scientific problems. Other food allergens may behave in quite different ways at different levels of immune responsiveness and responses.

Conformational allergenic determinants are probably more common than sequential ones. They are much more demanding with respect to characterization and synthesization. To me it is surprising that the codfish allergen model is—after 10 years—still the only one for which important epitopes have been defined. There are many other food allergens that most probably contain sequential epitopes that could be defined as well.

Allergens in hen's egg white, for example, are tempting targets for such studies. In fact, more than 75 years have elapsed since Schloss indicated this through his elegant investigations of the biochemistry of egg-white allergens (22). Availability of synthetic epitopes reacting with human IgE antibodies may provide tools for important research at the very basis of the immune reactions in question. Indeed, we need much more knowledge of this kind for all types of allergen, particularly in the confusing field of intolerance and allergy to food.

REFERENCES

1. Bleumink E. Food allergy. The chemical nature of the substances eliciting symptoms. *World Rev Nutr Diet* 1970;12:505–70.
2. King TP. Chemical and biological properties of some atopic allergens. *Adv Immunol* 1976;23: 77–105.
3. Aas K. Common characteristics of major allergens. In: Johansson SGO and Strandberg K, eds. *Molecular and biological aspects of the acute allergic reaction,* New York: Plenum, 1976:3–19.

4. Aas K. What makes an allergen an allergen. *Allergy* 1978;33:3–14.
5. Aas K. Die Natur der Allergene. *Die gelben Hefte* 1980;20:77–85.
6. Brostoff J, Challacombe SJ, eds. *Food allergy and intolerance.* London: Baillière Tindall, 1987.
7. IUIS Sub-Committee for Allergen Nomenclature: Allergen nomenclature. *Bull WHO* 1986;64:767–70.
8. DeBlas AL, Cherwinski HM. Detection of antigens on nitrocellulose paper immunoblots with monoclonal antibodies. *Ann Biochem* 1983;133:314–7.
9. Aukrust L, Aas K. A reference system in crossed radioimmunoelectrophoresis. *Scand J Immunol* 1977;6:1093–5.
10. Hoffman DR. Immunochemical identification of the allergens in egg white. *J Allergy Clin Immunol* 1983;71:481–6.
11. Langeland T, Aas K. Allergy to hen's egg white; clinical and immunological aspects. In: Brostoff J, Challacombe SJ, eds. *Food allergy and intolerance.* London: Baillière Tindal, 1987:367–74.
12. Blands J, Diamant B, Kallos P, Kallos-Deffner L, Løwenstein H: Flour allergy in bakers. I. Identification of allergenic fractions in flour and comparison of diagnostic methods. *Int Arch Allergy* 1976;52:392–406.
13. Theobald K, Thiel H, Kallweit C, Ulmer W, König W. Detection of proteins in wheat flour extracts that bind human IgG, IgE, and mouse monoclonal antibodies. *J Allergy Clin Immunol* 1986;78:470–7.
14. Baldo BA, Krilis S, Wrigley CW. Hypersensitivity to inhaled flour allergens. Comparison between cereals. *Allergy* 1980;35:45–56.
15. Bjørksten F, Halmepuro L, Hannuksela M, Lahti A. Extraction and properties of apple allergens. *Allergy* 1980;35:671–7.
16. Aas K. Fish allergy and the codfish allergen model. In: Brostoff J, Challacombe SJ, eds. *Food allergy and intolerance.* London: Baillière Tindal, 1987:356–66.
17. Aas K. Studies of hypersensitivity to fish. Allergological and serological differentiation between various species of fish. *Int Arch Allergy* 1966;30:257–67.
18. Lehrer SB. The complex nature of food antigens: studies of cross-reacting crustacea allergens. *Ann Allergy* 1986;57:267–72.
19. Dreborg S, Foucard T. Allergy to apple, carrot and potato in children with birch allergy. *Allergy* 1983;38:167–72.
20. Elsayed S, Apold J. Immunochemical analysis of cod fish Allergen M; locations of the immunoglobulin binding sites as demonstrated by the native and synthetic peptides. *Allergy* 1983;38:449–59.
21. Elsayed S. The native and synthetic peptides of codfish Allergen M. A short review. In: Bostrøm H, Epne H, Ljungstedt N, eds. *Theoretical and clinical aspects of allergic diseases.* Stockholm: Almqvist & Wiksell, 1983:237–53.
22. Schloss OM, Worthen TW. The permeability of the gastro-enterologic tract of infants to undigested protein. *Am J Dis Child* 1969;109:342–60.

DISCUSSION

Prof. Reinhardt: In the codfish model, the allergic molecule must not only fit into the IgE molecule but it must also create a cross-bridge between two IgE molecules. What is the cross-bridging in the cod? Is it due to two tetrapart peptides within the codfish structure, or what?

Dr. Aas: In most cases there will be two identical epitopes on the same molecule, but not necessarily always. They could be similar but not identical, binding to somewhat different IgE molecules on the mast cell. The distance between the epitopes may not be very important, because the electrophysical power field exerted by the two types of molecules (i.e., the antibody molecule on the mast cell and the epitope on the allergenic molecule) will make the IgE molecules move a little in the membrane of the mast cell, and possibly also induce slight changes in the conformation of the allergenic molecule, so that the molecules are drawn together, after which they are electrophysically "sucked" into place. It is interesting to study this point in the traditional Prausnitz-Küstner reaction. If you sensitize the skin with fish-allergic serum and then inject only about 50,000 molecules of the purified system into the other arm, you will get a strong reaction after 20 to 40 min, which shows how these molecules are rapidly distributed in body fluids and how, when a molecule reaches the sensitized site, it is stored there in a kind of "depot" until there is enough to make a visible reaction.

Dr. de Weck: What do you consider to be the minimum size of an antigenic epitope? In your studies and in previous classical studies it appears to be about three amino acids. However, there are indications from studies of allergy to chemicals that an antigenic or allergenic epitope may be much smaller—for example, the quaternary ammonium compounds or the $=N-O-CH_3$ side chains in cephalosporins, which are very small groupings but which can cause unexpected cross-reactions. Do you feel that sensitization to smaller epitopes might be a possible cause of unexpected cross-reactions in food allergy as well?

Dr. Aas: There is a considerable literature on the size of epitopes, and it is known that they may be quite large—for example, 8 to 12 amino acids in IgG antibody studies. I have no material to discuss specifically with regard to whether three amino acids is the minimum size, but when I read the literature I wonder what role is played by carrier substances in the material that has been used for the studies. With such a small number of amino acids in the epitope there is a good chance of cross-reactivities. For example, some of my patients who are allergic to codfish and salmon may also cross-react with a minor allergen in the salmon, while others have quite distinct IgE antibodies both to cod and salmon.

Dr. Guesry: I'd like to probe this point further. In the field of allergy to cow's milk it is said that in order not to be allergenic a molecule should be less than 5,000 daltons in size. You showed that a cod peptide of 16 amino acids—that is, about 2,000 to 2,500 daltons—is powerfully allergenic. Do you know the minimum size of the epitope of allergens such as casein and beta-lactoglobulin?

Dr. Aas: I think that some allergens of very small size present in cow's milk may be substances such as penicillin, and perhaps Professor de Weck may wish to comment on this. As far as native milk proteins go, there are always hydrolysates of milk of large enough size to carry two epitopes, which may be allergenic for the subgroup of patients who are allergic to the original molecule. However, I do not know their exact size, though from fish experiments allergenic hyrolysate peptides may be as small as 2,500 to 3,000 daltons in size, or even smaller.

Dr. de Weck: I cannot answer specifically about milk antigens, but experiments have shown that peptide molecules less than about 2,000 daltons in size are not usually very antigenic. However, there are exceptions, and a number of small molecules are known to be immunogenic, probably through covalent binding or very strong hydrophobic binding which enables them to bind to a cell membrane and thus be presented to T-cells. Such a molecule may elicit an immune response but may be too small to elicit an allergic reaction.

Dr. Walker: A clinical problem in the food allergy field is that the RAST test for the allergens is notoriously unreliable in making the diagnosis, especially in the case of milk proteins. Do you think that this is likely to be because the test involves the native protein rather than its digested product and that the process of digestion may expose certain epitopes or allergenic determinants which could, in turn, create an allergic reaction?

Dr. Aas: Küstner became world-famous because he was allergic to fish, and he was happy to have the collaboration of Prausnitz, who did the experiments! Küstner stated that he reacted only to cooked fish and never to raw fish, which would indicate that digestive denaturation had created an epitope to which he was reactive. I have never seen such a patient, and I believe that in Küstner's case there was probably a species difference, in that he ate some species raw and some cooked. I have no indication in the fish group that epitopes arise during digestion which represent something not found in raw fish. The difficulty in using RAST for diagnosis of fish allergy is that the commercial RAST uses a codfish allergen, so fish-allergic patients who are not allergic to codfish and do not have a true immunologic cross-reaction with cod-fish will have negative RAST. Another problem is that, even in the presence of persistent clinical fish allergy, the RAST results vary from highly positive to zero. A skin-prick test using the right sort of fish antigen in the correct concentration is more reliable.

Dr. Guesry: When you defined major and minor antigens you took the number of people reacting to these antigens as your guide, but if you look through the world literature you find huge discrepancies. For example, citrus fruit seems to be the most important allergen in Scandinavia, cow's milk in southern Europe, soya bean in the USA, and so on. Don't you think that exposure to an antigen in early life may be as important as its biochemical properties?

Dr. Aas: When I spoke about major allergens I was referring to the role of the different proteins within a certain group of allergic people. Thus if you take the fish-allergic population of Norway you find that cod is the major allergen, while in central Europe it is carp. However, they are completely identical with respect to the major allergens: They have the same epitopes. That means that when you use the system in the carp-allergic population you will find exactly the same basis for definitions of major, intermediate, and minor allergens as you do in the cod-allergic population. My own feeling is that it is not so much a question of what is in the food as of what is in the air: If you eat carp in your home I can find and define the major allergen of carp in your house dust.

Dr. Frick: Some earlier work by Berrens from Holland showed that sugar linkage onto proteins was an important factor in allergenicity, through the browning reaction. Nothing has been said about this. Could you comment?

Dr. Aas: I think the statement by Berrens about the importance of N-glycosidic bonding was probably an unjustified generalization from one finding, especially since that finding was based on an impure system. The codfish allergen has one sugar molecule, and we have been able to split it into two peptides, one with and one without sugar. The one without sugar is the most active. So I should warn against generalizations. There may be cases when N-glycosidic bonding is important, but it is not essential for allergenicity.

Dr. Wahn: I would like to comment briefly on the question of allergenic epitopes. There is a good deal of experimental evidence now that not only are there two different epitopes on one molecule but also that the two epitopes responsible for one single bridging of IgE antibodies may be different. For example, it has been shown that bivalent haptens do not have to be identical. It was a tantalizing idea that we might be able to find epitopes which could block anaphylactic reactions, as has been done by Dr. de Weck with penicillin, but since we now know that on one single molecule there may be 6, 8, or even 10 nonidentical determinants responsible for cross-linking in different combinations, I fear that we shall not be able to find blocking haptens.

Dr. Aas: I agree with your skeptical view about the results of epitope studies. I am equally skeptical about the use of the words "blocking antibody" in discussions concerning immunotherapy. This often-used term creates confusion in light of today's knowledge of allergenic molecules. You have to follow it with the question: What kind of epitope does it block? We have shown that IgG antibodies may react with the same epitope as IgE, but they may also react with quite different epitopes on the same molecule, yet they are all called "blocking antibodies." There are other ways of studying this, however, even if we are skeptical about the final aim of being able to block all types of allergens with single epitope substances. I think that *some* allergies may perhaps be blocked by a couple of epitopes—the major allergens of codfish, for instance—but epitopes could also be used to study the mechanisms of the reaction between receptors on antibodies or cells and the epitope—for example, by the use of cytotoxic agents to differentiate the cell stages during the process. Allergen research should now be allergen epitope research.

Food Allergy, edited by Eberhardt Schmidt.
Nestlé Nutrition Workshop Series, Vol. 17.
Nestec Ltd., Vevey/Raven Press, Ltd.,
New York © 1988.

Transmucosal Passage of Antigens

W. Allan Walker

Department of Pediatrics, Harvard Medical School, Boston, Massachusetts 02115; Chief, Combined Program in Pediatric Gastroenterology and Nutrition, Children's Hospital and Massachusetts General Hospital, Boston, Massachusetts 02115

An important adaptation of the gastrointestinal tract to the extrauterine environment is its development of a mucosal barrier against the penetration of antigens and antigenic fragments present in the intestinal lumen. At birth, the newborn must be prepared to deal with (a) bacterial colonization of the gut, (b) formation of toxic by-products of bacteria and viruses (enterotoxins and endotoxins), and (c) ingestion of antigens (milk and soy proteins) and their fragments. The potentially immunologic active substances, if permitted to penetrate the mucosal epithelial barrier under adverse circumstances (increased absorption of antigens or abnormal immune responsiveness), can cause inflammatory and allergic reactions, which may result in gastrointestinal and systemic disease states (1).

To protect against the potential danger of invasion across the mucosal barrier, the infant must develop an extensive system of defense mechanisms within the lumen and on the luminal surface; these mechanisms act to control and maintain the epithelial surface as an impermeable barrier to the uptake of antigens and large antigenic fragments. These defenses include a unique immunologic response (dimeric IgA antibody) to controlled penetration of luminal antigens, including production of local antibodies uniquely suited to (a) protection in the luminal environment (secretory component attached to dimeric IgA) and (b) the control of a systemic response (immune tolerance). The result of this physiologic immune response to luminal antigens is the absence of adverse immune reactions.

The purpose of this review is to (a) summarize the evidence for an altered mucosal barrier to proteins and protein fragments in human newborns, (b) consider factors contributing to mature mucosal barrier function in the human, and (c) stress the consequences (intestinal allergic reactions, etc.) of antigen penetration across an immature intestinal mucosa during infancy.

CONCEPT OF THE MUCOSAL BARRIER

As a result of a variety of recent observations (2) it is now apparent that nonimmunological processes working independently and in concert with the local mucosal immune system collectively comprise an effective barrier, the *mucosal barrier,* to the attachment and penetration of antigens and fragments present in the intraluminal environment. Table 1 lists some of the components that comprise the mucosal barrier. Of particular importance is our greater appreciation for the mucous coat overlying the microvillous membrane surface in this defense process. These aspects of intestinal host defense will be stressed. Other aspects have previously been reviewed (3).

Mucous Coat

The thickness and composition of the mucous coat overlying the microvillous surface contributes to the defense of mucosal surface against antigens and antigen fragment attachment and penetration. With increase of mucous discharge from goblet cells onto the mucosal surface, the physical thickness of the mucous coat can expand, providing a more extensive physical barrier to the diffusion of antigens from the lumen to the microvillous surface. This enhanced thickness of the mucous coat may be a contributing factor in the expulsion phenomenon for parasites and microbial antigens described by Miller and Nawa (4). Another protective property of mucus relates to the observation that microorganisms can attach to carbohydrate moieties (receptors) of glycoprotein components of the microvillous surface. Examples of this phenomenon are the mannose receptor (5) for *Escherichia coli* and the fucose receptor for *Vibrio cholera* (6). Recent studies from our laboratories (J. Snyder and W. A. Walker, *unpublished observations*) and others (7) suggest that mucus may contain similar carbohydrate moieties which can actually act as receptor inhibitors, thereby specifically interfering with the attachment of microorganisms and antigens to the microvillous surface. Interference with bacterial attachment by carbohydrate mucus inhibitors provides evidence for a specific protection against antigen penetration. Figure 1 depicts this concept with antigen-

TABLE 1. *Representative components of the mucosal barrier to antigens/fragments*

Nonimmunologic
   Intraluminal
      Gastric barrier
      Proteolysis
      Peristalsis
   Mucosal surface
      Mucosal coat
      Microvillous membrane
Immunologic
   Secretory IgA system
Combination of immunologic and nonimmunologic
   Immune-complex-mediated mucus release from goblet cells
   Immune-complex-facilitated mucosal surface proteolysis
   Kupffer cell phagocytosis of immune complexes

PHYSICAL BARRIER   LECTIN BINDING   ANTIGEN ALONE

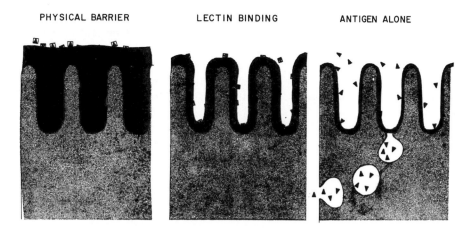

FIG. 1. Mechanism of mucus protection in small intestine (IgG complexes). Diagrammatic representation of intestinal secretions coating the intestinal surface as a mucosal barrier to intestinal allergens. Formation of antigen-antibody complexes results in increased release of mucus to form a physical barrier to allergen diffusion. These allergen-antibody complexes also bind to the mucous coat in lectin-like fashion to prevent penetration of the enterocyte. (From ref. 2.)

antibody complexes. Additional studies in this area are needed to further delineate this process.

Membrane Composition

The composition of the intestinal cell membrane changes as the epithelial cell migrates up the villus (8–10) and as the animal ages (11–13). Changes in membrane composition may determine whether antigen or fragments bind to the cell. Bresson et al. (14) have studied isolated microvillous membranes from the intestine of newborn and adult rabbits. They have shown that the membrane protein/phospholipid ratio is dramatically decreased in membranes of newborns as compared to those of adults. In addition, they noted increased cholera enterotoxin binding to microvillous membranes of newborns as compared to those of adults. These studies of the development of the intestinal surface may help us to better understand why antigen transport is greater early in life and why newborns have a high incidence of allergic diseases. In recent studies, a direct association between maturity of the microvillous membrane and antigen attachment has been demonstrated (Fig. 2) (15).

Immunologic Components of the Mucosal Barrier

The adequacy of local immune function in the gastrointestinal tract affects the attachment and penetration of ingested antigen and fragments. IgA is the immunoglobulin present in highest concentration in intestinal secretions (16,17). It has

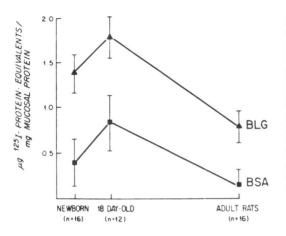

FIG. 2. Binding of ^{125}I-labeled bovine serum albumin (BSA) and beta-lactoglobulin (BLG) by the jejunal microvillous membrane in the rat, showing the effect of maturity. Numbers of animals *(n)* are given in parentheses. Means ±1 SD are shown. Protein concentration of BSA and BLG, 0.1 mg/ml; microvillous membrane protein concentration, 1.5 mg/ml. Differences in binding between 18-day-old and adult groups are statistically highly significant ($p < 0.0001$) for both proteins. (From ref. 15.)

been postulated that this immunoglobulin prevents the transport of antigen and antigen fragments by complexing with them in the lumen or within the mucous coat, thereby impeding adsorption (1,18). The concentration of IgA in saliva, stool, and serum of newborn animals and humans (19–22) is decreased, and it has been hypothesized that this transient deficiency can, in part, account for the increased attachment of antigens to the intestinal surface in newborn animals. This hypothesis is supported by studies of patients with selective IgA deficiency. These patients have circulating immune complexes and precipitating antibodies to absorbed bovine milk proteins (23). Again, when the sera of IgA-deficient individuals were studied for the appearance of complexes after the ingestion of milk, three of seven subjects had increases in antibody-antigen complexes, which peaked at 120 to 150 min (24). In another three subjects there was a tendency toward the formation of two peak concentrations of complexes: The first one was at 30 to 60 min; the second one occurred 120 to 150 min after drinking milk. Additionally, the circulating immune complexes found in some patients contained bovine milk proteins. Presumably the same process occurs in the transient IgA deficiency of the newborn as a contributing factor in the increased incidence of intestinal allergy (a common gastrointestinal disease occurring during infancy) and in the increased incidence of immune complex disease (nephritis, rheumatoid arthritis) in selective IgA-deficient patients.

Another important component of mucosal immunity is the access of intestinal antigens to lymphoid elements in Peyer's patches, a necessary first step in the secretory IgA cycle (18). Several researchers (25,26) have demonstrated that protein antigens can also traverse the epithelial barrier of the intestine. This occurs in the distal small intestine via specialized M (microfold) cells overlying Peyer's patches. Electron-microscopic studies of these cells indicate that they have few microvilli, a poorly developed glycocalyx, and an absence of lysosomal organelles. Using electron microscopy, Owen and co-workers have observed the uptake and processing of horseradish peroxidase by M cells (25,26). This type of antigen absorption in the gut has not yet been shown to occur via receptors, but it nonetheless appears to represent an important access route for the ingested antigens, fragments, and viruses (27) to reach lymphoid tissues and thereby stimulate the local and distant immune system. Figure 3 depicts our current concept of the IgA cycle in the gut (28). More research is needed to define the composition of the M-cell membrane

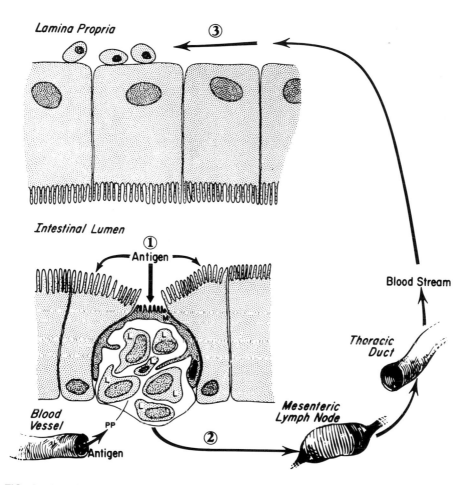

FIG. 3. IgA plasma cell cycle. Schematic representation of the cell for IgA-producing plasma cells populating the intestinal mucosa. Lymphocytes (L) within gut-associated lymphoid tissues (GALT), primarily Peyer's patches (PP) of the ileum, are stimulated by antigens entering from the intestinal lumen (**1**) via specialized epithelium (M cells), across conventional absorptive cells, or from the systemic circulation. Lymphoblasts migrate to mesenteric nodes for further maturation (**2**) and then enter the systemic circulation as plasmablasts to redistribute along intestinal mucosal surfaces (**3**) and produce secretory IgA antibodies in response to intestinally absorbed antigens. (From ref. 28.)

surface and to determine whether its composition is important in antigen/fragment attachment.

In summary, one can state that lymphoid elements in the gastrointestinal tract respond uniquely to luminal antigens, which are geared to optimize handling of these antigens. A physiologic immune responsiveness to mucosal antigens entails a two-part response, including the IgA response as discussed above and a preferential inhibition of systemic (IgE, IgG) responsiveness through the stimulus of T-suppressor-cell clones that act to modulate the conversion of lymphoblasts to plasma cells predisposed to producing systemic antibodies. This phenomenon, known as *tolerance,* seems to be uniquely the property of antigens or fragments crossing the mucosal surface (29). Figure 4 diagrammatically depicts this two-part response of intestinal lymphoid elements to luminal antigens.

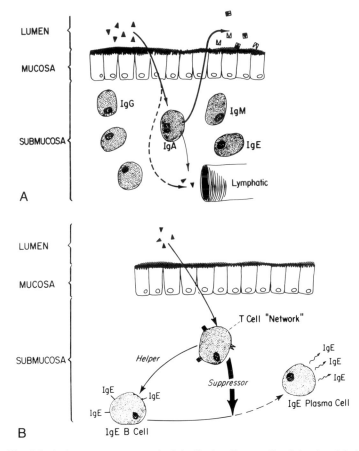

FIG. 4. Physiologic immune response to intestinal antigens stimulates local IgA-producing plasma cells previously primed by the IgA cycle (**A**). In addition, antigens and antigenic fragments can trigger a T-cell suppressor activity which presumably contributes to a tolerogenic IgE/IgG systemic response (**B**).

COMBINED EFFECT OF IMMUNOLOGIC AND NONIMMUNOLOGIC COMPONENTS OF THE MUCOSAL BARRIER

Several recent observations have suggested that the local immune process, in addition to its inherent protective actions, can also augment the protective capacity of the previously mentioned nonimmunologic components of the mucosal barrier (Table 1). Representative examples illustrate this phenomenon. In previous work (30) we reported that the proteolysis of intestinal antigens was considerably greater in immunized animals than in nonimmunized controls and that enhanced proteolysis most likely resulted from the interaction of immune complexes present in the mucous coat with pancreatic enzymes adsorbed onto the surface of the intestine after secretion into the lumen. A second example of combined protection is the mucous coat with pancreatic enzymes adsorbed onto the surface of the intestine after secretion into the lumen. A third example of combined protection is the enhanced discharge of goblet cell mucin occurring in intestinal anaphylaxis, as reported by Lake et al. (31). Using radiolabeled goblet cell mucus to quantify release, Lake showed that IgE-mediated mast cell discharge of histamine resulted in enhanced release of goblet cell mucus into the intestinal tract. This observation probably explains the expulsion of parasites associated with an increased mucous coat, described by Miller and Nawa (4), and may represent an important factor in host protection against parasitic infestation of the intestine.

A final example of the combined effect of immunologic and nonimmunologic processes in controlling host defense at the mucosal surface is the role of Kupffer cells in clearing immune complexes absorbed from the gastrointestinal tract. Several years ago in an animal model, we demonstrated that immune complexes to intestinal antigens formed on the intestinal surface or within the intestinal interstitium were cleared more readily by Kupffer cells in the liver than were antigens alone (32). This second line of mucosal defense may be important in preventing gram-negative microorganisms gaining access to the portal circulation and in the clearance of endotoxins and for antigens known to be taken up into the portal circulation.

DEFICIENCIES OF THE MUCOSAL BARRIER TO ANTIGENS AND THEIR FRAGMENTS

If the complex process of mucosal barrier defense is disrupted, or if specific deficiencies in components of barrier function exist, an increased incidence of antigen-induced intestinal diseases may ensue. Table 2 lists examples of circumstances that have resulted in disruption of mucosal barrier function and an increased incidence of gastrointestinal disease states. For discussion purposes, the immaturity of gastrointestinal barrier function will be used to illustrate this circumstance. Epidemiologic studies have shown a striking increase in allergic, infectious, and toxigenic diarrhea during infancy, particularly in premature infants (33).

TABLE 2. *Disruptions of mucosal barrier function
as causes of pathologic uptake
of antigens/fragment*

Immature gastrointestinal function
Malnutrition
Inflammation
Gastrointestinal anoxia
Transient/selective IgA deficiency

This increased incidence has been ascribed to immature mucosal host defenses against antigen attachment and penetration. A prototypic infectious disease occurring during this interval is necrotizing enterocolitis (NEC) (34), which is directly related to mucosal barrier deficiency.

During the last several years, a major thrust of our laboratory has been to define the developmental deficiencies in mucosal barrier function during the perinatal period. We have concentrated our efforts on the mucous coat and microvillous surface. Udall et al. (35) noted a striking increase in penetration of intestinal antigens in newborn animals as compared to adult animals (see Fig. 5). Subsequently, in comprehensive experiments by Pang et al. (36,37), striking differences in microvillous membrane composition and structure were demonstrated between newborn

ANTIGEN SPECIFIC

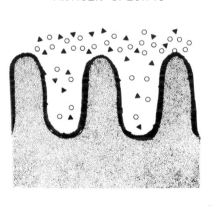

IMMATURE
GUT   SURFACE

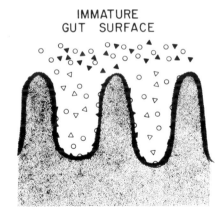

o Antigen A
▲ Antigen E

FIG. 5. Pathologic antigen interaction with intestinal surface. Intestinal antigens and their antigenic fragments may interact to a greater extent with the immature gut surface because of an absence of protective mucus and an immature composition of the mucosal surface. This enhanced interaction may account for increased antigen uptake in the small intestine of neonates. (o) Antigen A; (▲) antigen E.

and mature animals. Bresson et al. (14) showed that this immaturity could account for enhanced binding of cholera toxin to the microvillous surface, and Stern et al. (15) demonstrated increased antigen attachment at that site, suggesting an association between immaturity and the increased incidence of mechanisms of infectious/allergic disease. In additional studies from this laboratory, Shub et al. (38) have found striking differences in the carbohydrate composition of intestinal mucus from immature and mature rats which could account for the lack of mucus-specific receptor inhibition against bacteria in newborns. Obviously, more studies need to be done to show any specific effect of mucus composition and enhanced bacterial/antigen adherence to microvillous antigen uptake across an immature intestinal surface.

In addition to the immaturity of the intestinal surface of young infants, the mucosal response to antigens is abnormal; this abnormality is due to the developmental delay in local immune responsiveness. In the absence of enteric stimuli, principally by bacterial antigens, there is a paucity of IgA-producing plasma cells in the lamina propria. It requires weeks to months of extrauterine existence to establish protective levels in intestinal secretions (39). In addition, the suppressive T-cell function is necessary to control a systemic responsiveness rather than a state of systemic tolerance. Several studies have demonstrated that the normal response to enteric antigens is a systemic immune response occurring in infancy (40). Figure 6 depicts the pathologic local immune response to enteric antigens occurring in infancy.

EFFECTS OF IMMATURE ANTIGEN DIGESTION AND MUCOSAL BARRIER PENETRATION ON THE INITIATION OF IMMUNITY AND TOLERANCE

Identification of factors contributing to the elevated incidence of immune-mediated reactions to dietary antigens and their fragments in infants has been complicated by the array of changes that occur in the function and structure of the gastrointestinal and lymphoid systems throughout this period. Recent work in these areas has advanced from specifying and quantifying potentially relevant factors to defining model systems in which the impact of changes in those factors can be examined in terms of their direct influence on immune responsiveness in developing and mature animals. In particular, useful experimental systems would be (a) based on models that are well-characterized with regard to gastrointestinal and lymphoid maturation and (b) selected on the basis of evidence that early physiologic exposures to dietary antigens or fragments lead to enhanced specific immune responsiveness when compared with similar exposures in adults. One such system involves the feeding of ovalbumin, a potent immunogen, to experimental neonatal animals that are genetically defined ''high responders'' to this antigen (4). Initial studies of this model have demonstrated that newborn animals show enhanced specific responsiveness (''priming'') if fed 1 mg of ovalbumin per gram of body

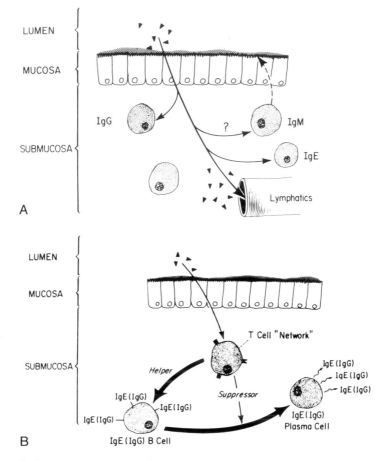

FIG. 6. Pathologic antigen interaction with the intestinal surface. Under circumstances of pathologic antigen interaction with the intestinal surface (IgA deficiency and/or decreased T-suppressor response), an abnormal immune response can occur. In the absence of a local IgA response (IgA deficiency) (**A**), no IgA antibodies are produced on antigen exposure and excessive antigens can be taken up into the systemic circulation. Alternately, the T modulation of B-cell response (**B**) can enhance the systemic IgE/IgG response resulting in adverse immune reactions, thus causing allergic disease.

weight within 2 to 3 days after birth. Weanlings and adults fed the same dose of antigen develop substantial depression of specific responsiveness (tolerance). These effects are expressed in both cell-mediated immune responses and antibody responses, including IgG and IgE antibody classes (41,42). Models of this kind should prove valuable in characterizing the influence of maturational events, at the lymphoid and gastrointestinal levels, upon tendencies toward increased or decreased immune responsiveness to specific dietary antigens. For example, initial dose-response studies led to the proposal of the hypothesis that infant mice, in which luminal digestive processes are poorly developed at birth, may respond to absorbed and injected antigens in a similar manner as determined by the systemic concentrations of antigen that are achieved, irrespective of the route of exposure.

This hypothesis, as well as the results of future testing, is likely to illuminate an as-yet poorly understood contribution of the maturation of gastrointestinal digestive processes and the mucosal barrier to differences between infants and adults in the character of absorbed antigens and in their immunomodulatory effects. Many investigators have shown that immunoreactive antigen—recognizable by specific antibodies—is taken up in greater amounts from neonates than from adults when both are fed under comparable conditions (see, e.g., refs. 36 and 41). Little is known, however, about whether the detectable antigenic materials represent molecular forms that are dissimilar or comparable (but absorbed in differing amounts) in neonates and adults. One might expect relatively inefficient luminal digestion and greater permeability of relatively intact fragmented antigen derivatives in neonates. As proposed in the above hypothesis, small or moderate amounts of antigen absorbed from neonatal gut would be expected to enhance specific responsiveness, whereas larger amounts would tend to tolerize, as observed when native antigen is injected parenterally into newborns (4). In contrast, the mature digestive capacity of adults would be expected to fragment proteins more effectively, encouraging a shift toward increased production of smaller derivatives which, by virtue of their size, could be taken up in significant amounts.

Support for the potential importance of intact antigen fragment ratios was obtained from a feeding study in which mice were injected parenterally with a small priming dose of native antigen (20 mg). Animals given both exposures showed neither tolerance nor priming, which suggested that systematic availability of small amounts of intact antigen overcame the effects of absorbed antigen by providing a positive stimulus of similar magnitude (43). Current studies in our laboratories show that acute prefeeding of a trypsin inhibitor to adult mice before a normally tolerizing feeding of antigen results in (a) substantial (12-fold) increases in the concentration of antigen-specific determinants in the serum and (b) a reversal in the immunologic effect of antigen feeding from tolerance to priming for specific antibody responses (D. Hanson et al., *manuscript in preparation*). While these observations have not yet been evaluated regarding the properties of antigen derivatives in the serum, they are consistent with the hypothesis that gastrointestinal processing and uptake of proteins can affect the immunologic outcome of antigen consumption by determining the influence of antigenic derivatives that reach the lymphoid tissues.

Exposure of local and systemic lymphoid cells to absorbed fragments of antigen may, in turn, be of considerable importance for understanding why protein feeding in adults is biased toward induction of tolerance rather than priming. Although a role of digestively produced protein fragments is not yet directly defined in the induction of priming and tolerance by ingested antigens, proteins that are denatured or fragmented *in vitro* are capable of inducing specific tolerance when injected parenterally (44,45). Some of these fragments (a) cannot be detected by traditional immunoassays that depend upon binding by antibodies specific to the native molecule and (b) have been shown to produce unresponsiveness through induction of suppressor T cells *in vivo*. A suppressor T-cell component has been identified in orally induced tolerance to several protein antigens (46–48). Antigen fragments that contain a specific epitope are also capable of depressing the response of specific helper T cells *in vitro* (49), consistent with other evidence that absorbed antigen may promote tolerance through more than one mechanism in fed animals (50).

Gastrointestinally processed protein fragments may achieve their effects by interacting differently than native molecules with the lymphoid and accessory cells that participate in immune responses. This is likely in view of studies indicating that B and T lymphocytes appear to bind conformational "determinants" associated with shapes found on exposed areas of the folded molecule. In contrast, the T-lymphocyte receptor is capable of recognizing "epitopes" on molecular fragments consisting of as few as 15 to 20 amino acids when the specific fragments are presented with appropriate histocompatibility markers on the surfaces of antigen-presenting cells (49,51). Whereas shape determinants are likely, in general, to be distorted or destroyed upon exposure to mature gastrointestinal processing that includes gastric acidity and luminal endopeptidase activity, the primary sequence of amino acids comprising an epitome may persist on fragments of various sizes until directly cleaved by endopeptidases or terminal peptidases. Differences in the degree and character of antigen fragmentation in neonatal and adult gut might therefore influence the stimuli available to specific B and T lymphocytes, hence modifying the pattern of later antibody and cell-mediated immune responses.

The ability of antigen fragments to interact with specific B lymphocytes is related to the retention of determinants that can bind surface immunoglobulin receptors. That retention probably varies widely for different antigens exposed to the same conditions of digestion. Fragments that possess two or more intact determinants can cross-link or "bridge" receptors on individual B cells, a critical event in the activation and clonal proliferation that underlie B-lymphocyte priming (52). Fragments that retain single determinants may have opposing effects, one of which is to "blockade" B-lymphocyte receptors by interfering with cross-linking by molecules that are more intact. Antigen fragments can also bind to endogenous plasma proteins after absorption (53); this might create "hybrid" molecules that could cross-link B-cell receptors if more than one fragment were present on the self-protein. Fragments that lack conformational determinants from the native molecules would be unable to interact with specific B lymphocytes but could retain short, primary sequence epitopes that permit (a) uptake by antigen presenting cells and (b) recognition by specific T lymphocytes (51). If absorbed in small amounts, such fragments are capable of specific T-cell priming, but larger quantities may be responsible for depressing helper T-cell responsiveness (49), thus leading to tolerance.

Additional study will be valuable in defining the components of luminal digestion and the properties of the mucosal barrier that jointly determine the stimulus characteristics of antigens and fragments that are taken up via the gut in infants and adults. Response to these materials will, in turn, depend on (a) the degree of maturation in lymphoid and accessory cells and (b) the pattern of distribution of these cells in gastrointestinal and other tissues.

ROLE OF HUMAN COLOSTRUM IN CLOSURE

As stated earlier, newborns lack many specific and nonspecific intestinal features that are necessary for protecting them adequately from the extrauterine environment. Fortunately, "nature" has provided an excellent substitute to protect the vulnerable neonate passively during this critical period. This substitute, human milk, contains many factors that can compensate for processes lacking in the infant and, at the same time, stimulate the maturation to the gut toward independent function.

It is increasingly apparent that human milk contains not only important nutrients and protective factors for the newborn but also factors that can facilitate intestinal maturation. Heird and Hansen (54) have reported that the ingestion of colostrum can facilitate the maturation of mucosal epithelial cells, enhance absorption of digested foods, and perhaps accelerate the development of an intact mucosal barrier. They have also shown that brush-border enzymes (lactase, sucrase, and alkaline phosphatase) are enhanced after the ingestion of colostrum (54). Udall et al. (55) have actually demonstrated a decrease in antigen penetration in newborns after colostrum feeding. These investigations have suggested that milk may contain "mucosal growth factor," which facilitates the early maturation of the gut (closure).

In addition to actively accelerating closure in the newborn, human colostrum/milk provides a passive protection of the gut surface while it is maturing. Specific secretory IgA antibodies exist in milk, and these exclude bacteria and luminal antigens. Also present are additional protective factors that contribute to the protection of the newborn. However, a more prolonged discussion of this topic is beyond the scope of this chapter.

CLINICAL CONDITIONS POSSIBLY ASSOCIATED WITH IMMATURE MUCOSAL BARRIER

Clinical conditions known to be associated with pathologic uptake of antigens are shown in Table 3. The pathophysiologic mechanism(s) of representative conditions discussed in this section will illustrate the association between antigen transport and clinical disease. A comprehensive review of all clinical conditions is beyond the scope of this chapter (18).

As a result of the pathologic transport of antigens across the small intestine, antigens may traverse the mucosal barrier and predispose to allergic and toxic reaction, thus leading to a number of gastrointestinal diseases. Those diseases possibly associated with antigen absorption are gastrointestinal allergy (56), inflam-

TABLE 3. *Clinical conditions possibly associated with immature mucosal barrier*

Newborn and early childhood (immediate clinical response)
  Necrotizing enterocolitis
  Gastrointestinal allergy
  Sudden infant death syndrome
  Dermatitis
  Toxigenic diarrhea
  Malabsorption
Later childhood and adulthood (delayed clinical response)
  Inflammatory bowel disease
  Chronic active hepatitis
  Nephritis
  Autoimmune (immune-complex-mediated disease)

---

matory bowel disease (57), celiac disease (58), toxigenic diarrhea (59), chronic hepatitis (60), necrotizing enterocolitis, and autoimmune disease (60). Because the evidence cited to support the hypothesis that intestinal permeability to antigens is involved in the pathogenesis of human disease is largely indirect, one should realize that these comments are somewhat speculative and still remain to be proved by more direct evidence. For purposes of this report, only gastrointestinal allergy will be discussed in detail as a prototype condition.

Gastrointestinal Allergy

Probably the most striking association between antigen handling and clinical disease is shown with gastrointestinal allergy. Several clinical symptoms of such allergy have been described, and these appear to relate specifically to the ingestion of specific foods (particularly cow's milk). These conditions may be localized to the gastrointestinal tract and present with diarrhea, gastrointestinal bleeding, or protein-losing enteropathy, or they may be represented by systemic manifestations of allergy ranging in severity from exanthem to anaphylaxis. The clinical expression of allergy may relate to the transport of antigens either into the lamina propria alone (local allergic reactions) or into both the lamina propria and systemic circulation (systemic allergic response). Factors that determine the nature of the allergic response are not entirely understood, but they undoubtedly are related to the degree of sensitivity of the allergic patient and/or related to the concentration of allergen ingested. Although the mechanism(s) of gastrointestinal allergy is presently obscure, it would appear that the intestinal transport of allergens is a necessary initial step in the process. In fact, it has been suggested that during the neonatal period, when increased antigen permeability exists, susceptible infants may become sensitized to specific ingested protein. With re-exposure at a time when much less macromolecular absorption is occurring, minute quantities of allergen may be absorbed and result in allergic symptoms. These symptoms can then be propagated by further uptake of allergens across a disrupted mucosal surface. In recent experimental studies from this laboratory (61), we reported that intestinal anaphylaxis can lead to increased uptake of nonspecific intestinal allergens, which consequently can evoke an IgG-mediated reaction leading to further propagation of disease. This secondary process occurring with classic IgE-mediated disease may be important in converting a self-limited process into a chronic disease state.

SUMMARY AND CONCLUSIONS

An important adaptation of the gastrointestinal tract to the extrauterine environment is its development of a mucosal barrier against the penetration of proteins and protein fragments. To combat the potential danger of invasion across the mucosal barrier, the infant must develop within the lumen and on the luminal mucosal surface an elaborate system of defense mechanisms that act to control and maintain the epithelium as an impermeable barrier to the uptake of macromolecular antigens. These defenses include a unique local immunologic system adapted to function in the complicated milieu of the intestine; they also include other nonimmunologic processes such as a gastric barrier, intestinal surface secretions, peristaltic movement, etc., all of which help to provide maximum protection for the intestinal surface.

Unfortunately, during the immediate postpartum period, especially for premature and "small-for-date" infants, this elaborate local defense system is incompletely developed. As a result of the delay in the maturation of the mucosal barrier, newborn infants are particularly vulnerable to pathologic penetration by harmful intraluminal substances. The consequences of altered defense are susceptibility to infection and the potential for hypersensitivity reactions and the formation of immune complexes. With these reactions comes the potential for developing life-threatening diseases such as necrotizing enterocolitis, sepsis, and hepatitis. Fortunately, nature has provided a means for passively protecting the "vulnerable" newborn against the dangers of a deficient intestinal defense system: human milk. It is now increasingly apparent that human milk contains not only antibodies and viable leukocytes but also many other substances that can interfere with bacterial colonization and prevent antigen penetration.

REFERENCES

1. Walker WA. Gastrointestinal host defense: importance of gut closure in control of macromolecular transport. *Ciba Found Symp* 1956;70:201–19.
2. Walker WA. Antigen absorption from the small intestine and gastrointestinal disease. *Pediatr Clin North Am* 1975;22:731–46.
3. Udall JN, Walker WA. The physiologic and pathologic basis for the transport of macrophages across the intestinal tract. *J Pediatr Gastroenterol Nutr* 1982;1:295–301.
4. Miller HRP, Nawa Y. Immune regulation of intestinal goblet cell differentiation. Specific induction of non-specific protection against helminths. *Nouv Rev Fr Hematol* 1979;21:31–45.

5. Boedeker EC. Enterocyte adherence of *Escherichia coli:* its relation to diarrheal disease. *Gastroenterology* 1982;83:489–92.
6. Jones GW, Freter R. Adhesive properties of Vibrio cholera: nature of the interaction with isolated rabbit brush border membranes and human erythrocytes. *Infect Immun* 1970;14:240–5.
7. Forstner G, Sturgess JM, Forstner J. Malfunction of intestinal mucus and mucus production. *Adv Exp Med Biol* 1976;89:349–58.
8. Quarone A, Kirsch K, Herscovics A, Iselbacher KJ. Surface-membrane biogenesis in rat intestinal epithelial cell at different stages of maturation. *Biochem J* 1980;192:133–44.
9. Raul F, Simon P, Kedinger M, Haffen K. Intestinal enzyme activities in isolated villus and crypt cells during postnatal development of the rat. *Cell Tissue Res* 1977;176:167–78.
10. Deboth NJ, Van Der Kamp AW, Van Dongen JM. The influence of changing crypt cells on functional differentiation in the small intestine of the rat. Nucleotide and protein synthesis. *Differentiation* 1975;4:175–82.
11. Lojda A. Cytochemistry of enterocytes and of other cells in mucosal membrane of the small intestine. In: Smyth DH, ed. *Biomembranes, Vol. 4A: Intestinal absorption.* London: Plenum Press, 1974:43–122.
12. Etzler ME, Branstratpr ML. Cell surface components of intestinal epithelial cells and their relationship to cellular differentiation. In: *Development of mammalian absorptive processes.* Amsterdam: Excerpta Medica (*Ciba Found Symp 70*), 1979:51–68.
13. Toofantan F, Kidder DE, Hill FW. The postnatal development of intestinal disaccharidases in the calf. *Res Vet Sci* 1975;16:382–92.
14. Bresson JL, Pang KY, Walker WA. Microvillus membrane differentiation: quantitative difference in cholera toxin binding to the intestinal surface of newborn and adult rabbits. *Pediatr Res* 1984;18:984–7.
15. Stern MS, Pang KY, Walker WA. Food proteins and gut mucosal barrier. II. Differential interaction of cow's milk proteins with the mucous coat and the surface membrane of adult and immature rat jejunum. *Pediatr Res* 1984;18:1252–7.
16. Tomasi TB, Lawson IM, Challacombe S, McNabb P. Mucosal immunity: the origin and migration pattern of cells in the secretory system. *J Allergy Clin Immunol* 1980;65:12–9.
17. Marsh MN. The small intestine: mechanisms of local immunity and gluten sensitivity. *Clin Sci* 1981;61:497–503.
18. Walker WA. Intestinal transport of macromolecules. In: Johnson LR, Christensen J, Grossman ML, Jacobson ED, Schultz SG, eds. *Physiology of the gastrointestinal tract.* New York: Raven Press, 1981:1271–89.
19. Allansmith M, McClellan BH, Butterworth M, Maloney JR. The development of immunoglobulin levels in man. *J Pediatr* 1968;72:276–90.
20. Selner JC, Merrill DA, Claman HN. Salivary immunoglobulin and albumin: development during the newborn period. *J Pediatr* 1968;72:685–9.
21. Haneberg B, Aarskog D. Human fecal immunoglobulin in healthy infants and children and in some with disease affecting the intestinal tract or the immune system. *Clin Exp Immunol* 1975;22:210–22.
22. Burgio GR, Lanzavecchia A, Pievani A, Hayakar S, Ugazio AG. Ontogeny of secretory immunity: Levels of secretory IgA and natural antibodies in saliva. *Pediatr Res* 1980;14:1111–4.
23. Cunningham-Rundels C, Brandeis WE, Good RA, Day NK. Milk precipitins, circulating immune complexes and IgA deficiency. *Proc Natl Acad Sci USA* 1958;75:2287–3389.
24. Cunningham-Rundels C, Brandeis WE, Good RA, Day NK. Bovine antigens and the formation of circulating immune complexes in selective immunoglobulin A deficiency. *J Clin Invest* 1979;64:272–9.
25. Owen RL, Jones AL. Epithelial cell specialization within human Peyer's patches: An ultrastructural study of intestinal lymphoid follicles. *Gastroenterology* 1974;66:189–203.
26. Owen RL. Sequential uptake of horseradish peroxidase by lymphoid follicle epithelium of Peyer's patches in the normal unobstructed mouse intestine: an ultrastructural study. *Gastroenterology* 1977;72:440–51.
27. Wolf JL, Rubin DH, Finberg R, Kauffman RS, Sharpe AH, et al. Intestinal M. cells: A pathway for entry of reovirus into the host. *Science* 1981;212:471–2.
28. Walker WA, Isselbacher KJ. Intestinal antibodies. *N Engl J Med* 1977;297:767–73.
29. Vaz NM, Maia LC, Hanson DG, Lynch J. Inhibition of homocytotropic antibody responses in adult inbred mice by previous feeding of the specific antigen. *J Allergy Clin Immunol* 1977;60:110–5.

30. Walker WA, Wu MM, Isselbacher KJ, Bloch KJ. Intestinal uptake of macromolecules. IV. The effect of pancreatic duct ligation on the breakdown of antigen and antigen-antibody complexes on the intestinal surface. *Gastroenterology* 1975;69:1223–9.
31. Lake AM, Bloch KJ, Sinclair KJ, Walker WA. Anaphylactic release of intestinal goblet cell mucus. *Immunology* 1979;39:173–8.
32. Walker WA. Role of the mucosal barrier in toxin/microbial attachment to the gastrointestinal tract. *Ciba Symp* 1985;112:34–47.
33. Virnig NL, Reynolds JW. Epidemiological aspects of neonatal necrotizing enterocolitis. *Am J Dis Child* 1974;128(2):186–90.
34. Lake AM, Walker WA. Neonatal necrotizing enterocolitis: a disease of altered host defense. *Clin Gastroenterol* 1977;6:463–80.
35. Udall JN, Pang K, Fritze L, Kleinman R, Trier JS, et al. Development of gastrointestinal mucosal barrier. The effect of age on intestinal permeability to macromolecules. *Pediatr Res* 1981;15: 241–4.
36. Pang KY, Bresson JL, Walker WA. Development of the gastrointestinal mucosal barrier. III. Evidence for structural differences in microvillus membranes from newborn and adult rabbits. *Biochem Biophys Acta* 1983;727:201–8.
37. Pang KY, Bresson JL, Walker WA. Development of the gastrointestinal mucosal barrier, V. Comparative effect of calcium binding on microvillus structure in newborn and adult rats. *Pediatr Res* 1983;17:856–61.
38. Shub MD, Pang KY, Swann DA, Walker WA. Age-related changes in chemical composition and physical properties of mucus glycoproteins from rat small intestine. *Biochem J* 1983;215:405–11.
39. Walker WA. Absorption of protein and protein fragments in the developing intestine: role of immunologic/allergic reactions. *Pediatrics* 1985;75(suppl):167–71.
40. Udall JN, Walker WA. Immunologic function of the developing gut. In: Warsaw J, ed. *Selected topics in developmental medicine*. New York: Elsevier, 1983:221–38.
41. Hanson DG. Ontogeny of orally induced tolerance to soluble proteins in mice. I. Priming and tolerance in newborns. *J Immunol* 1981;127:1518–24.
42. Strobel S, Ferguson A. Immune responses to fed protein antigens in mice. 3. Systemic tolerance or priming is related to age which antigen is first encountered. *Pediatr Res* 1984;18:588–94.
43. Hanson DG, Vaz NM, Rawlings L, Lynch JM. Inhibition of specific immune responses by feeding protein antigens. II. Effects of prior passive and active immunization. *J Immunol* 1979;122:2261–6.
44. Takatsu K, Ishizaka K. Reaginic antibody formation in the mouse. VII. Induction of suppressor T cells for IgE and IgG antibody responses. *J Immunol* 1976;116:1257–64.
45. Muckerheide A, Pesce A, Michael JG. Immunosuppressive properties of a peptic fragment of BSA. *J Immunol* 1977;119:1340–5.
46. Richman LK, Chiller JM, Brown WR, Hanson DG, Vaz NM. Enterically induced immunologic tolerance. I. Induction of suppressor T lymphocytes by intragastric administration of soluble proteins. *J Immunol* 1978;121:2429–34.
47. Miller SD, Hanson DG. Inhibition of specific immune responses by feeding protein antigens. IV. Evidence for tolerance and specific active suppression of cell-mediated immune responses to ovalbumin. *J Immunol* 1979;123:2344–50.
48. Silverman GA, Peri BA, Fitch FW, Rothberg RM. Enterically induced regulation of systemic immune responses. II. Suppression of proliferating T cells by and Lyt-1 + , 2 T effector cell. *J Immunol* 1983;131:2656–61.
49. Lamb JR, Skidmore GJ, Green N, Chiller JM, Feldmann M. Induction of tolerance in influenza virus-immune T lymphocyte clones with synthetic peptides of influenza hemagglutinin. *J Exp Med* 1983;157:1434–7.
50. Hanson DG, Miller SD. Inhibition of specific immune response by feeding protein antigens. V. Induction of the tolerant state in the absence of specific suppressor T cells. *J Immunol* 1982;128:2378–81.
51. Shimonkevitz R, Colon S, Kappler JW, Marack P, Grey HM. Antigen recognition by H-2-restricted T cells. II. A tryptic ovalbumin peptide that substitutes for processed antigen. *J Immunol* 1984;133:2067–74.
52. Pure E, Isakson P, Kappler J, Marrack P, Krammer P, Vitetta ES. T cell-derived B cell growth and differentiation factors: dichotomy between the responsiveness of B cells from adult and neonatal mice. *J Exp Med* 1983;157:600–12.
53. Udall JN, Pang KY, Scrimshaw NS, Walker WA. The effectuous peptide fragments to native

proteins: possible explanation for the overestimation of uptake of intact proteins from the gut. *Immunology* 1981;42:251–7.

54. Heird WC, Hansen IH. Effect of colostrum on growth of intestinal mucosa. *Pediatr Res* 1977;11:406.

55. Udal JN, Pang KY, Scrimshaw NS, Walker WA. The effect of early nutrition on intestinal maturation. *Pediatr Res* 1979;13:409.

56. Taylor B, Normal AP, Orgel HA. Transient IgA deficiency and pathogenesis of infantile atopy. *Lancet* 1973;2:111–3.

57. Ferguson A. Intraepithelial lymphocytes of the small intestine. *Gut* 1977;18:921–37.

58. Shiner M, Ballard J. Antigen-antibody reactions in jejunal mucosa in childhood coeliac disease after gluten challenge. *Lancet* 1972;1:1202–5.

59. Ogra PL, Karzon DT. The role of immunoglobulins in the mechanisms of mucosal immunity to viral infection. *Pediatr Clin North Am* 1970;17:385–9.

60. Walker WA. Antigen absorption from the small intestine and gastrointestinal disease. *Pediatr Clin North Am* 1975;22:731–46.

61. Kleinman RE, Bloch KJ, Walker WA. Gut induced anaphylaxis and uptake of a bystander protein: an amplification of anaphylactic sensitivity. *Pediatr Res* 1981;15:598.

DISCUSSION

Dr. Rieger: I would like to re-emphasize one aspect of your talk, which is that the passage of antigen through the mucosa is not the same as the passage of antigen into the blood; rather it is the passage of antigen into the local immune system of the gut or into the portal blood going to the liver. Nevertheless I think it is very important to measure circulating antigen; and everyone who is interested in this has the same problem, that of knowing the molecular size of the antigen. Do you have any new evidence as to the size of the molecules which are being absorbed?

Dr. Walker: There has certainly been some confusion in the literature because erroneously high values of circulating proteins have been reported when using radiolabeled proteins in animal models to measure absorption. What happens is that when the protein molecules are broken down in the gut, small fragments will be absorbed and will bind to endogenous circulating proteins, thus giving the erroneous impression that high-molecular-weight proteins have been absorbed. For this reason, most of us who have been looking at this problem have turned to radioimmunoassay to identify specific antigenic determinants. This does not entirely answer the question, because one can conceivably measure a large fragment, or even a small one, using this same technique. What we have done (and this is mostly the work of Dr. Kurt Bloch, who is a close collaborator) is to look at fractions of serum, separated by high-pressure liquid chromatography, from animals that have ingested various proteins. He has demonstrated a spectrum of fragments of low, intermediate, and high molecular weight with only a very small amount of native protein. I believe this is what usually happens during transport. A more important consideration is the amount of protein (or of fragments of protein) that retains antigenicity once it has been absorbed. We may be making a mistake in testing for native antigens when in fact the allergen is an entirely different molecule. If we could process the digested product we could perhaps get a more realistic appreciation of protein allergy in young infants.

Dr. Reinhardt: Is the binding of allergens to glycoprotein receptors on moieties of the microvillous membrane important for protection against proteolytic degradation, or is it a necessary binding process in a transport mechanism?

Dr. Walker: Our prejudice is that the attachment of these proteins to the immature intestine facilitates the engulfment of the protein by the enterocyte and its subsequent transport.

An association has been shown between attachment and the degree of uptake, and I believe that the attachment of antigens to receptors (I use the word "receptor" very loosely because we have not really demonstrated that there is a classic receptor to an adherence factor) seems to facilitate the cells' handling of the antigens for transport.

Dr. Cant: You ascribed a negative role to breast-milk antigens, but do you think that low levels of antigen in breast milk might induce tolerance and hence be beneficial?

Dr. Walker: I do not have evidence for this, though I agree it is possible. However, I should point out that we are seeing increasing numbers of breast-fed babies presenting with bloody diarrhea due to allergic colitis, whose mothers' milk contains small amounts of antigen.

Dr. Cant: But in my view the presence of food antigens in breast milk is a usual, rather than an unusual, finding.

Dr. Aas: I agree. The presence of food antigens in breast milk is a normal phenomenon, depending on the kind of food and the resistance to digestion. If you eat fish while lactating there will be fish allergens in your milk, but they will be small peptides. I think Dr. Walker has put his finger on the key point here, namely, the importance of the carrier substance. We should not only consider proteins in this respect. One of the most potent carrier molecules known in the body is heparin, and we should address the possibility that this transport molecule may also play a role in allergy.

Dr. Schmitz: Your data have been obtained predominantly in rabbits and cats, but human intestinal development is quite different, the human infant having a nearly mature intestine at birth. How relevant are your studies to the human?

Dr. Walker: It is axiomatic that you cannot do the same sort of studies on humans that you can on animals, and you use the animal model system to help interpret data in the human situation. We are currently looking at human fetal intestine in culture, and we have developed a system that allows us to follow its maturation. We are presently examining the effect of colostrum on this process. We can now say that some features of immaturity that are present in, say, the first 3 weeks of life in the rodent are present at a much earlier stage in the human (i e , 18–20 weeks' gestation). Since we now deliver so many babies prematurely, I think these animal findings are relevant to the potential for sensitization by food allergens in the immature human infant, though I accept that the animal work must be followed up with relevant human studies.

Dr. Revillard: You mentioned that some enterocytes may express IA (class 2) antigens, and there has been discussion in the literature about whether this expression may be associated with the capacity to present antigen to T cells. Could you speculate on the differences between (a) the handling of a protein by an enterocyte in the process of absorption and (b) the handling of that same protein by a macrophage or monocyte in terms of antigen presentation?

Dr. Walker: This is a very new area, so there are a lot of things we do not know. However, there have been a number of observations in the recent literature which are of relevance. For example, there has been evidence to suggest that the incubation of isolated enterocytes with T cells in the presence of specific antigen can act as a stimulus to the T cell (1); there has been an article suggesting that intraepithelial lymphocytes affect the expression of IA antigens and vice versa; and there is also some suggestion (2) that it may be in the nature of intraepithelial lymphocytes that they are predominately cytotoxic suppressor cells and that their association with IA expression may be a combined factor allowing the intestine to respond to the external environment. My particular interest is the effect which lymphokines and other factors such as γ-interferon, which are present in breast milk, may have on the expression of these factors in the human intestinal enterocyte.

Dr. Marini: Do you think that the type of delivery or the prenatal administration of drugs to the mother—steroids, for example—can influence the mucosal absorption of antigens?

Dr. Walker: This has interested me very much, and we have done a number of studies in which we have attempted to repeat the multicenter human trial carried out in the USA (3), which showed that antenatal administration of steroids to the mother caused a reduction in neonatal necrotizing enterocolitis. Using the same protocol on an animal model system with both low-dose cortisone and low-dose thyroxine, we have been able to reverse many of the observations we have reported as features of immature immunologic development, particularly the whole glycosylation process and the ability of certain lectins and toxins to bind under these circumstances. I believe that factors reaching the fetus transplacentally or given in breast milk may facilitate some of the steps which lead to maturation.

DISCUSSION REFERENCES

1. Bland PW, Warren LG. Antigen presentation by epithelial cells of the rat small intestine. I. Kinetics, antigen specificity, and blocking by anti-Ia antisera. *Immunology* 1986;58:1–7.
2. Bland PW, Warren LG. Antigen presentation by epithelial cells of the rat small intestine. II. Selective induction of suppressor T cells. *Immunology* 1986;58:9–14.
3. Bauer CR, Morrisson FC, Poole WK. A decreased incidence of necrotizing enterocolitis after prenatal glucocorticoid therapy. *Pediatrics* 1984;73:682–8.

Food Allergy, edited by Eberhardt Schmidt.
Nestlé Nutrition Workshop Series, Vol. 17.
Nestec Ltd., Vevey/Raven Press, Ltd.,
New York © 1988.

Regulation of Mucosal Immunity: An Overview with Special Emphasis on Secretory IgA Production and Oral Tolerance

J.P. Revillard, S. Lafont, and D. Kaiserlian

Pavillon P, Hôpital Edouard Herriot, 69374 Lyon Cedex 08, France

Mucosae represent (a) the main site of exposure of the immune system to environmental antigens and (b) one of the major routes of penetration of infectious agents into the body. Mucosal defense mechanisms involve cellular and humoral components, some of which are antigen-specific whereas others are nonspecific. A unified concept of mucosa-associated lymphoid tissue (MALT) was proposed by J. Bienenstock (1) to stress the structural and functional features common to gastrointestinal tract, upper and lower respiratory tract, mammary gland, eyes, ears, and urinary and genital tracts. Such distant anatomical sites not only share common immune effectors such as, for instance, secretory IgA antibodies, but they are interconnected by a traffic of lymphoid cells. Hence immunization by the oral route may induce the production of secretory antibodies at distant sites such as in the mammary gland. Furthermore, recent data suggest that tight regulatory pathways associate immune cells with other mucosal components by means of hormones and lymphokines.

Adverse reactions to food antigens may be analyzed within the general framework of the regulation of mucosal immunity. Indeed there is increasing evidence that oral administration of antigen results in the suppression of specific systemic immune responses, including delayed-type hypersensitivity and production of antibodies of the IgG and IgE classes, together with the development of a secretory IgA antibody response. The latter contributes itself to antigen exclusion (2). Systemic immune responses to food antigens are thus down-regulated upon repeated antigenic exposure. This process is likely to be defective during the postnatal period because of the delayed ontogeny of the mucosal immune system. Furthermore, it has been hypothesized that an early defect in the development of IgA response may be associated with an increased risk of allergic disorders (3). Although this hypothesis has received some support from clinical studies, it should be re-examined in light of recent data suggesting that, in humans, serum IgA and secretory IgA levels vary independently under distinct control pathways (4).

SECRETORY IgA

The major antibody class in secretory fluids is secretory IgA (sIgA) (5). It is made of dimeric or polymeric IgA, bound together by covalent association to a J chain and linked to a secretory component (SC). There are two isotypes, namely, sIgA1 and sIgA2. The former is highly susceptible to IgA proteases secreted by numerous pathogenic bacteria, whereas the latter can be split into Fc and Fab fragments by a unique protease from *Clostridium ramosum*. Antibodies to IgA proteases can be demonstrated in secretory fluids. Two iso-allotypes of IgA2 have been described: A2m(1), represented mostly among Caucasians; and A2m(2), represented mostly among other races. IgA2 accounts for less than 20% of serum IgA but accounts for 26% to 40% of sIgA. The SC glycoprotein is synthesized by various glandular and epithelial cells as a membrane poly-Ig receptor which ensures the transport of J-chain-containing Ig classes (IgM, IgA) to the apical pole of the cells (6). Both free and IgM- or IgA-associated SC are released into secretory fluids by proteolysis. Congenital defects of SC are extremely rare (7).

In the rat and other rodents, polymeric IgA contributes to 90% of the daily renewed circulating IgA. It is permanently cleared from the plasma and transported to bile by hepatocytes. In humans, however, polymeric IgA, which represents 10% to 15% of intravascular IgA, is cleared from plasma by internal catabolism (34 mg/kg/day), and not more than 1 mg/kg/day is transported into secretions (8). From these metabolic studies it can be concluded that most secretory IgA is produced by mucosal plasma cells. Considering that 60 mg/kg/day represents total IgA synthesis rate in adults, about one-third of this IgA originates from the bone marrow and is delivered to the circulating blood, whereas two-thirds of the IgA is synthesized in mucosae-associated plasma cells and is delivered to secretions.

These metabolic studies are of great significance with respect to clinical investigation. They suggest that secretory IgA antibody levels are unlikely to parallel those of serum IgA antibody, since they reflect IgA antibody production by two distinct compartments.

ISOTYPIC REGULATION

The generation of mature B cells involves a series of heavy-chain gene rearrangements that occur in a defined order in pre-B cells in hemopoietic tissues. Switching from expression of a μ chain to another one occurs by pairing tandemly repeated DNA sequences termed "S" and located 5' to each C_H gene except $C\delta$. The intervening DNA sequences may be deleted according to the loop and excision model of isotype switching (9). The isotype regulation of Ig production may therefore rely on two mechanisms: (i) switching of heavy-chain gene expression, and (ii) selective enhancement or suppression of clonal expansion of B cells committed for the expression of a given isotype. Depending on the timing of heavy-chain switch during B-cell ontogeny, regulatory signals triggered by antigenic stimulation or other environmental factors would act preferentially on one of these two mechanisms. T cells that can induce immunoglobulin class switch by sIgM B cells have been described in murine Peyer's patches (PP) (10) and in humans (11). However, most of the currently available models of isotype regulation concern the second pathway, which involves cell-surface receptors or soluble mediators that recognize Fc determinants of Ig at the B-cell surface, i.e., Fc receptors and Ig binding factors (Ig BFs) of defined class or subclass specificity (13).

Antigen feeding in mice induces differential isotype-specific immunoregulation in gut-associated lymphoid tissue (GALT). Peyer's patches from orally primed mice support in vitro antigen-specific IgA responses and contain T-helper cells that promote mainly IgA responses in normal splenic B-cell cultures. Among T-cell clones derived from PP, about 10% were found to support antigen-specific IgA responses by cooperating with sIgA$^+$ B cells. These T cells were Thy-1$^+$, Lyt-1$^+$2-, and L3T4$^+$, and they bear Fcα receptors. After fusion of these helper T cells with the R1.1 lymphoma, Kiyono and McGhee (14) obtained hybridoma which release IgA BFs that have been partially characterized. Such IgA BFs stimulate specific IgA antibody production by activated splenic B cells already committed for IgA production. After antigen feeding, IgA helper T cells migrate from PP to mesenteric lymph nodes (MLN) but not to the spleen (15). In addition to helper T cells, antigen feeding triggers the development of isotype-specific suppressor T cells, mainly IgG and IgE suppressor cells, which migrate to MLN, to spleen, and possibly to distant lymph nodes (16).

Class-specific suppression of Ig production can be achieved by T cells and Ig BF. Class- or subclass-specific Fc receptors can be induced on T cells in vivo by repeated injection of Ig (17). Similarly, release of subclass-specific suppressor Ig BFs can be induced by exposure of a T-cell hybridoma, T2D4, to the appropriate monoclonal Ig (18). In humans, two mechanisms of class-specific suppression have been demonstrated by our group (reviewed in ref. 19). First, exposure of T cells to aggregated IgG or IgA results in a selective reduction of the numbers of cells producing the matching Ig class among polyclonally activated B cells (20). Secondly, IgG BFs or IgA BFs, obtained by spontaneous release from T cells, B cells, or monocytes, selectively depress the generation of B lymphoblasts, thus producing IgG or IgA, respectively. In this model, suppression was shown to require CD8$^+$ radiosensitive T cells (19). The precise signals and mechanisms responsible for the triggering of isotype-specific suppressor cells in PP after antigen feeding are still poorly understood.

Most studies on isotypic regulation dealing with IgA do not take into account distinct regulation of IgA1 and IgA2 subclasses. In human newborns, peripheral blood mononuclear cells include lymphocytes bearing both sIgM and sIgA1 or sIgA2 in equal proportions, each cell being committed to a single IgA subclass (21). In infants, nearly all sIgA$^+$ B cells are of the IgA1 subclass; these cells also lack surface IgM, and many of them have a lymphoblastoid morphology. In adults, sIgA circulating B cells are small lymphocytes lacking sIgM; 80% of them are sIgA1$^+$, and 20% are sIgA2$^+$ (21). In cultures stimulated by the Pokeweed mitogen, IgA B blasts and plasma cells of each subclass are present in equal numbers, although IgA1 is secreted in much greater amounts than IgA2 (22). The relatively high number of IgA2 plasma cells is accounted for by the activation of a small subset of sIgM$^+$, sIgA2$^+$ B lymphocytes, but there is no switch from IgA1 to IgA2 (23). Most B cells express intracytoplasmic J chain, even when they produce monomeric immunoglobulins (24). In cell cultures, bone marrow and spleen cells were reported to secrete mostly monomeric IgA, whereas cells from lamina propria or peripheral blood mononuclear cells produced more polymeric than monomeric IgA (25). The relative proportion of polymeric IgA versus monomeric IgA was reported to increase with the duration of the culture period (26). From these data it appears that the terminal stages of B-cell maturation, including assembly of polymers and secretion of IgA by plasma cells, are regulated by as yet unknown mechanisms.

ANTIGEN-PRESENTING CELLS

In the GALT the elicitation of an immune response to luminal antigen requires the following sequence of events: (a) binding of antigen by enterocytes, particularly by specialized follicle-associated epithelial (FAE) cells (i.e., M cells); (b) endocytosis through M cells and transport to underlying PP lymphoid tissue; (c) antigen presentation by Ia$^+$ antigen-presenting cells (APC) to immunocompetent cells of the PP; (d) stimulation of antigen-specific T cells and induction of B-cell proliferation and/or differentiation. Based on the current knowledge of APC in spleen and peripheral lymph nodes contributing to systemic immune responsiveness, it appears that five main characteristics must be fulfilled for a given cell type to be a candidate for antigen presentation: (i) binding of antigen; (ii) processing of antigen; (iii) expression of Ia antigen; (iv) ability to migrate to distant lymphoid organs; (v) interaction with antigen-specific T cells involving the Ia-antigen complex and the T-cell receptor.

Macrophages

By analogy with the systemic immune response to a given antigen, PP macrophages were first candidates as APC in GALT. These cells populate the dome area and the germinal centers of PP and were also identified among intraepithelial lymphocytes (IEL). Despite their ability to phagocytose, to process antigen, and to migrate within GALT, their competence in the induction of humoral immunity has been questioned (27). Accessory cells with APC capacity were found in nonadherent Ia$^+$ PP cells (28) and in PP cells dissociated with collagenase (29) or dispase (30). However, in all these experiments, APC were not convincingly characterized as macrophages.

Absorptive Columnar Epithelial Cells and M Cells

Nonlymphoid cells in GALT, such as columnar epithelial cells (EC) of the villi and FAE cells of the PP dome (also called M cells), have been put forward as candidates for APC. In recent studies Bland and Warren (31) reported that columnar Ia$^+$ EC from the small intestine bind ovalbumin *in vitro* and induce antigen-specific T-cell proliferation upon 18-hr co-culture in the presence of antigen. Interleukin-1 or related factors are released by cultured rat EC (32). Interestingly, antigen-specific T cells with suppressive activity were generated during the induction phase by Ia$^+$ EC (32). IEL, which can modulate Ia expression on EC (33), may be the cells responding *in vivo* to antigen presented by absorptive EC and may be responsible for oral tolerance. However, the *in vivo* relevance of antigen presentation by columnar EC is still speculative, especially since EC are separated from lymphoid cells by the basement membrane.

M cells are specialized EC interspersed among other EC, including absorptive EC and goblet cells of the dome epithelium of PP. These cells transport antigen from the lumen to the lymphoid follicle of PP. From rat PP, Pappo et al. (34) isolated FAE cells bearing 2- to 10-fold more Ia antigen than nearby EC, and these FAE cells were able to endocytose antigens *in vitro*. Antigens may be preferentially absorbed by M cells and transferred to the lymphocytes enfolded by the M cells or transferred to the macrophages underlying the epithelium, which may present antigen to PP T cells.

Dendritic Cells

Ultrastructural and histochemical studies have shown that macrophage-like cells are present in the lamina propria and dome region of PP. Wilders et al. (35) reported that PP contains dendritic cells which are very similar to APC of the skin (epidermal Langerhans cells) skin lymph (lymph-born veiled cells), and lymph nodes (paracortical interdigitating cells). All these cells share common features: Ia antigen expression; ATPase positivity; absent or weak acid phosphatase activity; and comparable ultrastructural morphology. Furthermore, dendritic cells, such as veiled cells, form large moving cytoplasmic veils by which they make contact with other cells in their vicinity. It was therefore suggested that Ia$^+$ dendritic cells are involved in antigen presentation. Dendritic cells are localized in the lamina propria of small intestinal villi, as well as within PP where they are found in the subepithelial region of the dome, within the dome epithelium itself, and in the internodular T-cell areas (36,37). It has been recently proposed that the Ia$^+$ dendritic cells in the intestinal villi develop into a type of mononuclear cell which is mainly phagocytic rather than APC. In contrast, the Ia$^+$ dendritic cell accumulating in the PP evolves mainly into a cell type engaged in APC function (35). Furthermore, it is tempting to speculate that dendritic cells, distributed throughout the gut epithelium, could function as APC, highly efficient in the binding of randomly distributed luminal antigen, as compared to PP dendritic cells, which are confined to a discrete portion of the gut. Enzymatic dissociation of PP releases a cell population with accessory activity in oxidative mitogenesis; this cell population is nonadherent, Ia$^+$, and bears the 33D1 dendritic cell-specific determinant (38,39). Further dendritic cell clusters from PP provide the inducing stimulus for polyclonal IgA secretion (40). These cells are similar to epidermal Langerhans cells, which take up antigen and migrate through dermal lymphatics to regional lymph nodes where interaction with T cells and antigen presentation take place (41). One may propose that dendritic cells, after antigen uptake in the intestinal epithelium, migrate through the submucosae to MLN where they interact with T cells.

CELL TRAFFIC AND SELECTIVE HOMING TO MUCOSAL SITES

The selective homing of IgA plasma cells at various mucosal sites after antigenic stimulation in a defined site is still poorly understood despite extensive investigations. Neither the secretory component (which does not bind to IgA B-cell surface) nor the antigen itself can be regarded as appropriate homing signals. One may speculate that cytokines produced by epithelial cells or lymphokines released from antigen-activated intraepithelial T lymphocytes might be involved, but so far no data support this view.

After antigen feeding, immature B lymphocytes from PP can repopulate the small intestine of irradiated recipients with IgA plasma cells (42). PP blast cells migrate either to peripheral lymph nodes or to MLN, and most of those which settle in the intestine migrate through MLN and differentiate into IgA plasma cells. These transfer experiments indicate that PP contain B cells that are already committed for migration to MLN, mucosal homing, and differentiation into IgA plasma cells (43).

Circulation of T and B lymphocytes from one lymphoid organ to another is mediated by entry of the lymphocyte into the high endothelium venule (HEV) (44) of lymph nodes or PP. This interaction involves the expression of two sets of adhesion molecules, namely, the homing receptor of the lymphocyte and the HEV complementary structure. The latter has been characterized in mouse lymph nodes. It is a lectin that binds preferentially to mannose-6-phosphate present either as a single sugar or as part of a 6-phosphomannosyl-conjugated mannan on the lymphocyte homing receptor (45). Using cold incubation of lymphocytes with thin sections of lymphoid organs, it is possible to observe that only recirculating lymphocytes adhere to HEV and not to other blood vessels. Without exception, this assay correlates with lymphocyte homing *in vivo* (46). Two patterns of circulation have been described, each involving a distinct homing receptor. Guy-Grand et al. have shown that B and T lymphocytes from stimulated PP migrated to the thoracic duct before entering the circulation and returning to the lamina propria and intraepithelial regions (47,48). Recently, Stevens et al. demonstrated a preferential binding of T cells to lymph-node HEV and of B cells to PP HEV (49). A monoclonal antibody (MEL-14) directed against the mouse lymph-node homing receptor has been developed. This antibody prevents lymphocyte binding to lymph nodes but not to PP HEV (50). A monoclonal antibody specific for lymphocyte surface molecules mediating adhesion to rat PP HEV has been described (51). Most antigen-activated lymphocytes transiently down-regulate the expression of their homing receptor (52), presumably for a dual purpose: (i) to prevent inappropriate removal of these lymphocytes from the blood stream to lymphoid organs not draining the inducing antigen and (ii) to permit the localization of these effector lymphocytes in extralymphoid sites of antigen presentation.

REGULATION OF IMMUNE RESPONSE INDUCED BY ORAL ROUTE

Suppressor Mechanisms

The mucosae are in constant contact with a myriad of antigenic substances that have immunostimulatory or immunomodulatory properties, and within such an environment lymphoid tissue could conceivably undergo excessive stimulation. As a result, responses to potentially pathogenic stimuli might be preempted by responses to an overwhelming array of inconsequential materials. For this reason, it would not be surprising to find that the mucosal immune system had potent regulatory mechanisms allowing the development of local responses associated with a down-regulation of systemic reactions. Antigen feeding can induce local immunization with secretory immunoglobulin production and can simultaneously cause unresponsiveness (tolerance) to parenteral challenge with the same antigen (53). This state of oral unresponsiveness (oral tolerance) (54) can be observed as a reaction to both particulate (55,56) and soluble antigen (57–59).

The immune tolerance thus produced is specific and can be shown to affect cell-mediated hypersensitivity (56,60) as well as the production of specific antibody, including reaginic antibody (61). The relative contribution of antigen, antibody, immune complexes, and suppressor cells of various lineages and specificities to oral tolerance is still a matter of controversy.

Humoral Factors

Inhibitory serum factors (antibody or antigen antibody complexes) were reported in orally tolerized mice. Serum from mice that are intragastrically immunized with sheep red blood cells (SRBC) contains a very active antigen-specific tolerogen. The tolerogenic effect was demonstrated *in vivo* and could be related to immune complexes, with IgA as the antibody (54). Using the same antigen, other authors (62) have demonstrated suppressive effects of serum from intragastrically immunized mice or *in vitro* primary responses of normal spleen cells to SRBC. In this case, the suppressive factor was reported to be immunoglobulins of the IgG1 subclass.

Other serum factors can be incriminated: first, after administration, by stomach tube, of 25 mg bovine serum albumin (BSA), immunoreactive (and presumably intact) protein can be found in serum at concentrations ranging from 1 to 10 ng/ml; thus oral tolerance has some features in common with the state of tolerance induced by the parenteral administration of small amounts of antigen (low zone tolerance) (63). In serum transfer experiments, other authors (64) have shown that serum collected from mice 1 hr after a single intragastric dose of 25 mg ovalbumin could suppress systemic delayed-type hypersensitivity when injected intraperitoneally into recipient mice. This suppression was restricted to the cell-mediated limb of immunity and was antigen-specific. Absorption of tolerogenic serum from ovalbumin-fed mice with antiovalbumin antibody removed the tolerogenic moiety from the serum. Serum fractions lacking immunoreactive ovalbumin were not significantly tolerogenic *in vitro* (65). Thus the small intestine can deliver a tolerogenic antigen. It is not yet known whether this tolerance induction requires antigen processing with limited degradation and presentation by appropriate cell membranes or merely requires the delivery of very small amounts of intact molecules of soluble antigen. Moreover, oral tolerance to SRBC could be readily established in rats in which PP had been surgically removed (66).

Suppressor Cells

It has further been shown that antigen-specific suppressor T cells are formed after feeding with protein antigen (16,57), contact sensitizing agents (60), and particulate antigens (55). After 2 days of SRBC feeding in rats, PP and MLN contain suppressor cells that blocked IgM and IgG plaque-forming cell responses to SRBC in Mishell-Dutton cultures (55). After 4 days of feeding, suppressor cells were found in the thymus and spleen but not in the PP or MLN. Similar results were obtained with ovalbumin in mice (57,67). Feeding with the contact sensitizing agent oxazolone was associated with the presence of B and T suppressor cells in PP and MLN (60). By contrast, feeding with ovalbumin resulting in the suppression of systemic delayed-type hypersensitivity was associated with the presence of suppressor T cells in popliteal and inguinal lymph nodes (68). Thus suppressor B cells would appear to be a special feature of contact hypersensitivity.

Cellular Traffic and Suppressor Cell Interactions

Migration of PP lymphocytes (including suppressor cells) to MLN has been documented by injection of fluorescein isothiocyanate into PP and examination of fluorescent cells in lymphoid tissues. By using *in vivo* and *in vitro* transfer systems, Mattingly (69) demonstrated that, after SRBC feeding in mice, suppressor-inducer T cells were generated in PP and migrated to the spleen for the induction of effector suppressor cells. Suppressor-inducer T cells are Lyt-1$^+$ lymphocytes that are resistant to cyclophosphamide, whereas spleen suppressor T cells are cyclophosphamide-sensitive Lyt-2$^+$ lymphocytes. A comparable cascade of suppressor cells has been suggested in the model of suppression of contact sensitivity to trinitrochlorobenzene by feeding with the hapten (70). In this model, as well as in tolerance induced by intravenous administration of trinitrochlorobenzene, suppressor T effector cells were shown to produce a soluble suppressor factor that arms T acceptor cells, which in turn are triggered to release a nonspecific inhibitor that directly inhibits the function of delayed-type hypersensitivity T cells, regardless of their antigenic specificity. Development of suppressor T cells involved in oral tolerance can be prevented *in vivo* by treatment with cyclophosphamide or with 2'-deoxyguanosine (71).

Contrasuppressor Cells

A contrasuppressor cell circuit whose end-function is to antagonize the inhibitory action of suppressor T cells on the helper T-cell population has been described (72). Contrasuppressor T cells were recently described in the spleen of SRBC-fed mice (73,74). Contrasuppressor cells were obtained from the spleen of C3H/HeJ mice and were transferred to C3H/HeN mice made tolerant to SRBC by antigen feeding. As few as 5×10^4 transferred cells were sufficient to abolish the tolerance of recipient mice and to induce anti-SRBC antibody-forming cells of all major classes in the spleen. The same effect could be demonstrated *in vitro*. On the basis of various methods used to enrich or deplete inactive cells, it was concluded that contrasuppressor cells were Lyt-1$^+$, Lyt-2$^-$, and L3T4$^-$ and that they bear I-J^{k+} determinants and adhere to *Vicia villosa* lectin. These experiments would suggest that in orally tolerized mice, T helper cells are present but are controlled by suppressor cells.

Priming and Desensitization by Antigen Feeding

Depending on the nature and dose of the antigen used, the frequency and duration of antigen feeding, and the prior antigen exposure history of the host, antigen feeding may either (a) prime the animal for subsequent enteral or parenteral challenge or (b) induce the suppression of subsequent local and/or systemic antibody or delayed hypersensitivity responses (75). Using SRBC as antigen, it was shown that suppression of delayed-type hypersensitivity was achieved after 2 weeks and persisted up to 8 weeks after initiation of antigen feeding (76). Similarly, suppression of IgM anti-SRBC antibody-secreting cells in the spleen following intraperitoneal challenge started 2 weeks after SRBC feeding and was still profound after 52 weeks of feeding (77). However, in the same experiments it was found that IgA and IgG antibody-secreting cell number was increased during the first 2 weeks of feeding and then dropped after only 3 weeks. Nearly complete suppression of

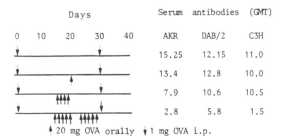

FIG. 1. Abrogation of antibody response by antigen feeding. (From ref. 78.)

FIG. 2. Amplification of antibody response to intraperitoneal immunization by prior administration of one oral dose of ova. (From ref. 78.)

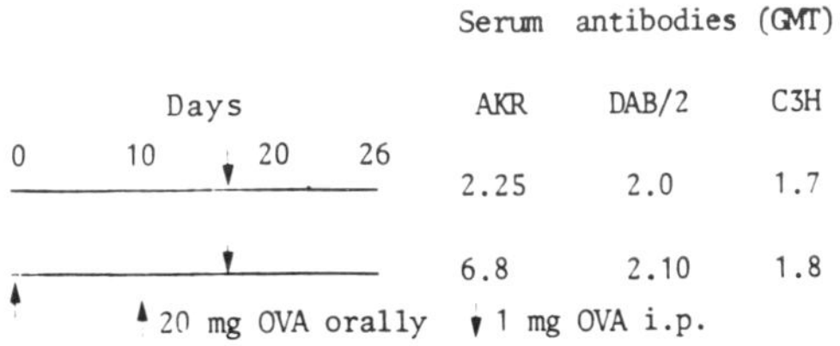

Serum antibodies (GMT)

Days			AKR	DAB/2	C3H
0	10	20 26	2.25	2.0	1.7
			6.8	2.10	1.8

⬆ 20 mg OVA orally   ⬇ 1 mg OVA i.p.

these two antibody classes was only achieved after 52 weeks of feeding (77). Lafont and co-workers showed that a single oral dose of ovalbumin was sufficient to prime AKR mice, but not C3H or DBA/2 mice, to induce a secondary serum antibody response to subsequent intraperitoneal challenge (Fig. 1) (78). In the same strains, the effect of antigen feeding on the suppression of an ongoing systemic antibody response to ovalbumin was investigated. Two intraperitoneal injections of 1 mg of this antigen at 1-month interval resulted in a strong antibody response, including reaginic antibodies (IgGl and IgE) demonstrable by passive cutaneous anaphylaxis. Antigen feeding prior to the intraperitoneal boost was shown to diminish serum antibody levels. The suppression increased with the repetition of ovalbumin feedings (Fig. 2) (78). The magnitude of the suppression varied according to the mouse strains, regardless of their H-2 haplotypes (79). Although it is difficult in some systems (80), suppression of an ongoing immune response in primed hosts by repeated oral administration of antigen may have important implications in allergic diseases.

CONCLUSION

We have attempted to delineate some of the critical steps involved in the regulation of secretory IgA production and suppression of systemic antibody and T-cell responses. Several other regulatory pathways could not be included in this brief survey—for instance, sex hormones, catecholamines, and neurointestinal peptides. One may expect that a better understanding of the nature and function of APC, homing receptors, and lymphokines with isotype-specific effects on the development of polymeric IgA1 and IgA2 antibodies will help to manipulate immunization by the oral route. Development of new adjuvants—for instance, cholera toxin or its B subunit—may improve the efficiency of oral immunization. Control of the resident bacterial flora by deliberate colonization of the gut may be an important factor in the development of the IgA secretory system. Major medical applications may be expected from progress in this field, which is concerned with immunization with nonreplicative antigens for the prevention of mucosal infections as well as the prevention of food allergy.

REFERENCES

1. Bienenstock J, McDermott M, Befus D. A common mucosal immune system. In: Ogra P, Dayton D, eds. *Immunology of breast milk*. New York: Raven Press, 1979:91–104.
2. Walker WA, Isselbacher KJ, Block KJ. Intestinal uptake of macromolecules: effect of oral immunization. *Science* 1972;177:608–10.
3. Buckley RH, Fiscus SA. Serum IgD and IgE concentration in immunodeficiency diseases. *J Clin Invest* 1975;55:157–67.
4. Kutteh WHS, Prince SJ, Mestecky J. Tissue origins of human polymeric and monomeric IgA. *J Immunol* 1982;128:990–5.
5. Underdown BJ, Schiff JM. Immunoglobulin A: strategic defense initiative at the mucosal surface. *Annu Rev Immunol* 1986;4:389–417.
6. Solari R, Kraehenbuhl JP. The biosynthesis of secretory component and its role in the transepithelial transport of IgA dimer. *Immunol Today* 1985;6:17–20.
7. Strober W, Krakauer R, Klaeveman HL, Reynolds HY, Nelson DL. Secretory component deficiency. A disorder of the IgA immune system. *N Engl J Med* 1976;294:351–6.
8. Delacroix DL, Hodgson HJF, McPherson A, Dive C. Selective transport of polymeric immunoglobulin A in bile quantitative relationships of monomeric and polymeric immunoglobulin A, immunoglobulin M and other proteins in serum, bile and saliva. *J Clin Invest* 1982;70:230–41.
9. Burrows PD, Cooper MD. The immunoglobulin heavy chain class switch. *Mol Cell Biochem* 1984;63:97–111.
10. Kawanishi H. Galtzman LE, Strober W. Mechanisms regulating IgA class-specific immunoglobulin production in murine gut-associated lymphoid tissues. I. T cells derived from Peyer's patches that switch sIgM B cells to sIgA B cells *in vitro*. *J Exp Med* 1983;157:433–50.
11. Mayer L, Posnett DN, Kunkel HG. Human malignant T cells capable of inducing an immunoglobulin class switch. *J Exp Med* 1985;161:134–44.
12. Ishizaka K. Regulation of IgE synthesis. *Annu Rev Immunol* 1984;2:159–92.
13. Daeron M, Fridman WH. Fc receptors as regulatory molecules. *Ann Inst Pasteur (Immunol)* 1986;136C:383–437.
14. Kiyono H, McGhee JR. Mucosal T cell networks: role of FcαR+ T cells and Ig BF in regulation of the IgA response. *Int Rev Immunol* 1986;2:99–124.
15. Richman LK, Graeff AS, Yarchoan R and Strober W. Simultaneous induction of antigenic-specific IgA, helper T cells and IgG suppressor T cells in the murine Peyer's patch after protein feeding. *J Immunol* 1981;126:2079–83.
16. Ngan J, Kind LS. Suppressor T cells for IgE and IgG in Peyer's patches of mice made tolerant by the oral administration of ovalbumin. *J Immunol* 1978;120:861–5.
17. Waldschmidt TJ, Williams KR, Lynch RG. Isotype-specific recognition and regulation by T cells studies with tumor models. *Int J Immunol* 1986;2:1–18.
18. Lowy I, Brezin C, Neauport-Sautes C, Thèze J, Fridman WH. Isotype regulation of antibody production: T cell hybrids can be selectively induced to produce IgG1 and IgG2 subclass-specific suppressive immunoglobulin-binding factors. *Proc Natl Acad Sci USA* 1983;80:2323–7.
19. Revillard JP, Millet I. Fc receptor bearing T cells and Ig binding factors as class-specific suppressors of polyclonally activated human B cells. *Int Rev Immunol* 1986;2:39–57.
20. Le thi Bich-Thuy, Revillard JP. Only T and T cells can be triggered by IgG or IgA to suppress the production of the matching Ig class. *Eur J Immunol* 1986;16:156–61.

21. Conley ME, Kearny JF, Lawton AR, Cooper MD. Differentiation of human B cells expressing the IgA subclasses as demonstrated by monoclonal hybridoma antibodies. *J Immunol* 1980;125:2311–6.
22. Conley ME, Doopman WJ. *In vitro* regulation of IgA subclass synthesis. I. Discordance between plasma cell production and antibody secretion. *J Exp Med* 1982;156:1615–21.
23. Conley ME, Bartelt MS. *In vitro* regulation of IgA subclass synthesis. II. The source of IgA2 plasma cells. *J Immunol* 1984;133:2312–6.
24. Kutteh WH, Moldoveanu Z, Prince SJ, Kulhavy R, Alonso R, Mestecky J. Biosynthesis of J chain in human lymphoid cells producing immunoglobulins of various isotypes. *Mol Immunol* 1983;20:967–76.
25. Kutteh WH, Prince SJ, Mestecky J. Tissue origins of human polymeric and monomeric IgA. *J Immunol* 1982;128:990–5.
26. Moldoveanu Z, Egan ML, Mestecky J. Cellular origins of human polymeric and monomeric IgA: intracellular and secreted forms of IgA. *J Immunol* 1984;133:3156–62.
27. Kagnoff MF, Campbell S. Functional characteristics of Peyer's patches lymphoid cells. *J Exp Med* 1974;139:398–406.
28. Barr WG, Challacombe SJ, Yem A, Tomasi TB. The accessory cell function of murine Peyer's patches. *Cell Immunol* 1985;92:41–52.
29. Richman LK, Graeff AS, Strober W. Antigen presentation by macrophage-enriched cells from the mouse Peyer's patches. *Cell Immunol* 1981;62:110–8.
30. Kiyono H, McGhee JR, Wannemuelher MJ, Frangakis MV, Spalding DM, Michalek SM, Koopman WJ. *In vitro* immune response to a T-cell dependent antigen by cultures of dissociated murine Peyer's patches. *Proc Natl Acad Sci USA* 1982;79:596–600.
31. Bland PW, Warren LG. Antigen presentation by epithelial cells of the rat small intestine. I. Kinetics, antigen specificity and blocking by anti-Ia antisera. *Immunology* 1986;58:1–7.
32. Bland PW, Warren LG. Antigen presentation by epithelial cells of the rat small intestine. II. Selective induction of suppressor T cells. *Immunology* 1986;58:9–13.
33. Cerf-Bensussan N, Quaroni A, Kurnick JT, Bhan AK. Intraepithelial lymphocytes modulate Ia expression by intestinal epithelial cells. *J Immunol* 1984;132:2244–52.
34. Pappo J, Ebersole JL, Taubman MA. Phenotypic analysis of Pcyer's patch epithelial cell population. *FASEB* 1985;886.
35. Wilders MM, Sminia T, Janse EM. Ontogeny of non-lymphoid cells in the rat gut with special reference to large mononuclear Ia positive dendritic cells. *Immunology* 1984;50:303–14.
36. Mayrhofer G, Pugh CW, Barclay N. The distribution, ontogeny and origin in the rat of Ia-positive cells with dendritic morphology and of Ia-antigen in epithelium with special reference to the intestine. *Eur J Immunol* 1983;13:112–22.
37. Kraal G, Breel M, Janse M, Bruin G. Langerhans cells, veiled cells, and interdigitating cells in the mouse recognized by a monoclonal antibody. *J Exp Med* 1986;163:981–97.
38. Spalding DM, Koopman WJ, Eldridge JH, McGhee, JR, Steinman RM. Accessory cells in murine Peyer's patch. I. Identification and enrichment of a functional dendritic cell. *J Exp Med* 1983;157:1646–59.
39. Nussenzweig MC, Steinman RM, Witmer MD, Gutchinov B. A monoclonal antibody specific for mouse dendritic cells. *Proc Natl Acad Sci USA* 1982;79:161–70.
40. Spalding DD, Williamson SI, Koopman WJ, McGhee JR. Preferential induction of polyclonal IgA secretion by murine Peyer's patch dendritic cell–T cell mixtures. *J Exp Med* 1984;160:941–6.
41. Bos JD, Kapsenberg ML. The skin immune system, its cellular constituents and their interactions. *Immunol Today* 1986;7:235–40.
42. Rudzik O, Clancy RL, Perey DYE, Day RP, Bienenstock J. Repopulation with IgA-containing cells of bronchial and intestinal lamina propria after transfer of homologous Peyer's patch and bronchial lymphocytes. *J Immunol* 1975;114:1599–1604.
43. Roux ME, Williams MM, Phillips-Quagliata JM, Lamm ME. Differentiation pathway of Peyer's patch precursors of IgA plasma cells in the secretory immune system. *Cell Immunol* 1981;61:141–53.
44. Stamper HB, Woodruff JJ. Lymphocyte homing into lymph nodes: *in vitro* demonstration of the selective affinity of recirculating lymphocytes for high endothelial venules. *J Exp Med* 1976;144:828–34.
45. Stoolman LM, Tenforde TS, Rosen SD. Phosphomannosyl receptors may participate in the adhesive interaction between lymphocytes and high endothelial venules. *J Cell Biol* 1984;99:1535–40.

46. Jalkanen S, Reichert RA, Gallatin WM, Bargatze RF, Weissman IL, Butcher EC. Homing receptors and the control of lymphocyte migration. *Immunol Rev* 1986;91:39–60.
47. Guy-Grand D, Griscelli C, Vassali P. The gut-associated lymphoid system: nature and properties of the large dividing cells. *Eur J Immunol* 1974;4:435–44.
48. Guy-Grand D, Griscelli C, Vassali P. The mouse gut T cell. Nature, origin and traffic in mice in normal and graft-versus-host conditions. *J Exp Med* 1978;148:1661–9.
49. Stevens SK, Weissman IL, Butcher EC. Differences in the migration of B and T lymphocytes: organ-selective localization *in vivo* and the role of lymphocyte-endothelial cell recognition. *J Immunol* 1982;128:844–51.
50. Gallatin WM, Weissman IL, Butcher EC. A cell-surface molecule involved in organ-specific homing of lymphocytes. *Nature* 1983;304:30–4.
51. Chin YH, Rasmussen RA, Woodruff JJ, Easton TG. A monoclonal anti-HEBF pp antibody with specificity for lymphocyte surface molecules mediating adhesion to Peyer's patch high endothelium of the rat. *J Immunol* 1986;136:2556–61.
52. Reichert RA, Weissman IL, Butcher EC. Germinal center B cells lack homing receptors necessary for normal lymphocyte recirculation. *J Exp Med* 1983;157:813–27.
53. Challacombe SJ, Tomasi TB. Systemic tolerance and secretory immunity after oral immunization. *J Exp Med* 1980;152;1459–72.
54. André C, Heremans JF, Vaerman JP, Cambisso CL. A mechanism for the induction of immunological tolerance by antigen feeding: antigen-antibody complexes. *J Exp Med* 1975;142:1509–19.
55. Mattingly JA, Waksman BH. Immunologic suppression after oral administration of antigen. I. Specific suppressor cells formed in rat Peyer's patches after oral administration of sheep erythrocytes and their systemic migration. *J Immunol* 1978;121:1878–83.
56. Kagnoff MF. Effects of antigen-feeding on intestinal and systemic immune responses. II. Suppression of delayed-type hypersensitivity reactions. *J Immunol* 1978;120:1509–13.
57. Hanson DG, Vaz NM, Maia LCS, Lynch JM. Inhibition of specific immune responses by feeding protein antigens. III. Evidence against maintenance of tolerance to ovalbumin by orally induced antibodies. *J Immunol* 1979;123:2337–43.
58. Swarbrick ET, Stokes CR, Soothill JF. Absorption of antigens after oral immunisation and the simultaneous induction of specific systemic tolerance. *Gut* 1979;20:121–5.
59. Vives J, Parks DE, Weigle WO. Immunologic unresponsiveness after gastric administration of human γ-globulin: antigen requirements and cellular parameters. *J Immunol* 1980;125:1811–6.
60. Asherson GL, Zembala M, Perera MACC, Mayhew B, Thomas WR. Producing of immunity and unresponsiveness in the mouse by feeding contact sensitizing agents and the role of suppressor cells in the Peyer's patches, mesenteric lymph nodes and other lymphoid tissues. *Cell Immunol* 1977;33:145–55.
61. David MF. Prevention of homocytotropic antibody formation and anaphylactic sensitization by prefeeding antigen. *J Allergy Clin Immunol* 1977;60:180–7.
62. Chalon MP, Milne RW, Vaerman JP. In vitro immunosuppressive effect of serum from orally immunized mice. *Eur J Immunol* 1979;9:747–51.
63. Thomas HC, Parrott MV. The induction of tolerance to a soluble antigen by oral administration. *Immunology* 1974;27:631–9.
64. Bruce MG, Ferguson A. Oral tolerance to ovalbumin in mice: studies of chemically modified and "biologically filtered" antigen. *Immunology* 1986;57:627–30.
65. Bruce MG, Ferguson A. The influence of intestinal processing on the immunogenicity and molecular size of absorbed, circulating ovalbumin in mice. *Immunology* 1986;59:295–300.
66. Enders G, Gottwald T, Brendel W. Induction of oral tolerance in rats without Peyer's patches. *Immunology* 1986;58:311–4.
67. Richman LK, Chiller JM, Brown WR, Hanson DG, Vaz NM. Enterically induced immunologic tolerance. 1. Induction of suppressor T lymphocytes by intragastric administration of soluble proteins. *J Immunol* 1978;121:2429–32.
68. Mowat A. McI. The role of antigen recognition and suppressor cells in mice with oral tolerance to ovalbumin. *Immunology* 1985;56:253–60.
69. Mattingly JA. Immunologic suppression after oral administration of antigen. III. Activation of suppressor-inducer cells in the Peyer's patches. *Cell Immunol* 1984;86:46–52.
70. Gautam SC, Battisto JR. Orally induced tolerance generates an efferently acting suppressor T cell and an acceptor T cell that together down regulate contact sensitivity. *J Immunol* 1985;135:2975–83.
71. Mowat A. McI. Depletion of suppressor T cells by 2'-deoxyguanosine abrogates tolerance in mice

fed ovalbumin and permits the induction of intestinal delayed-type hypersensitivity. *Immunology* 1986;58:179–84.
72. Green DR, Flood PM, Gershon RK. Immunoregulatory T cell pathways. *Annu Rev Immunol* 1983;1:439–63.
73. Suzuki I, Kitamura K, Kiyono H, Kurita T, Green DR, McGhee JR. Isotype-specific immunoregulation. Evidence for a distinct subset of T contrasuppressor cells for IgA responses in murine Peyer's patches. *J Exp Med* 1986;164:501–16.
74. Suzuki I, Kiyono H, Kitamura K, Green DR, McGhee JR. Abrogation of oral tolerance by contrasuppressor T cells suggests the presence of regulatory T-cell networks in the mucosal immune system. *Nature* 1986;320:451–4.
75. Kagnoff MF. Immunology of the digestive system. In: Johnson LR, ed. *Physiology of the gastrointestinal tract*. New York: Raven Press, 1981:1337–59.
76. Kagnoff MF. Effects of antigen-feeding on intestinal and systemic immune responses: II. Suppression of delayed-type hypersensitivity responses. *J Immunol* 1978;120:1509–13.
77. Kagnoff MF. Effects of antigen-feeding on intestinal and systemic immune responses: III. Antigen-specific serum-mediated suppression of humoral antibody responses after antigen feeding. *Cell Immunol* 1978;40:186–203.
78. Lafont S, André C, André F, Gillon J. Fargier MC. Abrogation by subsequent feeding of antibody response, including IgE, in parenterally immunized mice. *J Exp Med* 1982;155:1573–8.
79. André C, Lafont S, André F, Danière S. Induction de tolérance et désensibilisation par voie digestive. In: Revillard JP, Wierzbicki N, Voisin C, eds. *Mucosal immunity: IgA and polymorphonuclear neutrophils*. Paris: 1984:83–9.
80. Hanson DG, Vaz NM, Rawlings LA, Lynch JM. Inhibition of specific immune responses by feeding protein antigens. II. Effects of prior passive and active immunization. *J Immunol* 1979;122:2261–6.

DISCUSSION

Dr. Rossipal: You clearly showed the importance of IgA production in the gut for all immunizations. IgA deficiency is a common clinical condition, but does "deficiency" mean that there is no IgA production in the mucosa, or does it only mean that we cannot find IgA in the serum? And if there is no IgA in the mucosa, can IgM take over its function?

Dr. Revillard: It is true that serum IgA and secretory IgA are two compartments under separate control. However, despite the great heterogeneity of syndromes of IgA deficiency, nearly all patients with serum IgA levels below 10 mg/liter lack secretory IgA. The reverse situation defined by the absence of secretory IgA with normal serum IgA levels is extremely rare. A single case of deficiency in secretory component has been reported (1). IgA deficiency is usually associated with high secretory IgM levels, accounting for a rather low incidence of respiratory tract infections as compared with that of other antibody deficiencies.

Dr. Müller: In your scheme of isotype switching, you omitted IgE. Where is its place in the scheme?

Dr. Revillard: I could not cover all the literature on the regulation of IgE production, which is exceedingly complex. The question you ask is one of the most controversial in the field, but at the simplest level there are two possibilities. The first is that switching occurs at random very early in differentiation, with B-cells expressing the appropriate surface immunoglobulin at the pre-B stage. They are driven to multiply in an isotype-specific fashion. This is the selective theory. The second possibility is that switching is a late event and the regulation of switching is controlled by specific T cells which may signal the B cells, for example, to shut off a μ gene and use an α or ϵ gene instead. This is the instructive theory, but there is little experimental support for it (2,3).

Dr. de Weck: You have pointed out that IgA- and IgG-binding factors are important for regulating the differentiation of B cells. In the case of IgE-binding factors, there are supposed to be enhancing and suppressing factors in theory, at least in rodents, whose effect depends on their degree of glycosylation. Is there any evidence that there are enhancing factors in the IgA system, or are they always suppressive? Have they anything to do with the glycosylation of the factor?

Dr. Revillard: I do not think anybody has isolated and cloned an IgA-enhancing factor. In all models the amplification is achieved by T cells, which have been shown to bear Fc_α receptors. In terms of humoral mediators the IgA BFs which have been isolated have all been suppressive. The reason for this could be that we have not been using the appropriate cell source, since we have not started to work with human intestinal T cells. These could well be the source of T-cell clones producing enhancer or helper factors. Recently, two interleukins distinct from Ig BFs were shown to stimulate the production of IgE (interleukin-4) or IgA (interleukin-5) by mature human B cells. However, these lymphokines also display many other biological activities, and their present role in isotype regulation remains to be investigated (4).

Dr. Aas: There is much controversy in the literature with regard to the amount of IgE and IgA in intestinal secretions and fecal extracts. I believe this must be due, at least in part, to different immunoglobulin fragmentation procedures and also, of course, to methodologic differences. I know something about this from work on IgE in secretions and fecal extracts, where the choice of methods is very important for the proper quantification of results. What about IgA in this respect? Is there any chance of finding intact IgA molecules in secretions with antibody specificities that can be defined, and what are the main methodologic problems? There are some prominent pitfalls with regard to IgE, and there must also be some for IgA in this respect.

Dr. Revillard: This is a difficult problem. For example, we had a recent experience of studying a new cholera vaccine in collaboration with the Pasteur Institute in Paris. This produced a negligible effect on serum antibody titers and also produced apparently random variations in saliva antibodies. However, when we looked at jejunal fluid we found a nice rise in specific antibodies, but only after adjusting all the samples to a single IgA dimer standard and then testing for antibody activity in an ELISA solid phase system which revealed IgA binding, either by anti-α heavy chain or antisecretory component. This shows how difficult it is to demonstrate this type of specific secretory response. If we did not have access to jejunal fluid we would have wrongly concluded that the immunization had failed to induce an antibody response, and then if we had not standardized the fluids for the same arbitrary content of secretory IgA, we would not have been able to show a consistent rise in titer with immunization. Similar problems arise with all secretory fluids.

Dr. Strobel: I have two comments: The first is that you have compared animal studies which, in some cases, involved particulate antigens and, in others, involved soluble antigens. One must be very careful when extrapolating from particulate to soluble antigens, even in animal experiments. My second comment is that the HLA-DR or DP–DQ expression on epithelial cells is a normal phenomenon, and one must be wary of attributing increased or aberrant HLA-DR expression to these epithelial sites with a possible pathogenic mechanism. Cells carrying the HLA-DR/DP or DQ are only expressing class II antigens and do not necessarily take part in relevant antigen presentation. The article you quoted (5) is the only one reporting the presentation of antigen by epithelial cells, and there are many other studies where this could not be shown.

Dr. Revillard: I quite agree with your first comment, although one should emphasize that particulate antigens, which are always immunogenic by parenteral routes, may be tolerogenic by oral administration. It is assumed that digestion and absorption of those particulate antigens by enterocytes result in the presentation of soluble tolerogenic split products to the immune system. With respect to major histocompatibility complex class-II antigen expression by epithelial cells, it is clearly under the control of T-cell products (e.g., gamma interferon). Expression of these antigens is necessary but is not sufficient for any cell to process foreign antigens and present them to T cells.

DISCUSSION REFERENCES

1. Strober W, Krakaver R, Klaeveman HL, Reynolds HY, Nelson DL. Secretory component deficiency. A disorder of the IgA immune system. *N Engl J Med* 1976;294:351–6.
2. Kawanishi H, Saltzman LE, Strober W. Mechanisms regulating IgA class-specific immunoglobulin production in murine gut associated lymphoid tissues. I. T cells derived from Peyers patches that switch sIgM B cells to sIgA B cells *in vitro. J Exp Med* 1983;157:433–50.
3. Mayer L, Posnett DN, Kunkel HG. Human malignant T cells capable of inducing an immunoglobulin class switch. *J Exp Med* 1985;161:134–44.
4. Coffman RL, Ohara J, Bond MW, Carty J, Zlotnik A, Paul WE. B cell stimulatory factor-1 enhances the IgE response of lipopolysaccharide-activated B cells. *J Immunol* 1986;136:4538–41.
5. Bland PW, Warren LG. Antigen presentation by epithelial cells of the rat small intestine. I. Kinetics, antigen specificity and blocking by anti-Ia antisera. *Immunology* 1986;58:1–7.

Food Allergy, edited by Eberhardt Schmidt.
Nestlé Nutrition Workshop Series, Vol. 17.
Nestec Ltd., Vevey/Raven Press, Ltd.,
New York © 1988.

Comparative Studies of Specific IgG4 and IgE Antibody in Patients with Food Allergy

*Joseph A. Bellanti, **Ahmed El-Rafei, *Stephen M. Peters, and Nick Harris

*Departments of Pediatrics and Microbiology and the **International Center for Interdisciplinary Studies of Immunology, Georgetown University School of Medicine, Washington, D.C. 20007*

There has been considerable controversy concerning the possible pathogenetic role of various IgG subclasses in the pathogenesis of allergic disease. The IgG4 antibody has been found to be increased in atopic dermatitis (1) and asthma (2). Shakib and Stanworth (3) suggested the role of IgG4 in anaphylaxis. Gwynn et al. (4) suggested its involvement in asthmatics who had positive delayed-onset bronchial challenges. Vijay and Perelmutter (5) reported that human basophils have receptors for IgG4, can be passively sensitized with IgG4 antibody, and would subsequently release histamine on exposure to specific antigen. Fagan et al. (6) reported that white cells of 14 nonallergic subjects were induced to release histamine with monoclonal mouse anti-IgG4 antibody but not with monoclonal antibodies directed at the other three IgG subclasses. Similar findings were reported by Nagakawa et al. (7,8), who used flow cytometry to demonstrate degranulation of human basophils by anti-IgG4 but not by anti-IgG1, IgG2, or IgG3 antibodies.

Although IgG4 antibodies have been found to represent a class of reagenic antibodies, other investigators have not been able to confirm this possibility: van Toorenenbergen and Aalberse (9) concluded that there was too little evidence that IgG4 could function as a homocytotropic antibody in causing histamine release from human basophils, and Devey et al. (10) also could not demonstrate a pathogenetic role for IgG4. Van der Gieessen et al. (11) suggested that IgG4 may be involved in blocking activity, since IgG4 antibodies could increase dramatically following hyposensitization with pollen antigens.

In infants and young children, immediate-type hypersensitivity to foods is a common finding (12). IgG4 and IgG levels in atopics could be used to distinguish four groups of patients: (i) those high in both IgG and IgG4; (ii) those low in IgE and IgG4 levels; (iii) those high in IgE and low in IgG4; and (iv) those low in IgE and high in IgG4. The fourth group of atopic children was of particular interest and suggested that a role for IgG4 existed in these patients. Preliminary data on IgG4 RAST (radioallergosorbent test) to milk in some of these patients showed positive IgG4 RAST and negative IgE RAST to milk (13). This particular hypothesis seemed attractive because in many children with food allergy, no specific IgE antibodies can be detected and, hypothetically, food allergy could be related to the presence of IgG4.

The overall objective of this study was to evaluate the pathogenetic role of IgG4 antibody in food allergy and to determine its biologic function either as a blocking antibody or as an anaphylactic antibody. Specifically, IgG4 and IgE antibodies were measured in a group of children and adults with food allergy involving the skin, respiratory tract, and gastrointestinal tract, and these findings were correlated with history, skin testing, and the results of double-blind oral food challenge.

PATIENT SELECTION AND INCLUSION CRITERIA

The study population consisted of 25 children and adults, ranging from 6 years to 41 years of age, who had clinical symptoms of food allergy to one or more foods. Clinical symptoms included the following organ systems: (a) skin: urticaria, eczema; (b) respiratory tract: rhinorrhea, wheezing; and (c) gastrointestinal tract: vomiting, diarrhea. Shown in Table 1 are the inclusion criteria for the study.

EXPERIMENTAL DESIGN

Shown in Fig. 1 is a schematic representation of the experimental design of the study. Preliminary screening of all subjects consisted of history, skin testing, and *in vitro* tests to identify potential subjects for the study. If the subject met the entrance criteria, they were then assigned to an elimination diet for 3 weeks devoid of milk, egg, peanut, wheat, and corn. On the first clinic visit a history and physical was performed, and the suspected food allergen was ranked in order of proba-

TABLE 1. *Inclusion criteria for the food-allergy study*

1. Age: 6–40 years
2. Sex: male or female
3. Symptoms: tentative diagnosis of food allergy will include a history of one or more of the following symptoms following food ingestion: rhinorrhea, urticaria, eczema, asthma, diarrhea
4. Refrain from medications: antihistamines, tricyclic antidepressants, tranquilizers, antipsychotic agents (4 days); aminophylline, epinephrine, ephedrine (24 hr)
5. No beta-blocking agents
6. No dermatographism
7. Specific exclusions: other diseases or conditions, pregnant or lactating females, long-term steroids

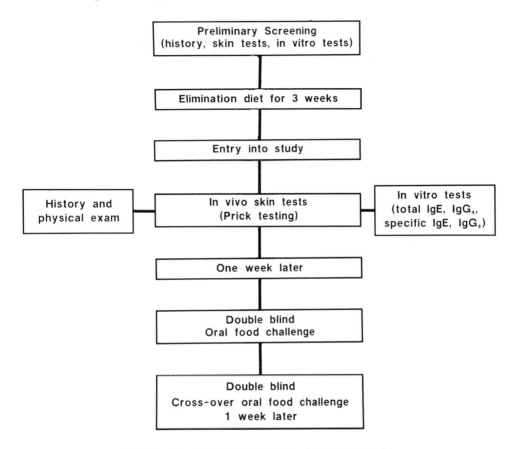

FIG. 1. Experimental design of the food-allergy study.

ble sensitivity. At this time a symptom score between 1+ and 4+ was established, based on the subject's verbal history of his or her problem; an assessment of the subject's clinical severity was also performed. This multiplicity of organ involvement, frequency, and duration of attacks allowed a symptom score assignment between 1+ and 4+. Blood specimens were also obtained at this time for the measurement of total IgE, specific IgE, specific IgG4, and total IgG4 antibody using the FluoroFAST procedures developed by 3M Diagnostic Systems. Standard skin-prick testing was performed, and a definite wheal or flare greater than 4 mm at 15-min intervals post-injection was considered positive. A positive control for the skin-prick test consisted of an injection of a 1% histamine solution containing 27.5 μg of histamine phosphate per milliliter of diluent; a negative control consisted of diluent solution containing 0.9% sodium chloride, 0.03% human serum albumin, and 0.4% phenol as a preservative in distilled water.

The Oral Food Provocation

Foods to be tested were administered in opaque tartrazine-free capsules. Approximately 8 g of dehydrated powdered food was administered in sequentially increasing amounts over a 1-hr period or until the patient showed signs of an allergic reaction. Milk, egg, peanut, wheat, and corn were used for both skin testing and for oral food challenge. The symptoms generally occurred within 10 to 16 min after initiating the challenge, although some reactions occurred as late as 12 to 24 hr later. These were arbitrarily designated immediate and delayed, respectively.

RESULTS

Presenting Symptoms in 25 Patients with Food Allergy

The presenting symptoms, as obtained by history, are shown in Table 2. It can be seen that cutaneous symptoms were observed in 13 of the patients; of these, five consisted of urticaria, four consisted of eczema, and four consisted of urticaria and eczema. Twenty-one patients presented with respiratory symptoms—either nasal symptoms, rhinorrhea, or wheezing. One patient presented with gastrointestinal symptoms.

Results of Skin-Prick Tests with Food Antigens

Shown in Table 3 are the results of skin-prick-test reactions to the food antigens employed in this study. The highest frequency of reactions were seen in response to milk, egg, and peanut, with fewer reactions in response to wheat and corn. This distribution of skin sensitivity is similar to findings described in other studies (14,15).

Comparison of Clinical History and Skin Testing with Results of Food Challenges

Of 67 food challenges performed, 35 were positive (Table 4). Of the positive reactions of food challenges, 10 of 35 (29%) were seen in skin-test-positive indi-

TABLE 2. *Presenting symptoms in 25 patients with food allergy*

Cutaneous symptoms, total		13
Urticaria	5	
Eczema	4	
Urticaria and eczema	4	
Respiratory symptoms: nasal symptoms, rhinorrhea, and/or wheezing		21
Gastrointestinal symptoms		1

TABLE 3. *Results of skin-prick-test reactions to food antigens*

Reagent	Number of positive tests	(%)	Number of negative tests
Milk	6	(26)	19
Egg	5	(22)	20
Peanut	5	(22)	20
Wheat	4	(17)	21
Corn	3	(13)	22
Subtotals:	23		102
		Total: 125	

TABLE 4. *Comparison of clinical history and skin testing with results of food challenges*

		Skin test positive				Skin test negative			
			Food challenge				Food challenge		
	Number	Sub-	Positive		Negative	Sub-	Positive		Negative	
Reagent	of food challenges	total	Hx+	Hx−	Hx+	Hx −	total	Hx+	Hx −	Hx+	Hx −
Milk	22	6	3	1	2	0	16	7	1	4	4
			4		2			8		8	
Egg	13	3	2	0	1	0	10	3	0	3	4
			2		1			3		7	
Peanut	11	4	2	1	0	1	7	2	2	0	3
			3		1			4		3	
Wheat	12	3	0	1	1	1	9	1	5	0	3
			1		2			6		3	
Corn	9	2	0	0	2	0	7	2	2	0	3
			0		2			4		3	
Totals:	67	18	10		8		49	25		24	

viduals; 25 of 35 (71%) were seen in skin-test-negative individuals. However, 22 of 35 (63%) were seen in history-positive individuals.

Of the 32 food-challenge negative reactions, eight of 32 (25%) were seen as skin-test-positive individuals; 24 of 32 (75%) were seen in skin-test-negative individuals. In 13 of 32 (41%) a positive history of food allergy was obtained, but only six skin-positive individuals were history positive.

Comparison of History, Skin Test, and IgE and IgG4 Responses of Three Patients with Positive Delayed Skin Reactions Following Food Challenge

Shown in Table 5 is a comparison of history, skin tests, and IgE and IgG4 responses in three patients who showed positive delayed reactions following food challenge. Each of these three patients had markedly elevated IgE (>200 IU/ml), and each of these patients showed a flareup of the skin following challenge to either peanut or milk. In patient 1, who showed a response to peanut, the IgE-specific antibody was nondetectable; however, a markedly elevated specific IgG4 of 34.4 µg/ml was detected. In patient 2 a positive response to milk challenge was seen, and a moderately elevated specific IgE (0.26 IU/ml) was observed with markedly elevated IgG4 (29.4 µg/ml). In patient 3 a positive challenge to milk was observed, and an elevated IgG4 of 5.8 µg/ml was seen with moderately elevated IgE of 0.13 IU/ml.

Comparison of History, Skin Test, and IgE and IgG4 Responses in Patients with Positive Immediate and/or Delayed Skin Reaction Following Food Challenge

Patient 4 showed an immediate oral food challenge to egg; this challenge consisted of coryza, wheezing at 1 hr, and a flareup of eczema at 2 hr. Patient 5 showed positive oral food challenge dermal responses consisting of immediate to milk (pruritis), delayed to wheat (flareup of eczema), and immediate to corn (flareup of eczema) (Table 6). Specific IgE responses to these various foods were elevated. In patient 5, elevated IgG4 antibody to milk and wheat (>40 µg/ml) but not to corn (<2µg/ml), was detected (Table 6).

Comparison of History, Skin Tests, and IgE and IgG4 Responses in Three Patients with Eczema Who Showed No Skin Reactions Following Food Challenge

Shown in Table 7 are the results of history, skin tests, and IgE and IgG4 responses in three patients with eczema who showed no specific flareup of the skin following food challenge. Patient 6 did not show a positive oral challenge to milk. Two of these patients, however, did show evidence of delayed reaction: Patient 7 exhibited coryza to wheat; patient 8, who showed a delayed reaction to peanut, exhibited an itchy throat and a tightness of the chest. Both of the patients did have elevations in their respective IgG4.

SUMMARY AND CONCLUSIONS

The results of these studies suggest a great heterogeneity in the clinical spectrum of atopic dermatitis. The double-blind oral food provocation protocol offers a reliable and objective method for making observations and correlations of specific IgE

TABLE 5. Comparison of history, skin tests, and IgG4 and IgE responses in three patients with positive delayed reaction following food challenge[a]

Patient	Sex	Age (years)	Symptoms	Symptom score	Food antigen	Skin tests					Oral food challenge			Total IgG4 (mg/dl) or total IgE (IU/ml)		Specific IgG4 (μg/ml) or IgE antibody (IU/ml)									
						M	E	P	W	C	Allergen	Imm.	Del.	IgG4	IgE	Milk		Egg		Peanut		Wheat		Corn	
																IgG4	IgE	IgG4	IgE	IgG4	IgE	IgG4	IgE	IgG4	IgE
1	Female	22	Eczema Urticaria Asthma Rhinorrhea	4	Peanut Corn Egg Milk Wheat	−	−	+	−	−	Peanut	−	+	60	>200	>40	0.02	32.8	0.02	35.4	0	36.2	0.1	12.2	0
2	Male	16	Eczema Urticaria	4	Milk	+	+	+	+	+	Milk	−	+	98	>200	29.4	0.20	9.6	0.03	26.8	0.03	19.6	0.06	<2	0.04
3	Female	22	Eczema	2	Milk	−	−	−	−	−	Milk	−	+	6	>200	5.8	0.13	2.6	0.1	<2	0.01	<2	0.06	<2	3.56

[a]M, milk; E, egg; P, peanut; W, wheat; C, corn; Imm., immediate; Del., delayed.

TABLE 6. Comparison of history, skin tests, and IgG4 and IgE responses in two patients with positive, immediate, and/or delayed dermal reactions following food challenge[a]

Patient	Sex	Age (years)	Symptoms	Symptom score	Food antigen	Skin tests					Oral food challenge			Total IgG4 (mg/dl) or total IgE (IU/ml)		Specific IgG4 (µg/ml) or IgE antibody (IU/ml)									
																Milk		Egg		Peanut		Wheat		Corn	
						M	E	P	W	C	Allergen	Imm.	Del.	IgG4	IgE	IgG4	IgE	IgG4	IgE	IgG4	IgE	IgG4	IgE	IgG4	IgE
4	Female	30	Rhinorrhea Eczema Wheezing	2	Egg	−	−	−	−	−	Egg	+	−	9	>200	<2	0.02	<2	0.01	<2	0.1	<2	0.31	<2	0.04
											Wheat														
											Placebo														
5	Male	27	Eczema Wheezing Rhinitis	4	Milk Egg	−	−	−	−	−	Milk	+	−	44	>200	>40	0.42	20.2	5.17	31.8	17.8	>40	35.6	<2	48.5
											Egg	−	−												
											Wheat	−	+												
											Corn	+	−												
											Peanut	−	−												
											Placebo	−	−												

[a]M, milk; E, egg; P, peanut; W, wheat; C, corn; Imm., immediate; Del., delayed.

TABLE 7. Comparison of history, skin tests, and IgG4 and IgE responses in three patients with eczema who showed no dermal reactions[a] following food challenge

Patient	Sex	Age (years)	Symptoms	Symptom score	Food antigen	Skin tests					Oral food challenge			Total IgG4 (mg/dl) or total IgE (IU/ml)		Specific IgG4 (μg/ml) or IgE antibody (IU/ml)										
						M	E	P	W	C	Allergen	Imm.	Del.	IgG4	IgE	Milk		Egg		Peanut		Wheat		Corn	
																IgG4	IgE	IgG4	IgE	IgG4	IgE	IgG4	IgE	IgG4	IgE
6	Male	11	Eczema Rhinorrhea	2+	Milk	+	+	−	+	−	Milk Placebo	−	−	610	>200	8.8	1.22	<2	0.01	2.6	0.01	<2	0.05	<2	0.07
7	Male	8	Rhinorrhea Urticaria Eczema	2	Milk	+	−	−	+	−	Milk Wheat Placebo	− − −	− + −	32	56.2	>40	0.01	<2	0	7.6	0	11.4	0	<2	0.01
8	Female	37	Asthma Urticaria Eczema	2	Peanut Egg	−	−	+	−	−	Peanut Egg Placebo Milk	− − − −	+ − − −	8	>200	14.4	0.01	<2	0.02	3	228	8.6	0	<2	0.01

[a]M, milk; E, egg; P, peanut; W, wheat; C, corn; Imm., immediate; Del., delayed.

and IgG4 antibodies with provoked reactions. The results thus far suggest a lack of correlation between skin tests and oral food provocation. There appears to be a better correlation, however, between history and food challenge. Although these preliminary studies demonstrate a lack of correlation between skin tests and the presence of specific IgE and IgG4 antibodies, some correlations can be made with "early" and "late" challenge responses with IgG4 and IgE. Thus there appears to be some evidence for a pathogenetic role of specific IgE and IgG4 antibodies in the provocation of both immediate and delayed homocytotropic reactions to these antibodies. Further studies will be required in order to draw definitive conclusions concerning (a) the biologic significance of IgE and IgG4 antibodies and (b) the role of these antibodies either as blocking antibodies or as anaphylactic antibodies.

REFERENCES

1. Shakib F, McLaughan P, Stanworth DR, Smith E, Fairburn E. Elevated serum IgE and IgG4 in patients with atopic dermatitis. *Br J Dermatol* 1977;97:59–63.
2. Gwynn CM, Smith JM, Leon GL, Stanworth DR. Role of IgG4 subclass in childhood allergy. *Lancet* 1978;1:910–1.
3. Shakib F, Stanworth DR. IgG4: a possible mediator of anaphylaxis in a hemophiliac patient. *Clin Allergy* 1979;9:597.
4. Gwynn CN, Ingram J, Almousaur T, et al. Bronchial provocation tests in atopic patients with allergen specific IgG4 antibodies. *Lancet* 1981;1:254–6.
5. Vijay HM, Perelmutter L. Inhibition of reagin-mediated PCA reactions in monkeys and histamine release from human leukocytes by human IgG4 subclass. *Int Arch Allergy Appl Immunol* 1977;53:78–87.
6. Fagan DL, Slaughter CA, Capra JD, Sullivan TJ. Monoclonal antibodies to IgG4 induce histamine release from human basophils *in vitro*. *J Allergy Clin Immunol* 1982;70:399–404.
7. Nagakawa T, Stadler BM, de Weck AL. Flow-cytometric analysis of human basophil degranulation. *Allergy* 1981;36:39–47.
8. Nagakawa T, Stadler BM, Heiner DC, et al. Flow-cytometric analysis of human basophil degranulation. II. Degranulation induced by anti-IgE, anti-IgG4 and the calcium ionophore A23187. *Clin Allergy* 1981;11:21–30.
9. Van Toorenenbergen AW, Aalberse RC. IgG4 and passive sensitization of basophil leukocytes. *Int Arch Allergy Appl Immunol* 1981;65:432–40.
10. Devey ME, Wilson DV, Wheeler AW. The IgG subclasses of antibodies to grass pollen allergens produced in hay fever patients during hyposensitization. *Clin Allergy* 1975;6:227–36.
11. Van der Giessen M, Homan WL, van Kernebeek G, et al. Subclass typing of IgG antibodies formed by glass pollen allergic patients during immunotherapy. *Int Arch Allergy Appl Immunol* 1976;50:625–39.
12. Bjorksten B, Ahlstedt S, Bjorksten F, Carlsson B, Fallstrom SP, Juntunen K, Kajosaari M, Kobes A. IgE and IgG4 antibodies to cow's milk in children with cow's milk allergy. *Allergy* 1983;38:119–24.
13. Perelmutter L. IgG4: Non-IgE-mediated atopic disease. *Ann Allergy* 1984;52:64–8.
14. Sampson HA, McCaskill CM. Food hypersensitivity in atopic dermatitis: Evaluation of 113 patients. *J Pediatr* 1985;107:669–75.
15. Sampson HA, Albergo R. Comparison of results of skin tests, RAST, and double-blind placebo-controlled food challenges in children with atopic dermatitis. *J Allergy Clin Immunol* 1984;74:26–33.

DISCUSSION

Dr. Rieger: I am very surprised at the high proportion of negative skin tests in your food-allergic patients. Previous studies have shown quite different correlations. How did you do your testing? And did you look for late reactions as well as for immediate reactions? Did you test with native foods or with a commercial extract?

Dr. Bellanti: We tested for immediate and delayed reactions, using a commercial extract and dried preparations. We, too, were surprised at the lack of correlation between allergic symptoms and skin testing, in both directions (i.e., false positives as well as false negatives).

Dr. Wahn: One problem may be the quality of the extracts. The standards by which we measure diagnostic extracts have become higher during the last few years, and some of the food allergen extracts supplied by the industry are terrible.

Dr. Urbanek: Do you think that it is satisfactory to use encapsulated antigens for oral provocation? Oral symptoms may be missed.

Dr. Bellanti: I agree; this is a good point. But however unsatisfactory, it is the only way we have to administer the antigen double-blind to avoid subjective symptoms. Certainly the antigen never comes in contact with the oral mucosa, where there could be significant absorption and symptoms. Also the dose of antigen is usually unnatural, and we may well not have achieved the normal dietary limits; and the quality of the antigen may be poor, as has already been said.

Dr. Aas: We do quite a number of double-blind oral challenges using capsules, and, when negative, we follow on with open challenge, using larger quantities. One of the problems with negative capsule tests is that the dose may have been too low in some patients. Also, I believe that natural food antigens are usually much better than manufacturers' preparations and lead to a better correlation with positive skin tests.

Dr. Bellanti: One other point should be made. The biologic half-life of specific IgE in the circulation is 1 to 2 days, and that of specific IgE on mast cells is approximately 14 days. Specific IgG (IgG4), however, has a circulation half-life of 21 days, so its residual time on mast cells, extrapolating from IgE, may be as long as 2 to 3 months. Thus tolerance, or the effect of challenges, may be crucially influenced by the timing of dietary management.

Food Allergy, edited by Eberhardt Schmidt.
Nestlé Nutrition Workshop Series, Vol. 17.
Nestec Ltd., Vevey/Raven Press, Ltd.,
New York © 1988.

Difficulty in Initiating and Maintaining Sleep Associated with Cow's Milk Allergy in Infants

*A. Kahn, *M.J. Mozin, *E. Rebuffat, *D. Blum, *G. Casimir, *J. Duchateau, **R. Jost, and **J. Pahud

*Pediatric Sleep Laboratory and Department of Immunology, Free University of Brussels, 1090 Brussels, Belgium and **Nestlé Research Department, Nestec Ltd., 1000 Lausanne 26, Switzerland; Dr. Kahn's present address is Hôpital Universitaire des Enfants, 1020 Brussels, Belgium

Persistent settling and waking difficulties, associated with disturbing behavior, restlessness, and intense crying, are encountered in up to 20% of infants under 1 year of age (1). The symptoms have been attributed to a variety of causes (2–6). In a preliminary study, we reported that the sleep of eight infants with chronic insomnia was normalized after these infants were fed a milk-free diet for a previously undiagnosed milk protein allergy (7). In the present study, we report on another group of patients with similar clinical symptoms and evolution.

PATIENTS AND INVESTIGATIONS

From July 1984 to July 1986, 71 infants were selected from an outpatient clinic and from the general pediatric ward. The infants were divided into three main groups according to the main complaints on presentation.

Group I: Insomnia

Of a total of 120 infants referred by their pediatricians for chronic waking and crying during sleep hours, 20 were selected because their sleep was severely disturbed, almost since the first days of life; an allergy to cow's milk protein was suspected because of family history of allergy and occasional mild episodes of diarrhea or skin rashes. An interview and a standard medical workup had failed to reveal any usual cause for the infant's poor sleep. An all-night polygraphic recording excluded further causes of arousals, such as obstructive sleep apneas (4) or esophageal reflux (5). The recordings were normal for each infant, except that it confirmed the frequent awakenings and short total sleep time reported by the parents. These infants were thus further subjected to a series of allergy tests.

All cow's milk was then removed from the diet by feeding the infants exclusively for 4 weeks with a new routine hypoallergenic infant formula based on enzymatically hydrolyzed cow's milk whey proteins (Nestlé). Follow-up interviews were conducted with the help of our dietician to evaluate the child's progress. During the treatment period the parents were asked to fill in a log describing the child's sleep schedule. After 4 weeks a second polygraphic recording was performed to confirm the reported increase in total sleep time and the decreased number of arousals. Milk was then reintroduced in the diet under close medical surveillance. The diagnosis of milk allergy was confirmed if sleeplessness and agitated behavior reappeared within 4 days. Cow's milk was then excluded again from the diet, and an improvement of the manifestations was to be obtained after the interruption of the milk challenge. Every infant in this group responded according to the protocol.

Group II: Milk Allergy

A group of 31 infants were referred with skin and digestive manifestations attributed to cow's milk allergy. After the introduction of cow's milk in their diet, these infants developed severe skin irritation, eczema ($n = 15$), repeated airway infections, vomiting, or diarrhea ($n = 28$). The symptoms were attributed to cow's milk allergy by their referring pediatricians, and the same series of allergy tests was performed. The diagnosis was confirmed when the symptoms disappeared after the infants were fed with the milk-free diet (Alfare). Although none of the parents spontaneously complained about their infant's sleep, they were asked to fill in a sleep questionnaire and a sleep log for 4 weeks after the exclusion of milk from the diet. According to this information the group was further subdivided into two subgroups. Eighteen infants with a normal sleep behavior formed the "good sleepers" subgroup; 13 with frequent awakenings and short sleep time formed the "poor sleepers" subgroup.

Group III: Control Infants

A group of 20 normal infants was selected among children hospitalized for minor interventions or examinations. Although none had a previous history of sleep disturbance and allergy-related symptoms, the parents allowed blood to be taken to test for allergy and to fill in a sleep questionnaire. No further investigations or regimen was instituted for these infants.

Hypoallergenic Formula Characteristics

NAN H.A. is a hypoallergenic formula intended for routine feeding of infants, particularly those with a positive family history of allergy. Basic composition is quantitatively identical to that of starter infant formula and complies with the most recent pediatric recommendations. NAN H.A. is composed of the following: a de-mineralized whey concentrate hydrolyzed by trypsin under specific conditions (8); palm olein, high oleic safflower oil, and coconut oil; malto-dextrin (+ lactose present in trypsin hydrolyzed demineralized whey); and minerals, vitamins, lecithin, and taurine additions.

Composition

The composition of NAN H.A., per 100 kcal, is as follows: protein, 2.46 g; fat, 5.1 g; carbohydrates, 11 g; minerals, 0.45 g; plus some vitamins and trace elements.

Hypoallergenicity

During the development of this formula, solid-phase radioimmunoassay was performed in order to detect traces of residual beta lactoglobulin. Furthermore, an oral sensitization test in animal models was used (9). Hypoallergenicity is controlled on each batch by the following biochemical tests:

1. Electrophoresis [Sodium dodecyl sulfate polyacrylamide gel electrophoresis (SDS-PAGE)]. This technique allows detection of intact proteins or of large molecular weight peptides (>10 kilodaltons)
2. Double immunodiffusion (Ouchterlony test). Each lot is routinely controlled by double immunodiffusion according to Ouchterlony. At a test concentration of 50 mg/ml, there must be absence of any precipitation lines with anti-beta-lacto-globulin, anti-bovine serum albumin, and anti-alpha-lactalbumin sera. Ouchterlony double diffusion detects approximately 10 μg/ml of beta-lactoglobulin or alpha-lactalbumin and 20 μg/ml of serum albumin.

RESULTS

The main characteristics of the 71 infants are shown in Table 1. The groups were comparable for age and sex of the infants. In group II, no family or personal characteristics differentiated the two subgroups of "good" and "poor sleepers," including the duration and apparent severity of their skin and digestive symptoms. The reported sleep duration significantly differentiated the three groups. The 20 infants in group I and the 18 "poor sleepers" in group II slept significantly less

TABLE 1. Characteristics of the 71 infants studied[a]

Group	Number of subjects	Main complaint on admission	Mean age (weeks)	Sex (male/ female)	Sleep duration (hours)	
					Nighttime	Daytime
I	20	Insomnia	25.5 ± 10.1	8/12	5.1 ± 1.0	1.0 ± 0.5
II	31	Milk allergy	31.5 ± 20.0	15/16		
		18 "poor sleepers"			5.9 ± 2.0	1.5 ± 1.0
		13 "good sleepers"			9.5 ± 1.5	3.0 ± 1.5
III	20	Controls	30.5 ± 16.5	12/8	9.9 ± 1.5	4.5 ± 2.4
		F-test:	NS[b]	NS	0.01	0.01

[a]The data are presented as absolute values, means, and standard deviations.
[b]NS, not significant.

than the remaining 33 infants. No difference in total sleep time was seen between the infants in group I and the "poor sleepers" in group II, or between the "good sleepers" in group II and the infants in group III. All infants in group I and 18 "poor sleepers" in group II had two to nine arousals per night. The "good sleepers" in group II and the infants in group III had no arousal during the night or only awoke occasionally. The tests for milk protein allergy were positive for the 38 infants in groups I and II but were not positive for any of the infants of group III (Table 2). Milk allergy was confirmed clinically by the favorable evolution during the exclusion diet for the infants in groups I and II and by the sleeplessness that followed the oral milk challenge in the infants in group I. Within 4 weeks of the milk-free diet, the sleep characteristics of all infants in group I and of the "poor sleepers" in group II normalized. Their sleep duration during the day, as well as during the night, could not be differentiated from that of the "good sleepers" in group II and of the control infants in group III (Table 3).

TABLE 2. Results of laboratory tests for allergy in the 71 infants studied[a]

Group	Number of subjects	Beta-lactoglobulin antibodies, titer (> 100 U)	High IgE, titer (> 10 U/ml)	High eosinophils, counts (> 400)
I	20	20/20	2/20	3/20
II	18	18/18	2/18	1/18
	13	13/13	3/13	1/13
III	20	0/20	0/20	1/20

[a]The figures represent the number of infants with results above normal values. Normal values are shown in parentheses for each test.

TABLE 3. *Effects of the milk-free diet on sleep duration*

Group	Before the diet	After 3 weeks of the diet	Probability, *p*
Group I—Insomnia (*n* = 20)			
Duration of daytime sleep	1 ± 0.5	3.0 ± 1.5	0.01
Duration of nighttime sleep	5.1 ± 1.2	9.9 ± 2.0	0.01
Group II—Milk allergy: "Poor sleepers" (*n* = 18)			
Duration of daytime sleep	1.5 ± 1.0	4.5 ± 2.4	0.01
Duration of nighttime sleep	5.9 ± 2.0	9.8 ± 1.0	0.01
Group II—Milk allergy: "Good sleepers" (*n* = 13)			
Duration of daytime sleep	3.0 ± 1.5	3.9 ± 1.6	NS[b]
Duration of nighttime sleep	9.5 ± 1.5	9.4 ± 1.2	NS

[a]During the day (from 7:01 A.M. to 7:00 P.M. and during the night (from 7:01 P.M. to 7:00 A.M.). Figures represent means and standard deviations. Statistics are done with the Wilcoxon's signed-rank test.
[b]NS, not significant.

DISCUSSION

In the infants with chronic sleeplessness, an allergy to cow's milk was suspected from each infant's history and was confirmed by (a) the improvement in symptoms after milk was avoided, (b) the recurrence of symptoms after an oral challenge with milk, and (c) a new improvement of sleep after a second trial of milk elimination. When cow's milk is eliminated from the diet, each infant's sleep time became similar to that of normal control children of the same age. Still, three caveats must be mentioned about possible limitations of the dietary treatment of sleep. First, the exclusion of all cow's milk protein can be a tedious procedure, since many food preparations contain beta-lactoglobulin and other milk protein antigens. The accidental reintroduction of only small quantities of cow's milk protein into the infant's diet can cause the return of poor sleep. Second, soya milk may not be the best choice for replacement of cow's milk, since up to 5% of allergic infants can also suffer from soya protein intolerance (10). In such a case the preference should be given to a hypoallergenic infant diet. Third, the diet should be maintained for at least 3 to 4 weeks before sleep normalizes. This implies that the families must be closely supported during the long treatment period. We don't know the prevalence of this cause of sleep disturbance in children, and we cannot yet explain the relation between milk allergy and sleeplessness. The poor sleep could be related to physical discomfort as well as to changes in metabolism of the central nervous system. We are unable to explain why 13 of the infants referred for atopy slept normally whereas 18 were poor sleepers. No significant difference was seen between the two groups of infants, either in their individual histories, clinically, or in laboratory tests. An immediate type of allergic reaction does not seem to account for the development of poor sleep, as indicated by the absence of elevated immunoglobin E levels in the blood of most infants. Further studies will be needed to clarify this question. We conclude that infants with clinically evident milk allergy may suffer from sleeplessness, although this sleep disturbance can be overlooked. Furthermore, when no evident cause for chronic insomnia can be found in an infant, the possibility of milk allergy should be given serious consideration.

ACKNOWLEDGMENTS

We wish to thank Prof. H.L. Vis for his encouragement; we also wish to thank Dr. I. Ingenbleek (NESTEC, Ltd.) for his continuing assistance.

REFERENCES

1. Bax MCO. Sleep disturbance in the young child. *Br Med J* 1980;5:1177–9.
2. Ferber R, ed. *Solve your child's sleep problems.* New York: Simon and Schuster, 1985.
3. Moore T, Ucko LE. Night waking in early infancy: Part I. *Arch Dis Child* 1957;32:333–42.
4. Guilleminault C, Anders TF. Sleep disorders in children. *Adv Pediatr* 1976;22:151–75.
5. Association of Sleep Disorders Centers and the Association for the Psychophysiological Study of Sleep: Diagnostic Classification of Sleep and Arousal Disorders (Roffward HP, chairman). *Sleep* 1979;2:21–57.
6. Jones NB, Ferreira MCR, Brown MF. The association between perinatal factors and later night waking. *Dev Med Child Neurol* 1978;20:427–34.
7. Kahn A, Mozin MJ, Casimir G, Montauk L, Blum D. Insomnia and cow's milk allergy in infants. *Pediatrics* 1985;76:880–4.
8. Jost R. Partial enzymatic hydrolysis of whey protein by trypsin. *J Dairy Sci* 1977;9:1387–93.
9. Pahud JJ, Schwarz K. Oral sensitization to food proteins in animal models. A basis for the development of hypoallergenic infant formula. In: *Production, regulation and analysis of infant formula, Proceedings of the Tropical Conference, Virginia Beach 1985.* Arlington: Association of Official Analytic Chemists, 1985:264–71.
10. Bahna, SL, ed. *Allergies to milk.* New York: Grune and Stratton, 1980.

DISCUSSION

Dr. Bellanti: As I understand it you had three groups: an insomniac group, an allergic group, and a control group. The control group slept, on average, 13.5 hr and the other groups slept a much shorter time. Then there was an intervention with a substitute formula, and the sleep times increased in the insomniac and allergic groups so that they were comparable to the controls. How do you know that there was not a psychological effect of the intervention? Did you control for this in any way?

Dr. Kahn: I should emphasize that the infants had already had a great deal of intervention without effect—drugs, food manipulations, behavior therapy, and so on—and none of it worked. We did not control specifically for possible psychological effects of our dietary treatment, but we had no reason to suspect that a psychological effect would be of primary importance. The children slept perfectly as soon as the diet was introduced, and when they went back to their former diet their sleep worsened again. Finally, sleeplessness reoccurred on several occasions, when the parents by accident reintroduced some milk proteins in the diet.

Dr. de Weck: How did you measure sleeping time?

Dr. Kahn: We measured it in three ways. First, we obtained records from the parents, who were highly motivated because they were so short of sleep themselves! Second, we did all-night polygraphic studies, which showed an 80% correlation between the sleep time observed in the laboratory and that reported by the parents from home. Third, we checked for possible bias using an accelerometer, which showed a good correlation with the definition of sleep stages obtained by polygraphic recordings in our laboratory.

Food Allergy, edited by Eberhardt Schmidt.
Nestlé Nutrition Workshop Series, Vol. 17.
Nestec Ltd., Vevey/Raven Press, Ltd.,
New York © 1988.

IgG and IgG Subclasses Response to Dietary Antigens in Patients with Immediate and Nonimmediate Food Allergy

*R. Urbanek and **M. D. Kemeny

*Universitäts-Kinderklinik Freiburg, 7800 Freiburg, West Germany and **Department of Internal Medicine, Guy's Hospital Medical School, London SE1 9RT, England

Adverse reactions to food are a common finding (1,2). Although an association between immediate hypersensitivity and the presence of specific IgE antibodies has been established (3–5), in many patients no IgE antibodies to nutritive proteins can be detected. In these individuals, adverse reaction to food might be related to the presence of antibodies from other classes.

Small amounts of antigenically intact food proteins can pass the enteric mucosa and reach the circulation. Although the quantities absorbed are nutritionally irrelevant, they are sufficient to immunize, thus inducing an immune response. Both humoral and cell-mediated reactions to dietary antigens have been described (6,7). In most normal children and adults, low-titer serum antibodies of different classes and subclasses against dietary proteins are present, without evidence of adverse reactions to the ingestion of specific food. Therefore, it is of interest to analyze the immunoglobulin class distribution of the antibodies produced in response to common dietary antigens in allergic disease, in patients with increased intestinal permeability, and in healthy controls.

In previous studies, accurate measurement of IgG subclass antibodies has been difficult because of the characteristics of the individual IgG subclass antibodies and the nature of the available subclass-specific antisera. The introduction of monoclonal antisera has, however, enabled us to develop more sensitive techniques (8). We studied the IgG subclass antibody response to dietary antigens in patients with the following defined types of adverse reactions to foods: (a) immediate-type allergy to milk proteins or egg proteins and (b) gliadin intolerance. The dietary antigens investigated were cow's milk casein, hen's egg ovalbumin, and wheat gliadin. The pattern of IgG subclass antibodies to these food proteins in patients with food allergy and celiac disease were compared with healthy control subjects.

MATERIALS AND METHODS

Subjects Studied

Twenty patients who had celiac disease were studied. Ten had been on a gluten-free diet for at least 6 months (treated) and 10 had not (untreated). A diagnosis of celiac disease was made in all using recommended criteria, including classic jejunal biopsy changes. Twenty-six patients with egg allergy were studied. Egg allergy was defined by history of adverse reaction to specific food and by a positive skin-prick test (>3 mm wheal) to dried egg solubilized in buffered sodium chloride solution. The controls were 26 healthy staff members who were not allergic to food and who had a negative skin-prick test and radioallergosorbent test. Blood samples were taken by venipuncture, and all serum samples were stored at $-20°C$ until used.

Reagents

Immulon 1 microtiter plates (M 129/A) and immuno 1 (Nunc) were purchased from Dynatech Inc. (USA) and Gibco Ltd. (UK), respectively. Horse serum was purchased from Sera Lab Ltd. (UK). Tween 20 and *p*-nitrophenyl phosphate were purchased from Sigma Inc. (USA). All other reagents were purchased from BDH Chemical Ltd. (UK).

Antigens and Antisera

Bovine casein, gliadin, and ovalbumin were purchased from Sigma Inc. in the purest form available. Monoclonal antibodies to human IgG and IgG subclasses 1 through 4 were purchased from Unipath Ltd. (UK). Affinity-purified alkaline phosphatase-conjugated rabbit anti-mouse IgG (AP anti-MIG) was purchased from Sigma Inc. and stored at 4°C until used.

Enzyme-Linked Immunosorbent Assay (ELISA)

IgG and IgG subclass antibodies were measured by ELISA as described elsewhere (8). Briefly, antigen (casein 1 μg/ml, ovalbumin 1 μg/ml, gliadin 10 μg/ml) was bound to microtiter plates (Nunc for casein and ovalbumin, Dynatech for gliadin) in pH 9.6 carbonate/bicarbonate buffer or 96% ethanol for gliadin. All incubation volumes were 100 μl at 4°C. Between each step, the plates were washed three times with phosphate-buffered saline (PBS), pH 7.4, 0.1 M containing 0.5% Tween 20. Test serum was then incubated with the antigen-coated plate at 1/200 to 1/10,000 dilution in assay diluent (PBS + 0.5% horse serum + 0.5% Tween 20) for 2 hr followed by monoclonal anti-IgG or IgG 1 to 4 at 1/1000 dilution for 1 hr and AP-anti MIG at 1/500 dilution for 1 hr. Substrate 1 mg/μl *p*-nitrophenyl phosphate in pH 9.8 diethanolamine buffer was added, and the reaction was stopped after 1.5 hr at 37°C by addition of 50 μl of 3 M NaOH. Optical density was measured in a titer-tek multiskan (Flow, UK) at 405 nm. Results were expressed as arbitrary units per milliliters by reference to an internal standard serum. Interassay variation expressed as coefficient of variation was 11% for casein, 2.3% for ovalbumin, and 5.8% for gliadin.

RESULTS

IgG Antibodies to Gliadin, Ovalbumin, and Casein

The concentration of IgG antibodies to gliadin, ovalbumin, and casein was measured by ELISA in patients with celiac disease or egg allergy and was compared with that of healthy control subjects (Figs. 1–3). There was considerable overlap between the IgG antibody levels in the different groups. Patients who had celiac disease had raised IgG antibody levels to all three dietary antigens tested, as compared with healthy control subjects (gliadin $p<0.001$, ovalbumin $p<0.01$, and casein $p<0.01$, as determined by the Mann-Whitney U test). There was no difference between the levels of total IgG antibody to any of the antigens in egg-allergic patients, as compared with those of healthy control subjects.

Untreated celiac-disease patients had higher levels of IgG antibodies to gliadin, as compared with those on a gluten-free diet ($p<0.001$, as determined by Student's t test). Indeed, treated celiacs had IgG antigliadin antibody levels that were indistinguishable from those of healthy control subjects. In contrast, there was no difference in the amount of ovalbumin or casein-specific IgG antibody in treated, as compared with untreated, celiacs.

Egg-allergic patients, who were expected to have increased IgG antibody to ovalbumin, did not differ from healthy controls.

IgG Subclass Distribution

IgG subclass antibodies to all three antigens were measured by ELISA. The relative amounts of each were determined by reference to a common standard curve of total IgG antibody. This was determined using a "pan-IgG" reactive monoclonal antibody to measure antibody in all four IgG subclasses. Dilutions of a pool of human sera which contained a high titer of IgG antibody were used to construct a reference curve, and the amount of IgG antibody in each subclass was expressed as arbitrary units per milliliter.

For all three antigens studied, the dominant subclasses were 1 and 4 (Fig. 4); IgG2 and IgG3 antibodies were usually at low or undetectable levels. All celiac disease patients had raised levels of IgG1 antibodies to gliadin ($p<0.001$, Mann-Whitney U test), ovalbumin ($p<0.001$, Mann-Whitney U test), or casein ($p<0.001$, Mann-Whitney U test), as compared with those of healthy control subjects. IgG4 antibodies in celiacs were the same as controls for gliadin and ovalbumin but were slightly raised for casein ($p<0.05$, Mann-Whitney U test).

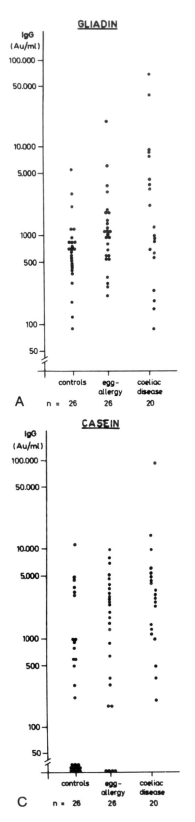

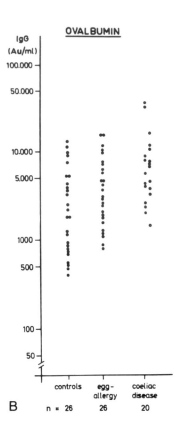

FIG. 1. IgG antibody to wheat gliadin (**A**), ovalbumin (**B**), and bovine casein (**C**) in patients with treated (●) or untreated (○) celiac disease, in egg-allergic patients, and in healthy control subjects.

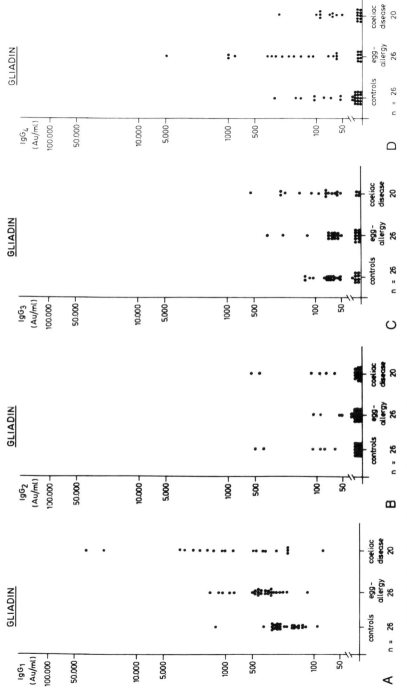

FIG. 2. The IgG subclass 1–4 response (**A–D**, respectively) to wheat gliadin in celiac-disease patients, in egg-allergy patients, and in healthy control subjects showing the predominance of IgG1 antibodies.

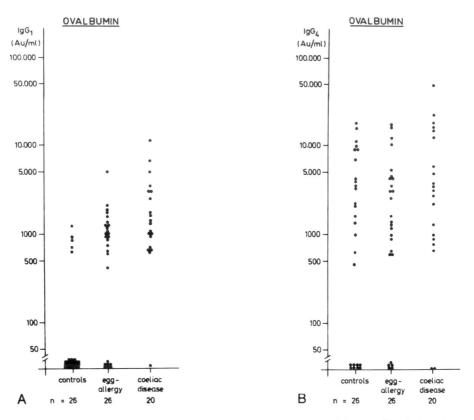

FIG. 3. The IgG subclass 1 and 4 response (**A** and **B**, respectively) to ovalbumin in celiac-disease patients, in egg-allergy patients, and in healthy control subjects. IgG2 and IgG3 antibodies were undetectable within the limits of the assay. The dominant subclass is IgG4.

Egg-allergic patients also had raised IgG1 (but not IgG4) antibodies to oval-bumin, as compared with those of healthy control subjects ($p<0.01$, Mann-Whitney U test).

DISCUSSION

The purpose of the study was to investigate the pattern of IgG antibody response in patients with adverse reactions to common dietary proteins. IgG antibodies to ingested proteins commonly develop early in life as a natural result of intestinal exposure (9,10). We have, therefore, limited our study to two types of adverse reactions to foods for which there are accepted criteria: immediate-type egg allergy (an IgE-mediated disorder) and celiac disease with its intolerance to gliadin.

Serum IgG antibodies to common dietary antigens were found in healthy indi-

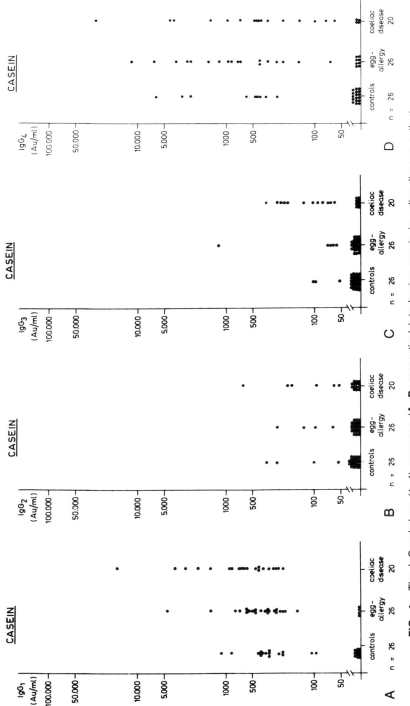

FIG. 4. The IgG subclass (1–4) response (**A–D**, respectively) to bovine casein in celiac-disease patients, egg-allergy patients, and in healthy control subjects. Levels of IgG1 and IgG4 antibodies were raised as compared with levels of IgG2 and IgG3 antibodies.

viduals as well as in patients with IgE-mediated allergy and celiac disease. For all antigens studied, the dominant subclasses were IgG1 and IgG4; IgG2 and IgG3 antibodies were usually at low or undetectable levels. Inhibition experiments with specific and unspecific antigens (results not shown) indicated that the antibodies were directed against the investigated dietary proteins.

Circulating antibodies to gliadin as well as to other food proteins have been reported previously in patients with celiac disease (11,12). Most importantly, we also found that persons with untreated celiac disease had elevated IgG antibody levels to food antigens, as compared with those of healthy controls or patients with immediate-type food allergy. However, antigliadin IgG antibodies in treated patients with celiac disease were lower as compared with those of untreated celiacs. Their antiovalbumin and anticasein IgG antibodies did not differ substantially.

Although we expected the highest antiovalbumin IgG antibodies in egg-allergic individuals, their IgG levels were in the range of healthy controls. A deliberate avoidance of egg may explain these results.

The relationship between IgG subclass and immunity was first investigated in patients with subclass deficiencies (2,13). IgG2 defect was reported in patients with chronic or recurrent bacterial infections. Low levels of IgG2 and IgG4 are frequently combined with IgA deficiency and were described in patients with ataxia-telangiectasia Louis-Bar. On the other hand, IgG subclass restriction to bacterial antigens, as well as to viral antigens and vaccines, was reported (14–17).

The finding of raised antibody levels of IgG1 subclass directed against food proteins such as gliadin, ovalbumin, and casein in celiac patients suggests a predominant subclass response to an antigenic stimulation, presumably caused by an increased penetration resulting from mucosal damage. Therefore, high levels of IgG1 antibodies to gliadin and common dietary antigens such as casein and ovalbumin appear as a valuable adjunct in the diagnosis as well as in the follow-up of patients with celiac disease.

Elevated levels of IgG1 antibodies (but not total IgG and IgG4 antibodies) to ovalbumin, as compared with the IgG1 antibody levels in healthy control individuals, had been detected in egg-allergic patients. This finding may also reflect recent changes in the gut mucosa associated with an increased absorption of specific dietary antigens and a predominent IgG1 immune response in this group.

IgG4 subclass antibodies have been reported as sensitizing antibodies mediating allergic disorders (18,19) as well as blocking antibodies after allergen immunotherapy (17,20). Our investigation demonstrates that IgG4 antibodies against food proteins occur in the same range in both healthy and diseased individuals. However, regarding our findings from successfully hyposensitized allergic patients, one can speculate that appropriate high levels of specific IgG4 in food-allergic persons may also be associated with some degree of protection. The good tolerance of milk in celiac patients having relatively high IgG4 levels in response to casein would support such an hypothesis.

In conclusion, physicochemical properties of dietary proteins, as well as the method of administration, determine the antigenic potency. Natural exposure to food proteins elicits a predominantly IgG1 antibody response. The magnitude of the immune response may also be influenced by the degree of antigen penetration due to mucosal damage. In addition, our findings suggest that the subclass of IgG antibody produced in response to dietary proteins is predominantly related to the antigen, not the disease.

REFERENCES

1. Jakobsson I, Lindberg T. A prospective study of cow's milk protein intolerance in Swedish infants. *Acta Paediatr Scand* 1979;68:853.
2. Schur PH, Bovel H. Gelfand E, Alper CA, Rosen FA. Selective gamma-G globulin and deficiencies in patients with recurrent pyogenic infections. *N Engl J Med* 1970;283:631–4.
3. Björksten B, Ahlstedt S, Björksten F, Carlson B, Fällström SP, et al. Immunoglobulin E and immunoglobulin G4 antibodies to cow's milk in children with cow's milk allergy. *Allergy* 1983;38:119–24.
4. Dannaeus A, Inganas M. A follow-up study of children with food allergy. Clinical course in relation to IgE- and IgG-antibody levels to milk, egg and fish. *Clin Allergy* 1981;11:533–9.
5. Kletter B, Gery I, Freier S, Noah Z, Davies MA, et al. Immunoglobulin E antibodies to milk proteins. *Clin Allergy* 1971;1:249–55.
6. Korenblatt RE, Rothberg RM, Minden P, Farr RS. Immune response of human adults after oral and parenteral exposure to bovine serum albumin. *J Allergy* 1968;41:226–36.
7. Rothberg RM, Farr RS. Anti-bovine serum albumin and anti-alpha lactalbumin in the serum of children and adults. *Pediatrics* 1965;35:571–88.
8. Kemeny DM, Urbanek R, Richards D, Greenall C. The development of a quantitative enzyme-linked immunosorbent assay (ELISA) for detection of human IgG subclass antibodies. *J Immunol Methods (submitted for publication)*
9. Barrick RH, Farr RS. The incidence of circulating anti-beef albumin in sera of allergic persons and some comments regarding the possible significance of this occurrence. *J Allergy* 1965;36:374–81.
10. Dannaeus A, Inganas M, Johansson SGO, Foucard T. Intestinal uptake of ovalbumin in malabsorption and food allergy in relation to serum IgG antibody and orally administered sodium cromoglycate. *Clin Allergy* 1979;9.263–70.
11. Bürgin-Wolf A, Singer E, Friess HM, Berger R, Birbaumer A, Just M. The diagnostic significance of antibodies to various cow's milk proteins. *Eur J Pediatr* 1980;133:17–24.
12. Stern M, Stupp W, Grüttner R. Kuhmilch-Antikörper in der Immunfloreszenz bei Kuhmilchproteinintoleranz and Kontrollen. *Monatsschr Kinderheilkd* 1982;130:556–61.
13. Yount WJ, Hong R, Seligmann M, Kunkel HB. Imbalances of gammaglobulin subgroups and gene defects in patients with primary hypogammaglobulinaemia. *J Clin Invest* 1970;49:1957–66.
14. Aalberse RC, van der Gaag R, van Leeuwen J. Serologic aspects of IgG4 antibodies 1. Prolonged immunization results in an IgG4-restricted response. *J Immunol* 1983;130:722–6.
15. Morell A, Roth-Wicky B, Skvaril F. IgG subclass restriction of antibodies against hepatitis B surface antigen. *Infect Immun* 1983;39:565–8.
16. Skvaril F, Joller-Jemelka H. IgG subclasses of anti-HBs antibodies in vaccinated and nonvaccinated individuals and in anti-HBs immunoglobulin preparations. *Int Arch Allergy Appl Immunol* 1984;73:330–7.
17. Urbanek R, Dold S. Schlüsselrolle der IgG4-Subklassenantikörper bei Schutzentstehung gegen allergische Reaktionen auf Insektenstiche. *Monatsschr Kinderheilkd* 1986;134:536–40.
18. Bruynzell PLB, Berrens L. IgE and IgG4 antibodies in specific human allergies. *Int Arch Allergy Appl Immunol* 1979;58:344–50.
19. Gwynn CM, Ingram J, Almousawi T, Stanworth DR. Bronchial provocation tests in atopic patients with allergen specific IgG4 antibodies. *Lancet* 1982;i:254–6.
20. Van der Giessen M, Homan WL, van Kernebeek G, Aalberse RC, Dieges PH. Subclass typing of IgG antibodies formed by grass pollen-allergic patients during immunotherapy. *Int Arch Allergy Appl Immunol* 1976;50:625–40.

DISCUSSION

Dr. Navarro: Is there a rapid change in IgG antibody response depending on whether or not gluten is present in the diet, and what are the correlations with the state of the intestinal mucosa?

Dr. Urbanek: The treated group had been on gliadin-free diet for at least 6 months and had not yet had repeat biopsies. But we can say from our previous experience that children who have been investigated during a gliadin-free diet show a decrease in both total IgG antibodies and IgG-1 antibodies to normal levels, which are maintained so long as the gliadin-free diet is continued. Thus it should be possible, at least in the majority of patients, to use IgG antibody levels to monitor the diet.

Dr. Rieger: You said that the IgG response is probably more closely related to the antigen than to the disease, and I completely agree with that. In a normal person there is a very close association between the amount of food eaten and the antibody response. How well are you able to monitor allergen intake or avoidance in an egg-sensitive individual, and how sure can you be of your interpretation of the antibody levels you measure?

Dr. Urbanek: I can only say that we have followed up some milk-allergic individuals over long periods (about 2 years), and with strict avoidance of cow's milk protein the level of IgG antibodies decreased, and in some cases the level of IgE antibodies decreased as well, where there was an IgE-mediated allergic response. However, there are some patients whose IgE antibodies persist but who are able to tolerate milk after 1 or 2 years' avoidance with no boost to their IgE levels.

Dr. Challacombe: In celiac disease at least one-third of the patients have bacterial overgrowth in the upper small intestine. I think it is possible that this might contribute to some of the abnormalities of the IgG results that you have described.

Dr. Scadding: Our further confounding factor could be that celiac disease is associated with the HLA B8 antigen and that people with this tend to have good antibody responses. Have you haplotyped your patients?

Dr. Urbanek: No, we have not. This is a very good point.

Dr. Hadorn: It is generally agreed that in celiac disease the younger the patient, the more pronounced the increase in antigliadin antibodies. Has this something to do with the permeability of the intestine?

Dr. Urbanek: We believe that increased permeability and the continuous administration of gliadin in the young child is likely to be the primary reason. Similarly, in egg allergy we assume that the increase in IgG antibodies to ovalbumin and to other dietary proteins occurs because there are mucosal changes.

Food Allergy, edited by Eberhardt Schmidt.
Nestlé Nutrition Workshop Series, Vol. 17.
Nestec Ltd., Vevey/Raven Press, Ltd.,
New York © 1988.

Antigens in Cow's Milk and Hen's Egg Allergy

U. Wahn

Children's Hospital, Free University of Berlin, 1000 Berlin 19, Federal Republic of Germany

Among alimentary allergen sources, cow's milk and hen's egg most frequently lead to hypersensitivity in children and give rise to allergic reactions. During recent years a number of proteins have been identified which have the ability to bind to IgE antibodies from sera of allergic infants and children and have the capacity to activate mediator-releasing cells (1–4).

COW'S MILK ALLERGENS

Thirty-six precipitates can be identified in bovine whey by means of crossed radioimmunoelectrophoresis (5). Among those proteins with the strongest IgE-binding capacity are alpha-lactalbumin, beta-lactoglobulin, bovine serum albumin (BSA), and immunoglobulin (6). Bovine whey is not the only protein that is composed of a large number of antigenic components. In the casein fraction of cow's milk, which constitutes about 80% of total milk protein, three antigenic fractions that strongly bind to IgE antibodies from human sera have been separated by crossed immunoelectrophoresis.

Radioallergosorbent-test (RAST) studies, utilizing purified cow's milk proteins that had been coupled to the solid phase, clearly showed that there are considerable variations in qualitative and quantitative IgE-antibody responses to milk proteins among cow's-milk-allergic children.

Similarly, when purified proteins from cow's milk are used in serial dilutions for *in vitro* incubation with actively sensitized basophils from cow's-milk-allergic children, the dose-response curves for histamine release indicate differences in the individual patterns of sensitization ("allergoprints"). In general, the majority of cow's-milk-allergic children release histamine in the presence of proteins from the casein fraction at a molar concentration ranging from 10^{-10} up to 10^{-7} M. At similar concentrations we were able to find sensitivities to BSA, beta-lactoglobulin, and alpha-lactalbumin as well as to gamma-globulin, though less frequently than to casein (Fig. 1).

Heating proteins from bovine whey leads to a significant decrease in their capac-

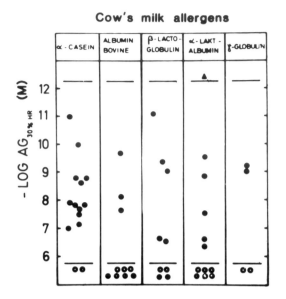

FIG. 1. Molar allergen concentrations necessary to induce 30% histamine release from washed leukocytes of 14 cow's-milk-allergic children.

ity to bind to human IgE antibodies as well as in their ability to release histamine from washed leukocytes *in vitro*. In contrast, proteins from the casein fraction retain their histamine-releasing ability even after boiling for 10 min.

HEN'S EGG ALLERGENS

Like cow's milk, hen's egg contains a variety of well-characterized proteins (7–12), some of which have recently been identified as allergenic molecules (Table 1). RAST studies, as well as histamine-release experiments using isolated proteins from hen's egg, have clearly shown that ovalbumin, the most abundant protein in

TABLE 1. *Cow's milk and hen's egg allergens*

Source/protein	Monomeric forms, MW × 10⁻³	pI	Percent carbohydrate	Percent of total protein
Cow's milk				
Casein	20–30	3.7–6.0		82
Beta-lactoglobulin	18.3	5.3	0.1	9
Alpha-lactoglobulin	14.2	5.1		3
Serum albumin	67	4.7		1
Immunoglobulin	160	5.6–6.0	2–12	2
Hen's egg white				
Ovalbumin	36		1	65
Ovomucoid	27	3.9	22.9	4
Ovotransferrin	78	6.1		?
Lysozyme				

When leukocytes of BSA-sensitive patients were preincubated for 10 min with the peptide at nonreleasing concentrations, and then BSA at an optimal histamine-releasing concentration was added to the test tubes, there was an inhibition of fragments BSA-$P_{307-582}$ and BSA-$T_{377-582}$ (Fig. 3). Therefore, these fragments serve as haptens inhibiting BSA-induced histamine release. Human IgE antibodies recognize only a single antigenic determinant on the second half of the BSA molecule.

We desensitized rabbit basophils for histamine release with peptide fragments to test for the presence of IgE antibodies recognizing unique or homologous sites. Desensitization occurs when the cells are exposed to an antigen under nonoptimal conditions such as the absence of calcium. With rabbit basophils, desensitization is antigen-specific. As expected, cells desensitized with BSA-P_{1-306} failed to release histamine when rechallenged with the desensitizing antigen (Fig. 4). There was also reduced reactivity on the desensitized cells when they were incubated with the other fragments. Desensitization with BSA-$T_{307-582}$ resulted in unresponsiveness to the desensitizing fragments without any change in the BSA-P_{1-306}-induced hista-

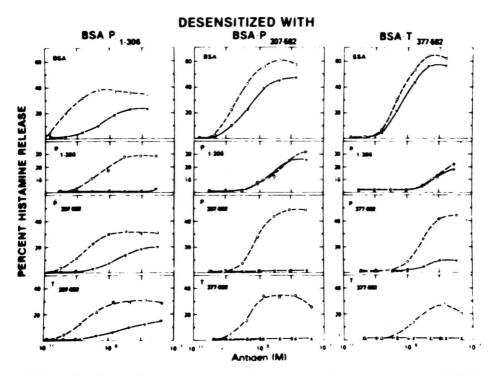

FIG. 4. Specificity of IgE-reactive antigenic determinants on bovine serum albumin. Rabbit basophils were desensitized with different fragments by incubation at 24°C in the absence of calcium. Control cells were preincubated in medium. After 60 min the cells were washed twice and challenged with BSA or the fragments, respectively. Each panel is a graph from a separate experiment.

mine release. These data indicate that there are unique IgE-reactive antigenic sites on each half of the BSA molecule. However, some of the sites on the COOH-terminal portion cross-reacted with antibodies directed toward the NH_2-terminal part of the molecule.

MODULATION OF THE ALLERGENIC ACTIVITY OF FOOD PROTEINS

The easiest way to reduce the allergenic activity of food proteins is heating. However, this will lead to tolerance only in those patients reacting to heat-labile allergens. Cleaving the molecules by enzymatic digestion may result in a marked reduction of allergenic activity due to (a) small fragments, which are not able to cross-link cell-bound IgE antibodies, or (b) smaller fragments with haptenic activity, which block IgE-mediated responses.

We were able to show, by histamine-release experiments with actively sensitized human basophils, that infants who are highly allergic to casein fail to release histamine from washed leukocytes on incubation with casein hydrolysate (Fig. 5). Theoretically, however, highly sensitive patients may still react to larger polypeptides or minute amounts of an intact protein molecule in casein or whey hydrolysates.

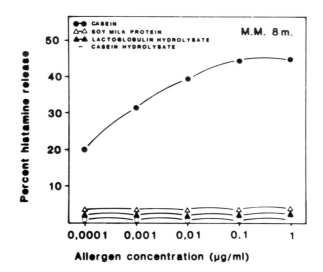

FIG. 5. Histamine release from washed leukocytes of an 8-month-old infant with cow's milk allergy utilizing casein soy milk protein and hydrolysates.

REFERENCES

1. Bahna SL, Heiner DC. *Allergies to milk.* New York: Grune & Stratton, 1980:202.
2. Bleumink E, Young E. Identification of the atopic allergen in cow's milk. *Int Arch Allergy Appl Immunol* 1968;34.521–43.
3. Bleumink E. Food allergy: the chemical nature of the substance eliciting symptoms. *World Rev Nutr Diet* 1970;12:505–70.
4. Goldman AS, Sellars WA, Halpern SR, et al. Milk allergy. II. Skin testing of allergic and normal children with purified milk proteins. *Pediatrics* 1963;32:572–9.
5. Lowenstein H. Quantitative immunoelectrophoretic methods as a tool for the analysis and isolation of allergens. *Prog Allergy* 1978;25:1–62.
6. Gjesing B, Osterballe O, Schwartz B, Wahn U, Lowenstein H. Allergen-specific IgE antibodies against antigenic components in cow's milk and milk substitutes. *Allergy* 1986;41:51–6.
7. Anet H, Back JF, Baker RS, Barnett D, Burley RW, Howden MEH. Allergens in the white and yolk of hen's egg. A study of IgE binding by egg proteins. *Int Arch Allergy Appl Immunol* 1985;77:364–71.
8. Feeney RE, Abplanalp H, Clary JJ, Edwards DL, Clark JR. A genetically varying minor protein constituent of chicken egg white. *J Biol Chem* 1963;238:1732–6.
9. Langeland T. A clinical and immunological study of allergy to hen's egg white. II. Antigens in hen's egg white studied by crossed immunoelectrophoresis. *Allergy (Copenh)* 1982;37:323–33.
10. Langeland T. A clinical and immunological study of allergy to hen's egg white. III. Allergens in hen's egg white studied by crossed radioimmunoelectrophoresis. *Allergy (Copenh)* 1982;37:521–30.
11. Langeland T, Harbitz O. A clinical and immunological study of allergy to hen's egg white. V. Purification and identification of a major allergen (antigen 22) in hen's egg white. *Allergy (Copenh)* 1983;38:131–9.
12. Tomimatsu Y, Clary JJ, Bartulovich JJ. Physical characterization of ovoinhibitor, a trypsin and chymotrypsin inhibitor from chicken egg white. *Arch Biochem Biophys* 1966;115:536–44.
13. Montreuil J, Castiglioni B, Adam-Chosson A, Caner F, Queval J. Études sur les glycoproteides. VIII. L'heterogenéité de l'ovomucoide. Étude critique des methodes de preparation de l'ovomucoide. *J Biochem* 1965;57:514–28.
14. Wahn U, Peters Th, Siraganian RP. Allergenic and antigenic properties of bovine serum albumin. *Mol Immunol* 1980;18:19–28.

DISCUSSION

Dr. Rieger: Crossed radioimmunoelectrophoresis (CRIE) is an interesting method, but as far as I know it is not very sensitive, so you need a lot of IgE to make it work. I would like to know if this is your experience too, and in how many of your allergic subjects were you able to demonstrate the offending allergen using this method?

Dr. U. Wahn: It is true that the cellular method and the basophil histamine-release test are more sensitive than CRIE. The problem with CRIE is that (a) the detection of allergens depends on rabbit antibody causing precipitates of the various antigens and (b) as far as cow's milk is concerned, there is a background IgE response using this method which is detectable in nonallergic serum. Therefore I think this is probably not the best method for testing large numbers of patients. However, we have tested about 20 sera, all RAST class 3 or 4, with CRIE and all were positive.

Dr. de Weck: In cases where you have a positive RAST and a positive histamine-release test but no provocation, have you looked to see whether these are patients who have a very high total IgE but a low ratio of specific IgE to total IgE? There are some skin-provocation data to support this possibility, which could be explained on the basis that the chance of the antigen bridging the basophils or other cells will be diminished if the relationship between specific and total IgE is low. Is that possible?

Dr. U. Wahn: This is quite correct. Our cases were mostly children with atopic dermatitis, who were polyvalently sensitive to many foods and, in general, had very high total IgE.

Dr. Bakken: You told us that you heated the antigen. How long did you heat it, and to what temperature? From a practical point of view when trying to reduce the chance of milk allergic symptoms, is it best to cook milk and for how long?

Dr. U. Wahn: We used several different temperatures, 56°C, 70°C, boiling, for different lengths of time. Even after mild heating, the heat lability of the whey proteins was obvious. However, this will only be relevant to a minority of milk-sensitive children. Many are sensitive to casein, which is not made less allergenic by heating.

Dr. Jost: Concerning your serum albumin experiments: You tested peptic and tryptic serum albumin fragments from Peters' laboratory in your histamine-release assay. Do you have evidence that the disulfide bonds in your fragments are in the initial position? This is especially important in the case of the tryptic fragments.

Dr. U. Wahn: Peters has been studying this for years, and he now has clear evidence that the disulfide bonds are intact.

Food Allergy, edited by Eberhardt Schmidt.
Nestlé Nutrition Workshop Series, Vol. 17.
Nestec Ltd., Vevey/Raven Press, Ltd.,
New York © 1988.

Antigen Presentation

S. Freier, M. Eran, and Y. Suranyi

Pediatric Research Laboratories, Shaare Zedek Medical Center, Jerusalem 91-000, Israel

With the increasing recognition of the clinical spectrum of food allergy in infancy, there is a growing need for a means of dealing with this problem adequately. It is now well established that the presence of foreign antigens in breast milk may be responsible for the manifestations of food hypersensitivity in nursing infants (1). After breastfeeding has been discontinued, food hypersensitivity is mostly dealt with by giving a substitute formula derived from soybean protein or a hydrolysate of cow's milk proteins. What is the nature of the antigens present in these preparations, and how likely are they to produce hypersensitivity phenomena? Furthermore, in the Western world today, the staple diet after the discontinuation of breastfeeding or in breastfeeding failure is a "modified" or "humanized" cow's milk formula. We still do not know if these formulae are capable of reducing the prevalence of cow's milk hypersensitivity. We should like to address some of the problems posed by the use of these foods in infancy.

FOREIGN ANTIGENS IN HUMAN MILK

It has long been known that human milk contains food antigens ingested by the mother (2). In the majority of infants these antigens produce no recognizable symptoms. However, some infants manifest hypersensitivity phenomena, not dissimilar to the symptoms produced by artificial feeds. These symptoms include colic, diarrhea (which may be watery, mucous or bloody), atopic dermatitis, and disease of the upper or lower respiratory tract. The fact that only nanogram quantities of foreign antigen are present does not detract from their potential allergenic effect. On the contrary, Jarrett (3) has shown in animals that small doses are more efficacious in producing immediate-type hypersensitivity than are large doses.

The factors that determine which infants will develop hypersensitivity reactions to foreign antigens in breast milk have not been completely unraveled. Obviously a predisposition to hypersensitivity reactions must be present. This is often genetic (4). Secondly, the properties of the mother's milk apparently play an important role.

This aspect has recently been investigated by Machtinger and Moss (5), who measured the amount of a cow's milk antigen, beta-lactoglobulin, in human milk. (Beta-lactoglobulin is not innate to human milk.) Other parameters that were measured included total breast milk IgA, IgA antibodies to whole cow's milk, and IgA antibodies to casein. These authors, who studied 57 nursing mother-infant pairs, found a highly significant correlation between the presence of symptoms suggestive of allergic disease in the infants and low total IgA in mother's milk. Similarly, a significant inverse correlation was found between symptoms and the presence of IgA antibodies specific to whole milk protein and to casein. If this study is proved correct, it leads to certain important conclusions regarding the interplay between the composition of mother's milk and foreign antigens. Firstly, IgA deficiency in mother's milk predisposes to hypersensitivity reactions in the infant. This observation is reminiscent of the studies of Soothill et al. (6), who claimed that transient IgA deficiency in infants is conducive to the development of infantile eczema. It may well be, therefore, that IgA in breast milk, as well as that produced by the infant's intestine, plays a preventive role in the development of food hypersensitivity. Secondly, the presence of cow's milk antibodies may also prevent the development of hypersensitivity phenomena. Presumably these antibodies may alter the allergenicity of the cow's milk proteins, possibly by complexing them or by preventing the penetration of the intestinal barrier, or by both these mechanisms.

Unfortunately, these conclusions can only be accepted with certain reservations, since several criticisms can be leveled at the study: Firstly, the population of infants studied was highly selected, although this is not stated in the communication. A family history of allergy in one or both parents was present in 63% to 73% of parents. This is far above the incidence of allergy in the general population. Secondly, the infants studied were not proven to have cow's milk protein hypersensitivity, but symptoms suggestive of allergic disease were observed. These criticisms notwithstanding, the observations are of interest and should stimulate further studies.

The amount of foreign antigens present in human milk is under the influence of a number of factors. In the experimental animal, it has been shown by Walker and co-workers (7) that macromolecular uptake from the intestine in lactating animals is decreased. The injection of prolactin in nonlactating animals has the same effect. Similarly, Walker and co-workers have shown that circulating maternal antibodies can limit the transfer of specific protein antigens via the mother's milk (8).

THE ALLERGENICITY OF PROTEIN HYDROLYSATES

Clinical experience has shown that formulae derived from protein hydrolysates are ideal foods for infants with hypersensitivity phenomena to cow's milk. There can be no doubt that these formulae have prevented considerable morbidity and mortality. A measure of their success is reflected in the fact that although one of us (S.F.) has been interested in the field of cow's milk protein hypersensitivity for 20 years, only two cases of adverse reactions to one of these hydrolysates have been encountered. These two cases presented with a history of hypersensitivity reactions to cow's milk. The administration of 15 ml of the casein hydrolysate formula diluted to 50 ml with water in both infants resulted in pallor, profuse vomiting for 12 hr, refusal to feed for 24 hr, and sleepiness. Challenge with the hydrolysate resulted in similar responses on two separate occasions in each infant. These two cases stimulated us to study some of the chemical and immunologic properties of the casein hydrolysate formula (9). As far as the molecular weight of these peptides in the hydrolysate is concerned, it was shown that 15% to 20% had a molecular weight above 3,850, and 35% to 42% had a molecular weight of 340 to 3,850. Injecting animals with one of these formulae showed that although it was believed to be solely casein hydrolysates, antibodies were also produced against beta-lactoglobulin, bovine serum albumin, and alpha-lactalbumin (Table 1). In spite of extensive breakdown, the antigenicity of the molecules is retained. Because the peptides studied were the result of *in vitro* peptic-tryptic digestion, they may well simulate the antigens normally present in the gastrointestinal tract following the ingestion of milk. It was therefore decided to study whether these hydrolysates were capable of giving rise to hypersensitivity phenomena in the intestine of experimental animals. Rats of the Charles River strain were used, weighing 170 to 215 g. Test animals received a subcutaneous and intraperitoneal injection of the commercial casein hydrolysate formula, together with *B. pertussis* adjuvant. Control animals received the adjuvant only. The animals were challenged with the formula on the 18th day in the following manner: At 0 min, the rats received 0.5 μci of ^{125}I-human serum albumin intravenously; at 15 min, 25 mg of the hydrolysate was given by stomach tube; and at 45 min, the rats were killed. Radioactivity was measured in the first and second 15-cm segments of the wall of the intestine, beginning at the pylorus (Table 2).

The experimental model we used was first proposed by Byars and Ferraresi (10). We modified this method and used a strain of rat more predisposed to developing hypersensitivity reactions. Evidence for hypersensitivity was obtained by a positive PCA reaction as well as by increased seepage of protein into the intestinal mucosa, as reflected by the higher radioactivity in the experiment cited here. This hypersensitivity phenomenon also results in a decrease in disaccharidases (11) as well as changes in electrolyte transport and increased histamine release (12). The conclusion therefore must be that although, from a clinical viewpoint, protein

TABLE 1. *Animals sensitized with casein hydrolysate*

Animal	Precipitating antibodies against:				
	Casein	BLG	BGG	BSA	ALA
Rabbit	0/2	0/2	2/2	2/2	2/2
Guinea pig	0/5	0/5	1/5	0/5	1/5

TABLE 2. *Hypersensitivity of intestine to casein hydrolysate formula*

Hypersensitivity, control group (n = 6)	Hypersensitivity, test group (n = 5)	p
Anterior segment		
2,987 ± 488 cpm/15 cm	3,663 ± 434 cpm/15 cm	< 0.05
3,861 ± 574 cpm/g	4,805 ± 732 cpm/g	< 0.05
Posterior segment		
2,542 ± 326 cpm/15 cm	3,130 ± 434 cpm/15 cm	< 0.05
2,815 ± 336 cpm/g	4,502 ± 627 cpm/g	< 0.05

hydrolysate formulae today are the best we have for the treatment of cow's milk hypersensitivity, they are theoretically, but rarely clinically, capable of producing allergic reactions.

THE ALLERGENICITY OF SOY FORMULAE

Some 15 years ago, we became aware of the fact that the use of soy-bean-based formulae for infants with gastrointestinal food allergy may result in a secondary soy protein allergy. The natural history of this phenomenon was usually that an infant suspected of suffering from cow's milk protein hypersensitivity was placed on a soy formula and showed initial improvement. About 2 weeks later, the infant developed increasing pallor, weight loss, and acidosis. The diarrhea may have gone unnoticed because of the bulky stools associated with soy formulae. The institution of protein hydrolysate usually returned the infant to health. It was our estimate that this phenomenon occurred in about 30% of infants fed with soy milk in the treatment of gastrointestinal cow's milk hypersensitivity. Our data were never published, but we know that other investigators had a similar clinical experience (J. Visakorpi, *personal communication*). On the basis of this observation, we do not recommend the use of soy formulae in infants under 6 months old suffering from cow's milk hypersensitivity with gastrointestinal manifestations. Because soy formulae are more palatable than protein hydrolysates, we do use them in infants over the age of 6 months and have not noticed any adverse effects.

The theoretical basis for these phenomena lies not only in the fact that affected infants usually have multiple food allergies. It has been shown that in the experimental sensitized animal, challenge with allergen will result in increased uptake of bystander antigens (13). It has been suggested, though this still remains to be proven, that this antigen uptake is ultimately responsible for sensitization of the intestine with the bystander antigen.

THE ANTIGENS IN MODIFIED MILKS

In spite of extensive experimental evidence which purports to show that heating and drying reduce the allergenicity of cow's milk protein, there is still no evidence that the use of modified formulae has reduced the prevalence of primary cow's milk protein hypersensitivity. In a study from Helsinki (14), it has been shown that the number of infants diagnosed as suffering from milk protein hypersensitivity has not decreased during a period when the majority of mothers using artificial milks have switched from commercial liquid cow's milk to one of the modified milks. The position may be different in the case of secondary, postenteritis, cow's milk protein-induced hypersensitivity. Thus it was shown that in children suffering from acute infectious gastroenteritis, the use of a high-protein, low-lactose milk resulted in the postenteritis diarrhea syndrome in 25% of patients. On the other hand, when infants received a protein hydrolysate formula or modified milk, only 5% suffered from postenteritis diarrhea. It is a reasonable assumption that in the first group of infants the high antigenic load resulted in secondary cow's milk protein hypersensitivity (15). Firer et al. (16) studied the effect of antigenic load on levels of immunoglobulins in infants allergic to cow's milk. Children allergic to milk who were breastfed and had had minimal exposure to cow's milk had decreased titers of IgG, IgA, and IgM milk antibodies as compared with infants allergic to milk, who, before diagnosis, had been fed substantial amounts of cow's milk. Furthermore, the breast-fed infants with minimal exposure to cow's milk showed vastly increased total milk-specific IgE antibodies.

Experimental studies relating to the effect of the amount and nature of the antigenic load in the animal are more abundant. We studied the effect of antigenic load in the mouse (17). In these experiments, one group of weanling mice was fed entirely on cow's milk while a second group was given a casein hydrolysate formula. Table 3 shows that mice receiving cow's milk have a much greater density of IgA-containing plasma cells than those receiving the hydrolysate. This study, as well as a recent study by Knox on human infants (18), suggests that there is a

TABLE 3. *Cell density index of IgA-containing plasma cells in mice fed cow's milk or nutramigen*

Food	Number of mice	Cell density index[a]	
		Jejunum	Duodenum
Cow's milk	5	557 ± 36	571 ± 51
Nutramigen	4	317 ± 21	342 ± 40
p		< 0.01	< 0.01

[a]Values are means ± SE.

direct relationship between the amount of antigen and the production of immuno-globulin-A-bearing plasma cells in the intestine. In allergic infants there is an inverse relationship between antigenic load and production of IgE.

The antigenicity of various milk preparations has been studied in the guinea pig (19). Heating cow's milk reduced the anaphylactogenic properties somewhat, whereas those of modified milks were abolished entirely. Animal experiments have allowed a more detailed study of how antigenic load affects the immune response. While the oral administration of antigen induces tolerance, different doses affect the humoral and cell-mediated immune response to different degrees (20). This subject is discussed in more detail elsewhere in this volume.

The question of whether modified formulae represent an advantage over cow's milk from the point of view of preventing cow's milk protein hypersensitivity reactions remains a moot point. It is possible that modified milk will have replaced pasteurized cow's milk before this question has been answered.

HUMORAL CONTROL OF ANTIBODY SECRETION

Little is known of the importance of local intestinal food antibodies in the handling of dietary antigens. Walker and Isselbacher (21) suggested that IgA might complex food proteins and anchor them to the mucosa, so as to permit more efficient proteolysis. Be that as it may, we have now obtained evidence that there is a synchronized outpouring of immunoglobulins at the time of food ingestion. Initially we showed that in humans the injection of cholecystokinin results in the outpouring of immunoglobulins A, M, E, and D (22,23). Subsequent experiments in rats have shown that, in addition to the biliary and pancreatic release of these immunoglobulins, there is a rise in the release of IgG and IgA antibodies through the intestinal wall following the administration of cholecystokinin intravenously. Finally, we have shown that the feeding of a protein hydrolysate formula also results in IgG and IgA release through the intestinal wall (24). Nervous impulses appear to control IgA release. Cholinergic agents such as pilocarpine, muscarine, and bethanechol significantly increased the release of IgA through the wall of the intestine (25). Atropine blocked the effect of pilocarpine and inhibited basal intestinal IgA secretion for 40 min after injection. These results further emphasize the fact that the secretion of secretory IgA is not a continuous process but is, instead, coordinated with digestive activity in the gastrointestinal tract.

In animal models, intestinal reaginic antibodies equivalent to human IgE have been studied. In the rat, reaginic antibodies to egg albumin have been found to correlate with gastrointestinal hypersensitivity to the protein (26). The local hypersensitivity response in the intestine is accompanied by enhanced mucus secretion and by an increase in vascular permeability. Mucus may then protect the mucosal surface against penetration of soluble antigens through the mucosa.

PATIENT VARIATION IN ANTIGEN HANDLING

In addition to the nature of the various antigens presented to the intestine, certain factors pertaining to the individual will influence antigen handling. In animals the phenomenon of closure has been demonstrated (27), but no evidence for this exists in the human gastrointestinal tract. Hypersensitivity phenomena in infants are rare in the first month of life. Their peak time of onset is at 4 to 6 weeks in formula-fed infants, and they disappear in the majority of infants by 2 years. We investigated this phenomenon in light of current concepts regarding defects in immune regulation as related to disease processes. We measured the activity of non-specific suppressor cells of peripheral blood lymphocytes in 22 patients with cow's milk hypersensitivity and compared the results with 26 age-matched controls (28). The patient's suppressor cell activity on donor cell proliferation was measured following concanavalin A stimulation. We found significantly reduced suppressor cell activity ($p<0.05$) in infants with cow's milk protein hypersensitivity. This activity progressively improved over the course of the first 20 months of life and ultimately reached normal levels. Infants not suffering from cow's milk protein hypersensitivity had normal suppressor cell activity. Stimulation of peripheral blood lymphocytes with beta-lactoglobulin resulted in increased stimulation of lymphocytes from sensitive subjects.

CONCLUSION

In addition to other considerations, breast milk is the preferred food for infants, from an immunologic point of view. Occasionally, breast-fed infants may manifest hypersensitivity phenomena to foreign antigens, and this may be related to the immune properties of the mother's milk. Protein hydrolysates are ideal foods for infants sensitive to cow's milk proteins, but they are expensive and therefore are not suitable as a routine food in normal infants. They, too, may produce hypersensitivity phenomena, but this is rare. Soy formulae are suitable for infants over 6 months old with cow's milk hypersensitivity; they are also suitable for individuals with extraintestinal hypersensitivity at any age. Whether modified cow's milk preparations present an immunologic advantage over unadulterated cow's milk has still not been clarified.

REFERENCES

1. Gerrard JW. Allergies in breast fed babies to foods ingested by the mother. *Clin Rev Allergy* 1984;2:143–9.
2. Kilshaw PJ, Cant AJ. The passage of maternal dietary proteins into human breast milk. *Int Arch Allergy Appl Immunol* 1984;75:8–15.

3. Jarrett EEE. Stimuli for the production and control of IgE in rats. *Immunol Rev* 1978;41:52–76.
4. Freier S, Finelt M, Seban A, Cohen T, Brautbar C. Genetic factors in food allergy of early childhood. In: Gerrard FW, *Food allergy: new perspectives*. Springfield: Thomas, 1980:3–24.
5. Machtinger S, Moss R. Cow's milk allergy in breast fed infants: the role of allergen and maternal secretory IgA antibody. *J Allergy Clin Immunol* 1986;77:341–7.
6. Soothill JF. The role of immuno-deficiency in allergy. *Clin Allergy* 1973;3:473.
7. Udall JN, Colony P, Fritze L, Trier JS, Walker WA. Development of gastrointestinal mucosal barrier. II. The effect of natural versus artificial feeding on intestinal permeability to macromolecules. *Pediatr Res* 1981;15:245–9.
8. Harmatz PL, Bloch KJ, Kleinman PE, Walsh MK, Walker WA. Influence of circulating maternal antibody on the transfer of dietary antigen to neonatal mice via milk. *Immunology* 1986;57:43–8.
9. Seban A, Konijn A, Freier S. Chemical and immunological properties of a protein hydrolysate formula. *Am J Clin Nutr* 1977;30:840–6.
10. Byars N, Ferraresi RW. Intestinal anaphylaxis in the rat as a model of food allergy. *Clin Exp Immunol* 1976;24:352–6.
11. Freier S, Eran M, Goldstein R. The effect of immediate type gastrointestinal allergic reactions on brush border enzymes and gut morphology in the rat. *Pediatr Res* 1985;19:456–9.
12. Perdue MH, Chung M, Gall DG. Effect of intestinal anaphylaxis on gut function in the rat. *Gastroenterology* 1984;86:391.
13. Bloch KJ, Walker WA. Effect of locally induced intestinal anaphylaxis on the uptake of a bystander antigen. *J Allergy Clin Immunol* 1981;67:312–6.
14. Verkasalo M, Kuitunen P, Savilahti E, Tiilikainen A. Changing pattern of cow's milk intolerance. *Acta Paediatr Scand* 1981;70:289–95.
15. Manuel PD, Walker-Smith JA. A comparison of three infant feeding formulae for the prevention of delayed recovery after infantile gastroenteritis. *Acta Paediatr Belg* 1981;34:13–20.
16. Firer MA, Hoskins CS, Hill DJ. Effect of antigen load on development of milk antibodies in infants allergic to milk. *Br Med J* 1981;183:693–6.
17. Sagie E, Tarabulus J, Maeir DM, Freier S. Diet and development of intestinal IgA. *Isr J Med Sci* 1974;10:532–4.
18. Knox WF. Restricted feeding and human intestinal plasma cell development. *Arch Dis Child* 1986;61:744–9.
19. McLaughlin PM, Anderson KJ, Widdowson EM, Coomlis RRA. Effect of heat on the anaphylactic-sensitizing capacity of cow's milk, goat's milk and various infant formulae fed to guinea pigs. *Arch Dis Child* 1981;56:165–71.
20. Mowat A McI, Strobel S, Drummond HE, Ferguson A. Immunological responses to fed protein antigens in mice 1. Reversal of oral tolerance to ovalbumin by cyclophosphamide. *Immunology* 1982;45:105–13.
21. Walker WA, Isselbacher KJ. Intestinal antibodies. *N Engl J Med* 1977;297:767–73.
22. Shah PC, Freier S, Park BH, Lee PC, Lebenthal E. Pancreozymin and secretin enhance duodenal fluid antibody levels to cow's milk proteins. *Gastroenterology* 1977;83:916–21.
23. Freier S, Lebenthal E, Freier M, Shah PC, Park BH, Lee PC. IgE and IgD antibodies to cow's milk and soy protein in duodenal fluid: effects of pancrozymin and secretin. *Immunology* 1983;49:69–75.
24. Freier S, et al. *(in press)*.
25. Dodd Wilson I, Soltis RD, Olson RE, Erandsen SL. Cholinergic stimulation of immunoglobulin A secretion in rat intestine. *Gastroenterology* 1982;83:881–8.
26. Bloch KJ, Lake AM, Sinclair K, Walter WA. IgE mediated alterations in intestinal permeability. In: *The mucosal immune system in health and disease. Proceedings of the 81st Ross conference on pediatric research*. Columbus, Ohio: Ross Laboratories, 1981:273–80.
27. Udall JN, Pang K, Fritze L, Kleinman R, Walker WA. Development of gastrointestinal muscosal barrier. 1. The effect of age on intestinal permeability to macromolecules. *Pediatr Res* 1981;15:241–4.
28. Weil S, Kuperman O, Ilfeld D, Finelt M, Freier S. Non-specific suppressor cell activity and lymphocyte response to beta-lactoglobulin in cow's milk hypersensitivity. *J Pediatr Gastroenterol Nutr* 1982;1:389–93.

DISCUSSION

Dr. Visakorpi: We always used to treat the severe forms of gastrointestinal allergy with human milk alone, and I now wonder why we never saw any reactions. Some patients were very sensitive indeed, and even a small drop of cow's milk would cause an enormous reaction, yet we never saw reactions to human milk. Of course we did not know then that there might be cow's milk in human milk, and maybe the patients did not know either! We always used pooled pasteurized human milk; perhaps pooling and heating introduce some inhibitory factors which reduce the likelihood of reactions. We used human milk not only because it was available to us but also because we saw a lot of reactions to soy milk, and I saw some reactions to Nutramigen as well. You mentioned the Helsinki report (1), which counted all the cases of intestinal cow's milk allergy over a long period of time, including those of abrupt onset before and after the introduction of commercially adapted formulas replacing the home-made formulas in 1972 to 1973 in Finland. In spite of this change in diet there was no change in the incidence of intestinal cow's milk allergy. However, there has been very great change in the type of reaction seen. The severe forms of enteropathies have completely disappeared, and this change seems to date from the time of the change of feeding to commercial formula. Of course there could be other reasons for this—for example, the increase in breast-feeding or the decline in the incidence of severe gastroenteritis among young infants.

Dr. Schmerling: I want to add to Professor Visakorpi's remarks. The situation is exactly the same in Zürich, in that the severe cases of pure gastrointestinal cow's milk intolerance have completely disappeared. However, we now have many more cases of young infants, mostly between 2 and 4 months of age, with severe generalized forms of cow's milk intolerance with cutaneous and respiratory manifestations, some of whom go into shock on contact with very small amounts of milk. I tried to correlate this change with alterations in feeding, and it seems that modified adapted formulas were introduced at about the same time, but there has also been an increase in breast-feeding, which confuses the picture. I think we have missed the point at which we could carry out a proper prospective study to provide the answers.

Dr. Freier: Another change that has occurred is the result of greater awareness of cow's milk hypersensitivity among pediatricians and general practitioners working in the periphery. In Jerusalem today there are many children who are not allergic to milk but who are given soy milk or Nutramigen for any untoward gastrointestinal symptom. This may be another reason why we no longer see children with such severe manifestations as we did in the late 1960s.

Dr. Guesry: I am somewhat confused at the assumption which has been made in this discussion, namely, that the new infant formulas are likely to be less allergenic to the gut than the old ones or unmodified cow's milk. In fact, the heat treatment of a modern infant formula, by spray-drying, is far less damaging to the protein than the old way of evaporating milk, or boiling milk in a pan in the kitchen for 10 min. Modern infant formulas should be at least as allergenic as the old ones.

Dr. Hadorn: I should like to ask the audience whether anyone is aware of a study in which the incidence of cow's milk intolerance was examined in children receiving adapted formulas versus hydrolyzed milks.

Dr. Van den Plas: We have done a study comparing infants fed on hypoallergic formulas, adapted formulas, and breast milk, with a 4-month follow-up. No infant on the hypoallergic formula developed symptoms of allergy, but several developed symptoms when changed to the adapted formula. Similarly, infants who developed symptoms on adapted formula improved when switched to hypoallergic formula. We have not yet published the results.

Dr. Cant: Returning to the subject of food antigens in breast milk, we have looked for beta-lactoglobin, ovalbumin, and ovomucoid in the milk of about 30 mothers and found that about two-thirds of the mothers passed these proteins into their milk. We found no relation between the presence of antigen and symptoms in the child or between the presence of antigen and the development of specific positive skin-prick tests. My colleague Dr. Kilshaw went on to look at IgA levels, but he found no correlation between IgA and the development of clinical features either, so I was surprised at the study that you mentioned by Machtinger and Moss (2), which apparently did show such a correlation. Was any account taken of the mothers' atopic status? If the mothers were atopic they might have had low serum levels of IgA, which would be an independent variable not related to the infant's symptoms.

Dr. Freier: I am sure that the Machtinger and Moss study needs to be repeated. I feel it was too good to be true. One of the criticisms that I had about the article was that the incidence of atopy among the parents was 63% to 73%, which obviously isn't the incidence in the general population. The use of such a selected group might well vitiate the results.

Dr. de Weck: Dr. Cant has nicely introduced the point I wanted to make. We speak often of the transfer of factors into breast milk, but always in terms of IgA or food antigens. It seems to me that we should at least consider other factors. What about the recent article showing that there may be IgE-binding factors in breast milk (3)? And what about the transfer of cells? Is it really a matter of indifference whether the mother who is breast-feeding is herself atopic? One could envisage that nonatopic mothers will have normal IgE-suppressing factors and will transmit them in their milk, whereas this may not be the case for atopic mothers.

Dr. Scadding: I should like to introduce one further possible confounding factor, which is maternal smoking. The incidence of women who smoke has increased in recent years, and there is quite a lot of evidence that smoke can predispose toward hypersensitivity to environmental allergens. This possibility needs to be explored.

DISCUSSION REFERENCES

1. Verkasalo M, Kuitunen P, Savilahti E, Tiilkainen A. Changing pattern of cow's milk intolerance. *Acta Paediatr Scand* 1981;79:289–95.
2. Machtinger S, Moss R. Cow's milk allergy in breast fed infants: the role of allergen and maternal secretory IgA antibody. *J Allergy Clin Immunol* 1986;77:341–7.
3. Sarfati M, Vanderbeeken Y, Duncan D, Delespesse G. Demonstration of IgE suppressor factors in human colostrum. *Eur J Immunol* 1986;16:1005.

Food Allergy, edited by Eberhardt Schmidt.
Nestlé Nutrition Workshop Series, Vol. 17.
Nestec Ltd., Vevey/Raven Press, Ltd.,
New York © 1988.

Developmental Aspects of Food Allergy

Stephan Strobel

*Department of Immunology, Institute of Child Health, University of London,
London WC1N 1EH, England*

It is a well-recognized fact that the risk of developing an immediate- or delayed-type food allergic disease is higher in children than in adults. This observation implies that developmental factors operative during gestation and after birth are likely to play an important, although as yet poorly defined, role in the development of food allergic disease. The present review will summarize clinical and experimental evidence and will outline the importance of pre-, peri- and postnatal host responses to fed antigens which are presented to the gut-associated lymphoid tissues (GALT) either directly or via the breast milk.

After a brief discussion of ontogenetic aspects of neonatal immunity, I will concentrate on the *afferent* part of the immune response (antigen handling and absorption) (Table 1) and will secondly focus on the *efferent* immune responses that are initiated *after* the antigen has reached the systemic circulation or the GALT. Furthermore, conditions that are likely to induce or interfere with the induction of oral tolerance (oral tolerance being defined as a specific hyporesponsive immunological state following the first antigen presentation via the gut and the GALT) will be outlined.

THE IMMUNE SYSTEM OF THE HUMAN NEONATE

Cell-Mediated Immunity (T-Lymphocyte Development)

T-cell-mediated immune responses are comparatively mature at birth, and responses to antigens have been documented with T lymphocytes of fetal tissue at 15 to 16 weeks of gestation (1). (Table 2). A well-known clinical example of the maturity of the T-cell system at birth is the mature immune response to early postnatal BCG vaccination. Human newborn cells show a mature proliferative response to mitogens and normal lymphokine production and are capable of cytotoxic activity. This contrasts with the functional immaturity of nonspecific systems such as phagocytosis, antigen-presenting activity, and activity of the complement system (2).

A unique suppressor cell function has been demonstrated by several investiga-

TABLE 1. *Factors influencing immune responses after oral antigen encounter*[a]

Lumen	Mucosa	Immune response
Afferent limb		**Efferent limb**
Motility	Digestion	Immunodeficiency
Colonization	Inflammation	Clearance
Mucus	Immaturity:	Circulating:
Digestion	binding	antibody
Antibody	uptake	antigen
	permeability	immune complexes
	Antibody	

[a]Immune responses after oral antigen encounter can be divided into an *afferent* limb and an *efferent* limb. The afferent limb includes a wide variety of luminal and/or mucosal factors which are often interdependent. After the antigen has gained access to the gut-associated lymphoid tissues (GALT), the efferent limb of the immune response will be initiated. A disturbance of the normal immune response at both levels could lead to food-related diseases.

TABLE 2. *Cell-mediated immunity of the human neonate*[a]

Mature at birth (BCG vaccination)
MLC/PHA: Responsive after 15 weeks of gestation
Nonspecific suppressor cells (cord blood):
    Inhibition of adult T-cells
    No effect on neonatal cells (prevention of GVHR?)

[a]Most of the cell-mediated immune responses are mature at birth, and lymphocytes respond—for example, in a mixed lymphocyte culture—or the lectin phytohemagglutinin (PHA) after 15 weeks of gestation. Phagocytosis and lymphokine production at birth are, however, reduced as compared with that of older children.

tors in the cord blood (3). These cells exert a cytostatic influence on adult T-cell functions but not on allogeneic (neonatal) cells. This antigen nonspecific suppression does not affect autologous B-cells and has been implicated in the prevention of graft-versus-host reactions (GVHR) after mutual lymphocyte exchange between mother and child during late pregnancy and birth. According to different authors, this nonspecific suppression lasts between 5 and 14 days after birth (4).

Humoral Immunity

It has been shown that B-cell functions are immature at birth (Table 3). *In vitro* studies measuring single-cell immunoglobulin production have indicated that the IgM production is fully mature at birth, whereas IgG and IgA production are not.

TABLE 3. *Humoral immunity of the human neonate*[a]

Immature B-cell function
IgA, IgG
Differential maturation of IgG
IgG1 + IgG3 < 12 months
IgG2 + IgG4 >24 months
Lack of T help for IgG (not suppression)

[a]B-cell functions are usually immature at birth (IgA, IgG), and the IgG subclass maturation extends well into infancy. Neonates born after 36 weeks of gestation are, for example, capable of producing anti-BSA and anti-beta-lactoglobulin antibodies. Under certain circumstances, specific IgE antibody production can be triggered *in utero* after prenatal sensitization.

Within 24 months, B-cell immunity has usually reached adult levels (IgA production may still be immature). IgG subclasses mature at different times; IgG1 and IgG3 responses reach adult levels within 12 months, whereas IgG2 and IgG4 may not have reached mature levels even 24 months after birth. The lack of T-cell help for the IgG production (90% of neonates) is not caused by active suppression (2).

DEVELOPMENTAL ASPECTS OF INTESTINAL PERMEABILITY AND ABSORPTION

The permeability of the intestine of the premature and term newborn to intact proteins (macromolecules) (5) and to inert sugar molecules (6) such as lactulose and rhamnose has been investigated for several years, yet there is still controversy as to how long the increased uptake of the cow's milk antigens bovine serum albumin (BSA) and beta-lactoglobulin (BLG) persists. Roberton et al. (5) presented data showing that infants born before 37 weeks of gestation demonstrate higher concentrations of BLG 5 days after birth than do infants of higher gestational age. A similar transitional period, from an increased to a normal sugar permeability at around 36 to 40 weeks of gestation, has been reported by another group (6). From these data, it seems that the gastrointestinal permeability of the premature infant (less than 36 weeks of gestation) is uniformly increased both to high- and low-molecular-weight marker molecules (Fig. 1).

Under different clinical conditions in later life, changes in permeability to sugars do not, however, necessarily reflect increased macromolecular absorption. Evidence that sugar permeability and macromolecular permeability of the gastrointestinal tract do not necessarily correlate—for example, during an immunologically mediated anaphylactic response—has been presented by Turner et al. in a rat model (7).

An important new dimension of macromolecular absorption has been presented

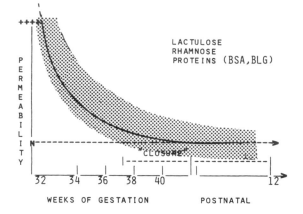

WEEKS OF GESTATION   POSTNATAL

FIG. 1. Changes in intestinal permeability. The intestinal permeability to lactulose, rhamnose, milk, and soy proteins and human lactalbumin in human neonates is increased before 36 weeks of gestation. According to most investigators, permeability reaches normal levels at 40 (±3) weeks of gestation. This reduction in permeability has been termed "gut closure," although there is no evidence of morphologic changes during that period in the human neonate.

by Müller et al. (9). Antigenic BLG and alpha-casein were measured in the serum of 45 5- and 10-day-old formula-fed infants born at 31 to 41 weeks of gestation. As expected, BLG was detected at 5 days of age in 14 of 19 infants born before 37 weeks of gestation but in only 1 of 10 infants born after 37 weeks of gestation. In contrast, however, casein was only present in 4 of 17 infants born before 37 weeks of gestation but in 10 of 12 infants of the more mature group.

If these observations are confirmed by other groups, these findings could point to a different (antigen-specific?) absorptive and/or clearing capacity of BLG and casein in premature and normal infants during the early postnatal period. Differential antigen handling at this age may be an important factor in modulating the immune responsiveness after ingestion. Although this study was well controlled for the presence of circulating (maternal) antibodies, specific immune complex formation could have affected their results. For obvious reasons, antigenic absorption in neonates is restricted to the measurements of cow's milk or soy proteins. The advantage of using a normal dietary antigen is reduced by the influences of passive and/or active immunity transferred during birth and/or lactation.

A different approach was taken by a Swedish group (10) that measured the serum concentration of human lactalbumin, which is a normal constituent of human milk and is taken up unaffected by local or systemic immune responses. Levels of human lactalbumin have been demonstrated to be 10 times higher in premature infants (26–31 weeks of gestation). Serum concentrations fell to normal levels at approximately 39 weeks (10). It remains to be proven whether this reflects increased uptake or delayed clearance.

To test the interesting hypothesis that an increased uptake of macromolecules may lead to food allergic disease (8) (Fig. 2), it would be important to investigate, in a prospective study, the incidence and prevalence of food allergic disease in premature, artificially fed infants. Alternatively, it is equally possible that the increased intestinal permeability is not sufficient (on its own) to induce a sensitization. Other genetic factors—for example, those affecting the antigen-processing

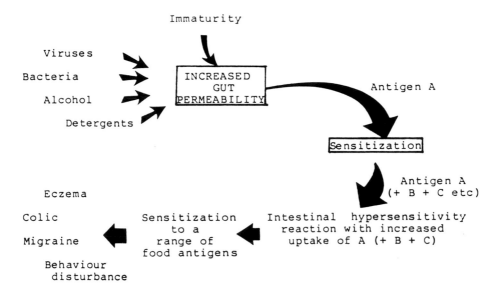

FIG. 2. Hypothetical role of an increased intestinal permeability on subsequent development of food-induced hypersensitivities (I). An increased intestinal permeability to macromolecular antigens may lead to sensitization to antigen A. Continuing administration of A further increases the permeability based on an immunologic mechanism to antigen A but also to the unrelated antigens B, C, etc. This chain of events may lead to sensitization to a wide range of food antigens. This mechanism could explain the existence of multiple food allergies but does not explain the initial event that leads to sensitization to antigen A.

capacity and/or the immune responsiveness of the host (I-r genes)—may play a more important role in tipping the balance toward sensitization (Fig. 3).

EFFECTS OF HUMAN MILK AND IMMUNITY OF LACTATION

Generally, human milk is the normal infant food; it represents optimal nutrition and transfers active and passive protective immunity for the neonate. Paul Ehrlich (11) demonstrated in 1892 that immunity could be transferred by breast milk (in mice), and later studies clearly demonstrated that human colostrum (and milk) provide important immune defenses during early neonatal development. Among the substances transferred are nonspecific agents such as: lysozyme; lactoferrin; specific secretory antibodies (and possibly antiidiotypic antibodies) against viruses, bacteria, and food antigens; and immunocompetent cells (macrophages, T- and B-lymphocytes) (12–14). High levels of IgA antibodies in human milk prevent bacterial attachment and may also protect against potentially harmful immune responses to ingested antigens (15). On the other hand, human milk has been known for a long time to contain food antigens (such as milk proteins, wheat, and ovalbumin) (16,17), which may also trigger food allergic symptoms in the infant; sensitization

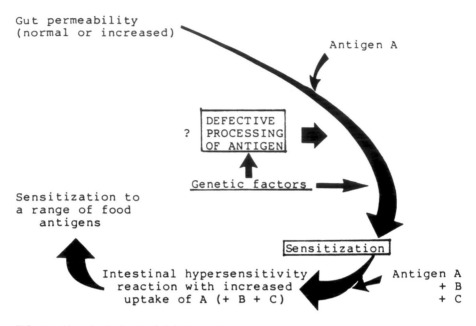

FIG. 3. Hypothetical role of defective antigen processsing and/or genetic factors in the development of food-induced hypersensitivities (II). Regardless of changes in intestinal permeability, alterations in the antigen handling and processing mechanisms of the gut-associated lymphoid tissues (GALT) could lead to sensitization to a variety of food antigens. The immune responsiveness is likely to be governed by genetic factors, and the increased incidence of atopic diseases in children with a parental history of allergy points in this direction. An increased macromolecular permeability may be necessary but is not sufficient on its own to cause a sensitization.

via breast milk has also been described (18,19). These observations would suggest that dietary manipulations in the mother might be helpful in preventing food allergic disease in the neonate. Early clinical studies seem to point to a protective role of antigen avoidance during pregnancy (20). These studies, however, need confirmation.

On balance, it still seems that breast-feeding is not an important source of sensitization in a population at risk, and it is more likely to protect the population of infants against food allergic and infectious diseases (21–23).

A recent study (24) casts some doubts on the beneficial effects of prolonged breast-feeding (>3 months) on the reduction of allergic symptoms in infants at risk of developing an allergy (family history of allergy). This study, however, also demonstrates that breast-feeding reduces diarrheal episodes in infancy. Further studies are needed, and this study certainly cannot be taken as an argument against breast-feeding.

EFFECTS OF IMMATURITY AND LACTATION ON INTESTINAL ANTIGEN HANDLING

In vitro studies, using the everted gut-sac technique, demonstrated that intestinal antigen handling and uptake was changed during the lactation period in the rat. Observed changes were reversible at the end of lactation and could be reproduced by the injection of an equivalent amount of the hormone prolactin. Details will be discussed by W. A. Walker (*this volume*).

The same group demonstrated an increased binding of BSA and BLG and an increased uptake in newborn animals using microvillous membrane preparations (25). These microvillous membranes of newborn animals also showed a decreased protein breakdown capability which could account for this phenomenon. However, it remains to be proven whether these disturbances in the immunophysiology of antigen handling alone might increase the susceptibility to develop adverse reactions to foods in the early postnatal period. Further work is clearly needed to clarify whether this potentially important and complementary mechanism of the regulation of macromolecular antigen uptake exists in humans too and whether it is of physiological importance.

EFFECTS OF PASSIVELY TRANSFERRED ANTIBODY ON THE HUMORAL IMMUNE RESPONSE

Placental transfer of specific antibodies protects the human neonate effectively against pathogenic organisms and toxins before he or she is capable of producing an active humoral immune response. It was tempting to speculate that a high level of circulating antifood antibody may similarly be protective against potentially hazardous oral sensitization in the neonate. High levels of IgG antibodies to milk and egg in cord sera reflect the maternal concentration, and there is a slight correlation with protection against atopic (IgE-mediated) disease during the first 2 years of life (26,27). The influence of circulating antibody on the transfer of antigen into milk in mice has been studied in animals. The findings suggest that circulating maternal antibodies can limit the transfer of a dietary protein from mother to newborn (28). However, it remains to be established whether the reduction of "maternally processed" antigen in this experimental system has beneficial effects on the offspring in reducing the chances of sensitization, or whether the presentation of small amounts of antigen is necessary for the induction of tolerance. Further studies are needed in order to answer these questions.

Studying the effects of passively transferred maternal anti-BSA antibodies on the development of anti-BSA antibodies in the human neonate (29) (with and without passively transferred antibody), Rieger's group showed, over a 6-month period, that there was no difference in either group. This was also true when high and low BSA intake (via cow's milk formulas) was taken into account (30).

These findings suggest that the initiation of IgG + IgM antibody formation to ingested antigens occurs relatively unaffected by the presence of circulating maternal antibodies (31). This important observation is at variance with the well-known fact that circulating antibodies can modulate systemic immune responses to *parenterally* administered antigens (see, for example, the effects of circulating specific antibodies on the reduced "take rate" after diphtheria and measles vaccinations in the young infant). This further highlights the important differences observed in immune responses following *enteral* or *systemic* antigen administration.

NEONATAL CAPACITY TO PRODUCE SPECIFIC ANTIBODY

Because of obvious ethical restrictions, the neonate's capacity to produce specific antibody has mainly focused on the capacity to produce BSA or BLG antibodies after oral administration of a cow's-milk-containing formula. The highest incidence of anti-BSA antibodies (above 80%) was found in children between the age of 4 months and 5 years (32). Premature infants born at around 35 to 36 weeks of gestation were able to produce detectable anti-BSA antibodies (33,34). The authors hypothesized that the failure of B cells to respond to ingested antigens in infants born before 30 weeks of gestation may represent the functional immaturity of the B-cell system and that antigens reaching the Peyer's patches before the 34th week may preferentially stimulate the suppressor T-cell system, which would then suppress the systemic B-cell response (34). The above observations, however, lend themselves to a variety of different explanations, which will be discussed later. The hypothesis does not take the digestive, immunologic, and mucosal immaturity, as well as the existence of a nonspecific suppressor cell population (around birth), into account. It has also been shown that fetal B and T lymphocytes at 14 to 15 weeks of gestation are capable of responding to mitogens and to HLA-DR antigens (1–3). The capacity of the neonate to respond to ingested antigens will be discussed below.

PERINATAL INFLUENCES ON IgE RESPONSES

Limited studies in humans have demonstrated that circulating maternal anti-BSA antibodies (IgG or IgM) have no effect, in the child, on the further development of the immune response to ingested antigens of the same type (30,31,34). However, this phenomenon may not be true for the regulation of immunoglobulin E (IgE) synthesis. Evidence to support a different way of immune regulation for IgE has been presented by the work of the late E. Jarrett and her group (35–38). In a series of experiments, rats were used to explore factors influencing the development of IgE regulation during early life, when the immune system of the neonate most probably differs intrinsically from that of mature animals.

Stimulation of adult rats with antigens, whether injected or fed, led more often to *reduced*, as opposed to enhanced, IgE responses to subsequent challenge. This

TABLE 4. *Perinatal influences on IgE responses*[a]

Suckling mother	Neonate
Immunized with OVA	IgE low
Control	IgE high
Cross-foster control neonates	
Immunized with OVA (lactating)	IgE low
IV antibody (lactating)	IgE low
	(Jarrett)

[a]This table summarizes the work of the late E. Jarrett in rodents. If pregnant animals are immunized with hen's egg albumin (ovalbumin), the IgE responses in the neonate will be suppressed. Normal neonates cross-fostered by lactating animals previously immunized (OVA) or injected with specific anti-OVA antibodies also show a reduced IgE response, and the subsequent suppression is suggestive of an IgG-mediated mechanism. (A similar IgE regulatory mechanism has not been established in humans.)

capacity to suppress IgE production is activated by even minute amounts of antigen (nanogram quantities) which are frequently absorbed via the gastrointestinal tract. It was hypothesized that this would maintain the down-regulation of the IgE response in the neonatal rat (35). Further experiments demonstrated that there is a marked suppression of IgE responsiveness in the offspring of parenterally immunized female rats and that this state of suppression in the neonatal rat persists even when the circulating maternal antibody is no longer detectable (36,37). This protective effect could also be produced by injection of a small amount of antigen-specific IgG after birth and would suggest that transferred maternal antibody can suppress and modulate IgE responsiveness of neonatal rats. To summarize, it seems that both specific maternal IgG and specific antigen have a profound effect on the regulation of the IgE response (38) (Table 4). It has to be stressed that the existence of a similar regulating pathway for human IgE responses has not been established.

IMMUNE RESPONSES TO INGESTED ANTIGENS

An antigen can be defined as any substance (bacterial, viral, food) that elicits a specific immune response when introduced into the tissues of a person or animal. Single-protein molecules may have several antigenic determinants, and any antigen may evoke several immune responses that are not mutually exclusive. In the case of antigen administered via the gut, both systemic and mucosal immune reactions occur, and there may be either induction or suppression of a particular immune response (antibody-mediated or T-cell-mediated) (39–41). Active immunity, in which antigen-reactive cells and specific antibody develop, must be distinguished from immunologic tolerance, which is a specific immune response leading to a specific hyporesponsiveness if the antigen is subsequently given parenterally (39,42). Active immune responses can readily be detected and measured in humans and in animals. The phenomenon of immunologic tolerance to ingested proteins has been studied mainly in small laboratory rodents (39,42–44), although circumstantial evidence implies that it also exists in humans (45,46). The experiments described below illustrate how the pattern of immune responses to ingested antigens of an individual animal, or possibly of a person, is critically dependent on the route of first exposure. An irreversible chain of events is set in motion, depending on the primary presentation of an antigen. The subsequent immune response may be modified, but never completely reversed, as a result of further antigen exposure or by the use of cytotoxic drugs (42). Chronic antigen exposure after initial immunization can, however, modulate the immune response, which has been shown in adult (47) and neonatal animals (48), but this treatment does not usually reinduce a complete state of tolerance. There is, however, some preliminary evidence (49) that mice immunized with ovalbumin in complete Freund's adjuvant and re-fed 1 week after immunization show a substantial reduction of their cell-mediated immune responses to ovalbumin ($p<0.01$) as well as reducing serum antibody levels to a lesser extent ($p<0.05$). The above-mentioned observations stress the fact that the humoral and cell-mediated limbs of the immune system are under different control and are also affected differently by oral antigen exposure (50,51).

Crucial for the understanding of the immunologic events triggered by oral antigen exposure is the knowledge of the recirculation pathway of (Peyer's patch) lymphocytes and of immune regulation within the GALT. This will not be discussed in detail here, but it has been the subject of recent reviews (52,53). Briefly, immune responses that develop after gastrointestinal antigen exposure are associated with stimulation of several types of immune regulatory T-lymphocytes in the GALT. Within the Peyer's patches and other organized lymphoid tissues of the gut, antigen-specific T-helper and T-suppressor cells are activated. There appears to be a dual activation of the T-lymphocytes which regulate the B-lymphocyte population; there seems to be an induction of T-helper cells for the IgA system and suppressor cells for IgM and IgG synthesis (41,54). Activation of antigen-specific T-helper cells for IgA probably leads to stimulation of B-lymphocytes which have recirculated to the mucosa and produces a mucosal IgA response. The simultaneous induction and activation of T-suppressor cells for IgG and IgM leads to the specific systemic tolerance. At the same time, T-suppressor cells for suppression of cell-mediated immune response in the gastrointestinal tract are also induced. Several groups have shown that the administration of antigens at an early stage in the postnatal development can cause diarrheal diseases, which are probably due to a cell-mediated immune response within the gastrointestinal tract. The sensitizing capacity of antigen administration has been shown in the preruminant calf, in piglets, and in mice (55–57).

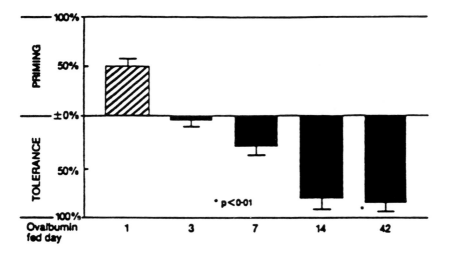

FIG. 4. Age-dependent modulation of the immune response after feeding ovalbumin to mice. Percentage suppression of systemic immune responses compared to saline fed controls. (From ref. 60.)

EXPERIMENTS IN NEONATAL MICE

Based on clinical experience that suggests a vulnerable period in the human neonate within the first 4 to 6 weeks of life, potentially hazardous effects of early antigen administration on the development of food allergic disease have been investigated by studying the effects of age at first feed on the development of subsequent specific systemic immunity (in mice). Suppression (tolerance) or priming (enhancement of the immune response) of the immune system was investigated in animals that had been fed at various times after birth (1–42 days). Full details of the methods and results have been published (48,57,59). All animals were age-matched and were fed 1 mg of antigen ovalbumin per gram of body weight. Control animals were handled the same way but were given water instead. The findings are summarized in Fig. 4. Mice that had been fed OVA at ages 1, 3, 7, 14, and 42 days were immunized with ovalbumin and an adjuvant 28 days later. Animals fed at 14 and 42 days were tolerant (as expected); however, as shown in Fig. 4, animals fed OVA between age 1 and 7 days after birth did *not* develop oral tolerance, and mice fed on the day of birth repeatedly and consistently developed signs of priming, both for antibodies and cell-mediated immunity. This priming was always consistent in a series of experiments but did not reach significant levels within any individual experiment. Thus we argued that antigen administration, even earlier in life, may increase the priming effect.

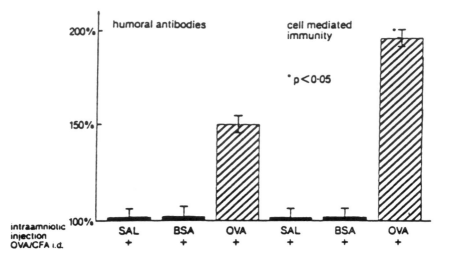

FIG. 5.   Effects of prenatal antigen (OVA) exposure. Percentage antigen-specific enhancement of systemic immune responses after intra-amniotic exposure. (From ref. 60.)

PRENATAL ANTIGEN EXPOSURE

Based on the above-mentioned results, we exposed individual fetuses to 1 mg of OVA by intra-amniotic injection. Controls were injected with either saline or, as an unrelated antigen, BSA (Fig. 5). After the mice were born and normally reared, they were systemically immunized at 28 days of age (following the normal experimental protocol). Significant priming, both for antibody and DTH responses, was obtained in mice fed OVA before birth. No effects on the fetus were seen after systemic antigen exposure of only the mother on the 19th day of gestation.

EFFECTS OF WEANING ON THE INDUCTION OF TOLERANCE TO OVA

Usually by the time the mice were 14 days of age, the magnitude of immunologic suppression was as complete as in adult animals. This pattern was shortly disturbed when the animals were fed during the weaning period. In an experimental design in which the separate effects of age and weaning could be examined, animals were fed OVA or saline on the day of weaning as well as 3 and 7 days before or after the weaning day. The results are summarized in Fig. 6. When mice were weaned at 28 days of age and given a feed of OVA on that day, they showed no subsequent oral tolerance for antibody responses and less than usual suppression of cell-mediated immune responses. However, when littermates were weaned 3 days after a feed of ovalbumin or were fed OVA 3 days after weaning, they had

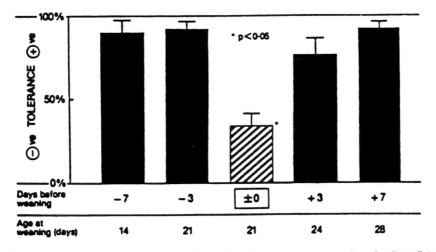

FIG. 6. Effects of weaning on tolerance induction. Percentage suppression of cell-mediated immune responses after an OVA-feed. Effects are not age-related but seem to be dependent on the weaning process. (From ref. 60.)

normal oral tolerance for both limbs of the immune system. Mice fed 7 days before or after the weaning day became tolerant in the normal way. It seems, therefore, that the transient reduction of oral tolerance was not age-related but was, instead, the result of the weaning process.

INDUCTION OF MUCOSAL CELL-MEDIATED IMMUNITY BY NEONATAL FEEDING

Administration of OVA to the gut of neonatal animals failed consistently to induce a mucosal cell-mediated immune response in the gut. However, feeding neonatal animals on day 1, followed by a challenge at 28 days of age, led to an increase in intraepithelial lymphocytes within the jejunal mucosa. This finding suggests induction of mucosal cell-mediated immune response (Fig. 7).

CONCLUSION

As briefly outlined, our knowledge about developmental aspects of food allergy is still scanty, and the conclusions drawn from published reports of animal and human studies are sometimes contradictory, if not confusing. It is, however, obvious that immune responses after oral antigen encountered in the neonate (or young infant) are different from adult immune responses, and they cannot be dissociated from developmental aspects. The final (immunologic) outcome after antigen pre-

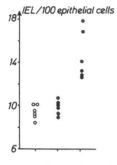

FIG. 7. Effects of a neonatal ovalbumin feed and an ovalbumin challenge in mice. Animals were fed either water or OVA on the first day of life and were challenged for 10 days with OVA or water when they were 4 weeks of age. Only animals fed *and* challenged with OVA exhibited a significantly increased intraepithelial lymphocyte count (IEL, $p<0.01$) compatible with a cell-mediated immune response in the gut.

sentation to the GALT is an equation with a variety of interrelating variables, some of which are listed below:

1. Genetic background (parental history of atopy).
2. Environmental factors (e.g., smoking, pollution).
3. Time of intestinal antigen exposure.
4. Immaturity of digestion (creation of tolerogens versus immunogens?).
5. Immaturity of gut-associated immune regulation (e.g., HLA-DR expression).
6. Effects of breast milk on the neonate's immune system.
7. Age-related differences in binding, uptake, and mucosal permeability of macromolecules.
8. Immunosuppressive effects of (virus) infections.

For didactic reasons, the events that finally lead to oral sensitization or oral tolerance can be divided into an *afferent* limb (antigen binding uptake, digestion, processing, and permeability) and an *efferent* limb (which comprises the subsequent immune response). The final immune response can also be modulated by circulating antibodies.

The transmission of antigen and antibody via breast milk is likely to affect both limbs. It remains to be proven whether the reduction of antigen transmission into breast milk, be it through circulating maternal antibodies or by antigen avoidance, has a protective effect on the human neonate at risk (21,24). Early clinical reports investigating the effect of antigen avoidance during pregnancy are, however, encouraging but need confirmation on a larger scale (20).

ACKNOWLEDGMENTS

I am grateful to Dr. Anne Ferguson, Western General Hospital, Edinburgh, for continuing support and critical discussions during the experimental work of this chapter. I am also grateful for the financial support provided by Action Research, by the MRC, and by the Deutsche Forshungsgemeinschaft (STR 210 1-2). I also thank Miss Faith Hanstater for expert preparation of the manuscript.

REFERENCES

1. Hayward AR. Development of lymphocyte responses and interactions in the human fetus and newborn. *Immunol Rev* 1981;57:39–60.
2. Andersson U, Bird AG, Britton S, Palacios R. Humoral and cellular immunity in humans studied at the cell level from birth to two years of age. *Immunol Rev* 1981;57:5–38.
3. Miyawaki T, Moriya N, Nagaoki T, Taniguchi N. Maturation of B-cell differentiation ability and T-cell regulatory function in infancy and childhood. *Immunol Rev* 1981;57:61–88.
4. Murgita A, Wigzell H. Regulation of immune functions in the fetus and newborn. *Prog Allergy* 1981;219:54–113.
5. Robertson DM, Paganelli R, Dinwiddie R, Levinsky RJ. Milk antigen absorption in the preterm and term neonate. *Arch Dis Child* 1982;57:369–72.
6. Beach RC, Menzies IS, Clayden GS, Scopes JW. Gastrointestinal permeability changes in the preterm neonate. *Arch Dis Child* 1982;57:141–5.
7. Turner MW, Boulton P, Shields JG, Strobel S, Gibson S, Miller HRP, et al. Uptake of ingested protein from the gut, changes in intestinal permeability to sugars and release of mast cell protease II in rats experiencing locally induced hypersensitivity reactions. 1986. In: Chandra K, ed. *Food allergy*, St. Johns, Newfoundland, Canada: Nutrition Research Education Foundation, 1987:79–93.
8. Walker WA, Isselbacher KJ. Uptake and transport of macromolecules by the intestine—possible role in clinical disorders. *Gastroenterology* 1974;67:531–50.
9. Müller G, Bernsau I, Müller W, Weisbarth-Riedel E, Natzschka J, Rieger CHL. Cow's milk protein antigens and antibodies in the serum of premature infants. *J Pediatr* 1986;109:869–73
10. Jacobsson I, Liudberg T, Lothe L, Axelsson I, Benediktsson B. Human alpha-lactalbumin as a marker of macromolecular absorption. *Gut* 1986;27:1029–34.
11. Ehrlich P. Über Immunität durch Vererbung und Säugung. *Z Hygiene Infektionskr* 1892;12:183–203.
12. Ogra SS, Ogra PL. Immunologic aspects of human colostrum and milk. I. Distribution characteristics and concentrations of immunoglobulins at different times after onset of lactation. *J Pediatr* 1978;92:546–9.
13. Ogra SS, Ogra PL. Immunologic aspects of human colostrum and milk. II. Characteristics of lymphocyte reactivity and distribution of E-rosette forming cells at different times after onset of lactation. *J Pediatr* 1978;92:550–4.
14. Hanson L, Ahlstedt S, Andersson B, et al. Protective factors in milk and the development of the immune system. *Pediatrics* 1985;75(Suppl):172–5.
15. Svanborg-Eden C, Carlsson B, Hanson L, et al. Anti-pili antibodies in breast milk. *Lancet* 1979;ii:1235.
16. Jacobsson I, Lindberg T. Cow's milk as a cause of infantile colic in breast-fed infants. *Lancet* 1978;ii:437–9.
17. Kilshaw PJ, Cant AJ. The passage of maternal dietary proteins into human breast milk. *Int Arch Allergy Appl Immunol* 1984;75:8–14.
18. Warner JO. Food allergy in fully breast-fed infants. *Clin Allergy* 1980;10:133–6.
19. Gerrard JW. Allergies in breast fed babies to foods ingested by mothers. *Clin Rev Allergy* 1984;2:143–9.
20. Chandra RK, Puri S, Suraiya C, Cheema PS. Influence of maternal food antigen avoidance during pregnancy and lactation on incidence of atopic eczema in infants. *Clin Allergy* 1986;16:563–9.
21. Björksten B. Does breast feeding prevent the development of allergy? *Immunol Today* 1983;4:215–7.
22. McLelland DBL, McGrath J, Sambon RR. Antimicrobial factors in human milk. *Acta Paediatr Scand (Suppl)* 1978;271:1–20.
23. Gillin FD, Reiner DS, Wang CS. Human milk kills parasitic intestinal protozoa. *Science* 1983;221:1290–1.

24. Savilhati E, Tainio V-M, Salmenpera L, et al. Prolonged exclusive breastfeeding and heredity as determinants in infantile atopy. *Arch Dis Child* 1987;62:269–73.
25. Stern M, Pang KY, Walker WA. Food proteins and gut mucosal barrier. II. Differential interaction of cow's milk proteins with the mucous coat and the surface membrane of adult and immature rat jejunum. *Pediatr Res* 1984;18:984–7.
26. Dannaeus A, Inganäs M. A follow-up study of children with food allergy. Clinical course in relation to serum IgE and IgG antibody levels to milk, egg and fish. *Clin Allergy* 1981;11:533–9.
27. Dannaeus A, Johannson SGO, Foucard T. Clinical and immunological aspects of food allergy. II. Development of allergic symptoms and humoral immune response to foods in infants of atopic mothers during the first 24 months of life. *Acta Paediatr Scand* 1978;67:715–8.
28. Harmatz PR, Bloch KJ, Kleinman RE, Walsh MK, Walker WA. Influence of circulating maternal antibody on the transfer of dietary antigen to neonatal mice via milk. *Immunology* 1986;57: 43–8.
29. Rieger CHL, Kraft SC, Rothberg RM. Lack of effect of passive immunization on the active immune response to an ingested soluble protein antigen. *J Immunol* 1980;124:1789–93.
30. Müller W, Lippmann A, Rieger CHL. Oral immunization to milk protein in human infants in the presence of passive antibody. *Pediatr Res* 1983;17:724–8.
31. Kobayashi RH, Hyman CJ, Stiehm ER. Immunologic maturation in an infant born to a mother with agammaglobulinaemia. *Am J Dis Child* 1980;13:942–5.
32. Rothberg RM, Farr RS. Anti bovine serum albumin and anti alpha lactalbumin in the sera of children and adults. *Pediatrics* 1965;35:371–6.
33. Rieger CHL, Rothberg RM. Development of the capacity to produce specific antibody to an ingested food antigen in the premature infant. *J Pediatr* 1975;87:515–8.
34. Rothberg RM, Rieger CHL, Silverman GA, Peri BA. Antigen uptake and antibody production in the human newborn. In: Ogra PL, Bienenstock J, eds. *The mucosal immune system in health and disease. First Ross Conference.* Columbus, Ohio: Ross Laboratories, 1981:57–62.
35. Jarrett EEE. Stimuli for the production and control of IgE in rats. *Immunol Rev* 1978;41:52–76.
36. Jarrett EEE, Hall E. Selective suppression of IgE antibody responsiveness by maternal influence. *Nature* 1979;280:145–7.
37. Jarrett EEE, Hall E. IgE suppression by maternal IgG. *Immunology* 1983;48:49–58.
38. Jarrett EEE. Perinatal influences on IgE responses. *Lancet* 1984;ii:797–9.
39. Tomasi TB. Oral tolerance. *Transplantation* 1980;29:353–6.
40. Strober W. The regulation of mucosal immune system. *J Allergy Clin Immunol* 1982;70:225–30.
41. Challacombe SJ, Tomasi TB. Systemic tolerance and secretory immunity after oral immunization. *J Exp Med* 1980;152:1459–65.
42. Strobel S, Mowat AMcI, Pickering MG, Ferguson A. Immunological responses to fed proteins in mice. 2. Oral tolerance for CMI is due to activation of cyclophosphamide sensitive cells by gut processed antigen. *Immunology* 1983;49:451–6.
43. Vaz N, Maia L, Hanson DG, Lynch J. Inhibition of homocytotropic antibody responses in adult inbred mice by previous feeding of the specific antigen. *J Allergy Clin Immunol* 1977;60:110–5.
44. Wannemuehler MJ, Kiyono H, Michalek SM, McGhee JR. Lipopolysaccharide (LPS) regulation of the immune response: LPS converts germ free mice to sensitivity to oral tolerance induction. *J Immunol* 1982;129:959–65.
45. Korenblatt PE, Rothberg RM, Minden P, Farr PS. Immune responses of human adults after oral and parenteral exposure to bovine serum albumin. *J Allergy* 1968;41:226–35.
46. Lowney ED. Immunologic unresponsiveness to a contact sensitiser in man. *J Invest Dermatol* 1968;51:411–7.
47. Lafont S, André C, Gillon J, Fargier MC. Abrogation by subsequent feeding of antibody response, including IgE in parenterally immunized mice. *J Exp Med* 1982;152:1573–8.
48. Strobel S. Modulation of the immune response to fed antigen in mice. Ph.D. thesis, University of Edinburgh, 1984.
49. Peng H-J, Strobel S. Unpublished observation, 1987.
50. Mowat AMcI, Strobel S, Drummond HE, et al. Immunological response to fed proteins in mice. I. Reversal of oral tolerance to ovalbumin by cyclophosphamide. *Immunology* 1982;45:105–13.
51. Strobel S, Ferguson A. Persistence of oral tolerance in mice fed ovalbumin is different for humoral and cell mediated immune responses. *Immunology* 1987;60:317–8.
52. Parrott DMV. The gut as a lymphoid organ. *Clin Gastroenterol* 1976;5:211–28.

Food Allergy, edited by Eberhardt Schmidt.
Nestlé Nutrition Workshop Series, Vol. 17.
Nestec Ltd., Vevey/Raven Press, Ltd.,
New York © 1988.

Epidemiology of Food Allergy

N.-I. Max Kjellman

Department of Pediatrics, Linköping University Hospital, 58185 Linköping, Sweden

Milk allergy, whose existence was known in ancient Greece, was the first of all food allergies to be described in modern literature by Hamburger in 1901 (for review, see ref. 1).

Despite many recent studies within the field of food allergy, there is still no agreement on its frequency (2). These differences in opinion are due to differences in (a) definitions and (b) the criteria for the diagnosis and its assessment. Some authors present data on prevalence, whereas others present data on accumulated incidence. Differences may also depend on (a) whether the material consists of infants/children at risk of allergy or unselected subjects, (b) their age at study, and (c) whether the study is prospective or cross-sectional. Habits and socioeconomic status of the study group may also be important.

The *ideal* study on food allergy still remains to be performed: It should be prospective, in an unselected population that is large enough to allow conclusions, documenting heredity and exposure as well as symptoms and signs, with blinded evaluation including objective data, especially provocation tests, performed under *double-blind* conditions, and with repeated assessments to find out the *true* prevalence at various ages. Such a study would, of course, be time-consuming but would still not be relevant for all parts of the world because of the great differences in feeding habits and exposure to adjuvant factors.

Because almost any food may elicit any symptom from almost any organ by various mechanisms, and many factors may influence the outcome, the history alone is not generally reliable. Double-blind provocation tests may also incur pitfalls and may not be the final "gold standard" for the evaluation of food allergy. There are crucial points such as the way of intake, state of the food, adjuvant factors, and time of exposure, all of which may give false-negative provocation tests. For the present review, *food reaction* is defined as any type of reaction occurring at least twice after ingestion of the same food, whereas the term *food allergy* is used only for food reactions based upon immunologic mechanisms. Only well-conducted, prospective studies are considered.

HOW COMMON IS FOOD ALLERGY?

Few studies allow estimation of the true incidence of food allergy. Kajosaari (3) found, in a total of 866 Finnish children aged 1 to 6 years—on the basis of history, elimination, and challenge at home with fish, egg, and citrus fruits—a total prevalence of *food reactions* of 19% at 1 year of age, peaking at 3 years at 27% and decreasing to 8% at 6 years of age. The most common causes of these reactions were citrus fruits, tomatoes, egg, strawberry, and fish. The majority of sensitive children only reacted to a single food, but 10% of them reacted to more than three foods. Food allergy was verified after elimination and provocation, albeit open, in about 50% of children in the younger age group but in *all* children 6 years of age with a history of food allergy. This higher incidence of a verified history in older children is in accordance with the experience of others (4); one of several explanations is that older children are more often exposed to foods by curiosity or mistake than are younger children, who often are overprotected by their family, giving a more relevant history with increasing age. Negative provocation tests at a certain age, even if performed properly, do not, of course, preclude the presence of a relevant allergy at a younger age.

The true prevalence of food allergy in adults is unknown. In the northern parts of Europe, where birch allergy is found in 10% to 15% of teenagers and young adults, the occurrence of allergy toward birch-associated allergens in nuts, apples, cherries, etc., alone accounts for a prevalence of about 5% (5).

DEVELOPMENTAL ASPECTS

The development of *immediate*-type food allergy (as opposed to late-onset allergy) is closely associated with the development of atopic disease later on (6). There is also a definite genetic influence on the development of food allergy (Table 1) (7).

Maternal IgG antibodies to foods, transferred via the placenta (8) or food-specific secretory IgA antibodies in the breast milk (9), may modify the immune

TABLE 1. *Cumulated history of repeated food reactions in the skin before 7 years of age in comparison with the family history of atopic disease (number of parents suffering from atopic disease)[a]*

Atopic parents	Number of children	Total (%)	Egg (%)	Fish (%)
2	48	58	15	13
1	58	29	14	5
0	38	13	5	0

[a]Data are from ref. 7.

response of the fetus and infant when exposed to foreign food directly or to foods hidden in the breast milk (10).

It is important to know that production of food-specific IgE antibodies at introduction of, for example, cow's milk and egg into the diet is a phenomenon also seen in nonatopic infants (11). These infants may show low concentrations of IgE antibodies during a limited period of time, whereas atopic subjects tend to have higher concentrations and seem to have difficulties in turning off the production of IgE antibodies.

It is also important to realize that even high concentrations of IgE antibodies *do not prove* current allergy but *do indicate* that the subject is atopic by constitution and may or may not have a manifest allergy toward the particular allergen.

The time of introduction of the food is important for the immunologic, as well as the clinical, responses: Lower IgG class antibody concentrations are produced when, for instance, cow's milk is introduced *after*, rather than before, 6 months of age (12,13). Fewer subjects with IgE antibodies to cow's milk were found following late (5%), rather than early (16%), introduction in allergy-risk infants (14). A lower incidence of cow's milk reactions before 1 year of age has been reported in children who started on cow's milk after 6 months of age as compared to children who were introduced to cow's milk at an earlier age (15). The findings are probably explained by maturation of gut barrier properties and of the immune system. In long-term follow-up studies, however, the prevalence of sensitization against, for example, fish was only slightly lower in children with late, as compared to those with early, introduction of these foods (16). The preventive effect regarding specific sensitization thus seems to be only temporary. Because sensitization also has an adjuvant effect with regard to further sensitization (17,18), it seems worthwhile to recommend preventive measures, such as late introduction of potent allergens into the diet, from an immunologic point of view (19) as well as for psychologic reasons. Late introduction of foreign food ("beikost") is also supported by other studies (20,24).

EFFECT OF MANIPULATION OF MATERNAL DIET (PRELIMINARY RESULTS)

Maternal abstention of cow's milk and egg during the last trimester of pregnancy (25) does not seem to reduce the risk for early sensitization against these two foods (cow's milk allergy was found in 2%, and egg allergy was found in 8%, according to provocations) nor does it seem to reduce the development of IgE or atopic disease up to 18 months of age. In this prospective, randomized, and blind evaluated study of 209 allergy-risk pregnancies the atopic score of the children, the total IgE concentration and the results of skin-prick tests and radioallergosorbent tests were almost identical in the study group and in the control group. Furthermore, no food-specific IgE antibodies were found in cord blood. Both groups had the same recommendations regarding maternal food intake, infant feeding, and home sanitation after delivery. However, the diet mothers continued, by their own choice, to keep to their diet slightly more often ($p<0.05$) during the first 3 months of lactation, indicating a lower postbirth risk for exposure to cow's milk and egg in the study group. This would have been expected to reduce the risk for sensitization and the development of atopic disease in this group. The negative findings in the 180 mother-child pairs, fulfilling all the requirements of the study protocol, might be due to the fact that low-dose exposure can be even more sensitizing than high-dose exposure, as demonstrated in animals. Jarrett and Hall (22), on the basis of their experiments in rats, suggested *high* maternal intake of allergens as a means of immunization, leading to induction of tolerance in the offspring.

Preliminary results from a presently ongoing Swedish study, where mothers with allergic respiratory disease were randomized at week 25 to *increased* or low intake of cow's milk and egg, show no significant difference between the groups in the prevalence of atopic disease at 18 months of age (26). Thus, there seems to be no reason to manipulate maternal food intake during pregnancy; it does, however, seem reasonable to recommend a nutritionally adequate intake of food, excluding only foods that cause symptoms in the mother.

Maternal abstention from eating potent allergens (egg, fish, cow's milk) during lactation seems worthwhile according to preliminary results of a presently ongoing study from our group (27). Symptoms tended to start later and were milder in babies of diet mothers than in babies of control-group mothers. A very recent study by Chandra et al. (23) also lends support to maternal diet during lactation. However, maternal intake of nutrients and calcium has to be monitored if the diet is restricted during lactation.

NATURAL HISTORY AND PROGNOSIS

It is well known that food allergy tends to resolve with time, but there are differences between foods: For example, allergy to fish, nuts, and peanuts is more likely to persist for a longer period of time than allergy to cow's milk and egg (4,24). The computed mean "survival" of food allergy in the study of Esteban et al. (24) was 71% after 3 years, 50% after 6 years, and 28% after 9 years. Similarly, after 3 years, 50% "survival" was found for cow's milk allergy; after 5 years, 50% of egg allergy was still present; and after 8 years' follow-up, 80% of fish allergy "survived." In this series, age at onset of symptoms and clinical features had little influence on the persistence of clinical sensitivity.

Food allergy in children with severe atopic dermatitis resolved, on an appropriate elimination diet, in 40% of the children already over the first year of antigen avoidance (28). The highest rate of disappearance of food allergy is found in children younger than 3 years of age (4). In children with positive double-blind provocation tests as the criterion for food allergy, followed for up to 7 years, tolerance developed in 44% of those younger than 3 years of age at the start of the study but developed in only 19% of children older than 3 years of age at the start of the study.

Milk allergy is recognized in about 2% of infants (29), but tolerance is achieved by 3 years of age in 60% of these children. Egg allergy has been reported in 4% of unselected infants (3) and was found in 8% of allergy-risk infants (25). Tolerance developed in about 70% of the unselected children by 6 years of age. Fish allergy was also found in about 4% of the unselected Finnish infants (3), but at 6 years of age less than 1% were still fish-intolerant.

HOPE FOR THE FUTURE

There is reason to hope that future or ongoing studies will give us a better understanding of the epidemiology of food allergy as well as more efficient methods for preventing its development. In particular, the importance of various adjuvant factors, such as the gut flora, needs to be evaluated. Better understanding of mechanisms involved will also allow more specific treatment and, hopefully, a more rapid induction of tolerance.

REFERENCES

1. Businco L, Benincori N, Cantani A. Epidemiology, incidence and clinical aspects of food allergy. *Ann Allergy* 1984;53:615–22.
2. Andersson J A, Sogn DD, eds. *Adverse reactions of foods*. AAAI and NIAID Report, NIH Publication No. 84-2442, 1984.
3. Kajosaari M. Food allergy in Finnish children aged 1 to 6 years *Acta Paediatr Scand* 1982;71:815–9.
4. Bock S A. The natural history of food sensitivity. *J Allergy Clin Immunol* 1982;69:173–7.
5. Ericsson NE. Allergy to pollen from different deciduous trees in Sweden. *Allergy* 1978;33:299–309.
6. Van Asperen PP, Kemp AS, Mellis CM. A prospective study of the clinical manifestations of atopic disease in infancy. *Acta Paediatr Scand* 1984;73:80–5.
7. Kjellman N-IM. Development and prediction of atopic allergy in childhood. In: Boström H, Ljungstedt N, eds. *Skandia International Symposia. Theoretical and clinical aspects of allergic diseases*. Stockholm: Almqvist & Wicksell, 1983;57–73.
8. Casimir G, Gossart B, Vis HL. Antibody against beta-lactoglobulin (IgG) and cow's milk allergy. *J Allergy Clin Immunol* 1985;75:206.
9. Machtinger S, Moss R. Cow's milk allergy in breast-fed infants: the role of allergen and maternal secretory IgA antibody. *J Allergy Clin Immunol* 1986;77:341–7.
10. Gerrard J, Perelmutter L. IgE-mediated allergy to peanut, cow's milk and egg in children with special reference to maternal diet. *Ann Allergy* 1986;56:351–4.
11. Hattevig G, Kjellman B, Johansson SGO, Björkstén B. Clinical symptoms and IgE responses to common food proteins in atopic and healthy children. *Clin Allergy* 1984;14:551–9.
12. Eastham EJ, Lichauco T, Grady MI, Walker WA. Antigenicity of infant formulas: role of immature intestine on protein permeability. *J Pediatr* 1978;93:561–4.
13. Kjellman N-IM, Johansson SGO. Soy versus cow's milk in infants with a biparental history of atopic disease: development of atopic disease and immunoglobulins from birth to 4 years of age. *Clin Allergy* 1979;9:347–58.
14. Hamburger RN. Diagnosis of food allergies and intolerances in the study of prophylaxis and control groups in infants. *Ann Allergy* 1984;53:673–7.

15. Halpern SR, Sellars WA, Johnsson RB, et al. Development of childhood allergy in infants fed breast, soy, or cow's milk. *J Allergy Clin Immunol* 1973;51:139–51.
16. Saarinen UM, Kajosaari M. Does dietary elimination in infancy prevent or only postpone a food allergy? *Lancet* 1980;i:166–7.
17. Robert SA, Soothill JF. Provocation of allergic response by supplementary feeds of cow's milk. *Arch Dis Child* 1982;57:127–30.
18. Reinhardt MC, Paganelli RP, Levinsky RJ. Intestinal antigen handling at mucosal surfaces in health and disease; human and experimental studies. *Ann Allergy* 1983;51:311–4.
19. Burr ML. Does infant feeding affect the risk of allergy? *Arch Dis Child* 1983;58:561–5.
20. Kajosaari M, Saarinen UM. Prophylaxis of atopic disease by six months total solid food elimination. *Acta Paediatr Scand* 1983;72:411–4.
21. Fergusson DM, Horwood LJ, Beautrais AL, Shannon FT, Taylor B. Eczema and infant diet. *Clin Allergy* 1981;11:325–31.
22. Jarrett EE, Hall E. The development of IgE-suppressive immunocompetence in young animals: influence of exposure to antigen in the presence or absence of maternal immunity. *Immunology* 1984;53:365–73.
23. Chandra RK, Puri S, Suraiya C, Cheema PS. Influence of maternal food antigen avoidance during pregnancy and lactation on incidence of atopic eczema in infants. *Clin Allergy* 1986;16:563–9.
24. Esteban MM, Pascual C, Madero R, Diaz Pena JM, Ojeda JA. Natural history of immediate food allergy in children. In: Businco L, Ruggieri F, eds. *Proceedings of the first Latin food allergy workshop, Rome, June 28–29 1985*. Rome: Fisons SpA, 1985:27–30.
25. Fälth-Magnusson X, Kjellman N-IM. *(to be published)*.
26. Lilja G, et al. *(to be published)*.
27. Hattevig G, et al. *(to be published)*.
28. Sampson HA. IgE in eczema [abstract]. In: *Third international symposium on immunological and clinical problems of food allergy, Taormina (Italy), October 1–4, 1986.*
29. Wood CBS. How common is food allergy? *Acta Paediatr Scand* 1986;323:76–83.

DISCUSSION

Dr. Lenard: I think it is clear that stress is an important adjuvant for the appearance of atopic disease, but it was new to me that perinatal stress is considered a possible adjuvant. Do you have any hard evidence that problems during birth affect the occurrence of allergic disease?

Dr. Kjellman: There are two studies showing that perinatal stress influences the development of allergic disease, mainly of the respiratory tract (1,2). Both showed an increased risk if the child had an abnormal delivery or if the mother had a perinatal illness such as toxemia. We have recently shown that beta-blocking agents given to the mother during late pregnancy enhance the development of atopic symptoms up to 1 year of age. Recent studies have also shown high IgE concentrations in neonates whose mothers smoked as compared to neonates of controls, and smoking seems to be a definite risk factor.

Dr. Frick: We have been interested in the effects of stress on immune mechanisms. Our studies involve an animal stress model, where we separate newborn rabbits from their mothers and compare them with control littermates. Separated pups have a marked reduction in concanavalin A and PHA stimulation index. A parallel series of experiments has shown that the separated animals have a very striking reduction in PHA response to low-dose somatostatin but have an increased response to high-dose somatostatin. Thus there is a prominent immunologic effect in these animals which we believe is related to stress.

Dr. Kjellman: I am convinced that we are going to find many connections between neuropeptides and allergic symptoms, so why not in the neonatal stage?

Dr. de Weck: You have alluded to the possibility that it may be sensible to try to reduce the load of allergens in breast milk, but don't you think that maybe this policy is doomed since it seems, experimentally at least, that the lower the dose of allergen, the greater the chance to sensitize an atopic child. Has anybody ever tried the reverse, i.e., to inundate the child with a very high dose of antigens from an early age? There are some Swiss data to support this idea, showing that rural children with heavy pollen contact (mainly farm children who helped with hay gathering) rarely develop hay fever, while children from the same area who had much less grass contact developed hay fever in a high percentage.

Dr. Kjellman: It is certainly possible that if lactating mothers eat antigen in only very small quantity, this may increase the risk for the infant. This is why we are confining our recommendations on allergen avoidance during lactation to small print! As to early high-dose allergen, this study has been done, unintentionally initially, in Sweden (3), where neonates were given early formula-feeding to try to reduce the incidence of jaundice. After a time it became apparent that these children had fewer allergic symptoms, so a randomized study was begun, and preliminary results seem to indicate that allergic symptoms develop in a lower proportion of the at-risk infants who had early exposure to cow's milk. The study has not yet been published.

Dr. Leroy: I am disturbed by the vagueness with which genetic factors in allergy are treated. All too often we pronounce the truism that all phenomena are somehow genetically determined, yet we make little attempt to identify the genetic factors. In none of the studies mentioned has anything been said about the father's genotype. I feel strongly that studies which are not controlled for the father's genotype related to atopy are seriously deficient as attempts to identify the genetic factors properly.

Dr. Kjellman: In all our studies we monitor the father's atopic status as well as the mother's, using IgE and skin-prick tests. There is very little difference in outcome with regard to whether the father or the mother is atopic with a particular symptom.

Dr. Revillard: I wish to comment on the question of *in utero* sensitization as a possible determinant of allergic disease. To my knowledge there is no strong evidence for the passage of protein antigens from the maternal to the fetal circulation. However, there is very good evidence that anti-idiotype IgG antibodies cross the placenta and represent the first contact between the fetal immune system and the mother's internal image of the environmental antigens. Therefore, before attempting to assess clinically the effect of antigen avoidance during pregnancy, which is extremely difficult to do, it would be better to obtain more information on the balance of anti-allergen and anti-idiotype antibodies during pregnancy, depending on the degree of exposure to any particular antigen. With this knowledge, and knowing the isotype of the anti-idiotype, one may have better grounds for speculating about the possible effect of the immune system on the fetus. Do you agree?

Dr. Kjellman: I fully agree that we must learn more about the effect of anti-idiotypes.

Dr. Rieger: I think Dr. Revillard has addressed a very important point. There are data from Lars Hanson's group, for example, suggesting that anti-idiotypic antibodies may play a role as antigens for early sensitization.

Dr. Aas: I have some comments on the question of *in utero* sensitization. Sensitization in the IgE system seems to be particularly dependent on low-dose stimulation, and I think it is most important not to overlook inhaled allergens in this respect. In any sample of house dust it is possible to demonstrate all the food antigens we have discussed in this meeting. Thus most people inhale low-dose food antigens continuously from birth, acting on a very sensitive and sensitizable system. *In utero* sensitization cannot be deduced, as many have done, from the occurrence of a fierce reaction at the time of the apparent first introduction of a food in infancy. It can only be demonstrated by immunologic methods *in utero* or in correctly taken cord blood samples. You mentioned that contamination accounted for some of the cases where you found IgE antibodies in cord serum. This is an important point in studies using cord serum. However, in a large prospective study which we are carrying out at the moment, we have found two instances of IgE-positive cord blood, one to egg and the other to cow's milk, where we do not believe there was any contamination with mother's blood. This suggests to us, without proving anything, that there may be occasional instances of intrauterine sensitization, such that the fetus produces IgE antibodies in late gestation.

Dr. Kjellman: May I just comment that in the literature there are less than 10 studies showing intrauterine sensitization and that in our latest study on cord blood IgE concentrations, using three methods of control, we found up to 10% contaminated.

Dr. von Giser: How do you collect cord blood? And how do you assess contamination?

Dr. Kjellman: Because we collect cord blood routinely, we do not do it by venipuncture. We simply wipe the cord thoroughly, cut it, and allow the blood to flow freely into a container. We control for contamination by simultaneously checking maternal serum for IgE antibodies to see, in the next step, whether the mother's major IgE antibodies are also present in cord blood. We also measure IgA concentrations and we look at IgE again on day 5 to 7, if necessary.

Dr. U. Wahn: It is clear from the results of screening procedures that there are two populations of at-risk infants: those with a two-parent family history and those with high cord blood IgE. However, there appears to be very little overlap between these two groups. Will you please comment on this?

Dr. Kjellman: We do see a definite overlap between these two populations, but unfortunately there are high IgE producers among those infants with no family history of atopic disease who have the same high risk of developing atopic disease later on. For screening purposes I think at present that it is best to obtain both IgE measurements and the family history.

Dr. Rieger: One final point: You said or implied that it is a totally different thing looking for specific igE in a 9-month-old infant as compared with a 3-year-old child, since many infants of 9 months have specific IgE which is later turned off. Did I understand you correctly?

Dr. Kjellman: IgE antibodies in very low concentration, usually below RAST class 1, are produced by 70% of normal subjects for a short period, which peaks at about 8 months of age.

DISCUSSION REFERENCES

1. Salk L, Grellong BA: Perinatal complications in the history of asthmatic children. *Am J Dis Child* 1974;127:30–3.
2. Johnstone DE, Roghmann KJ, Pless IB. Factors associated with the development of asthma and hay fever in children: the possible risk of hospitalization, surgery and anaesthesia. *Pediatrics* 1975;56:398–403.
3. Lindfors A, Enocksson E. Development of allergic symptoms after early neonatal exposition to cow's milk based formula. An 18 month prospective study. Abstract 54, Annual Meeting of the European Academy of Allergology and Clinical Immunology, Stockholm, June 2–5, 1985.

Food Allergy, edited by Eberhardt Schmidt.
Nestlé Nutrition Workshop Series, Vol. 17.
Nestec Ltd., Vevey/Raven Press, Ltd.,
New York © 1988.

The Symptomatology of Food Allergy

Andrew J. Cant

Department of Paediatrics, Guy's Hospital Medical School, London SE1 9RT, England

Although the fundamental immunology underlying allergic diseases is now being elucidated, there are still few useful diagnostic tests. Thus the recognition and treatment of these disorders continues to be based mainly on clinical skills and, in particular, on the taking of a careful history. This means that observer bias can be a significant factor, and so whether or not the diagnosis is made may depend on a clinician's preconceptions. Furthermore, the large public interest in the subject, often highlighted by extravagant and poorly substantiated claims, has tended to polarize medical opinion between "believers" and "nonbelievers." Some pediatricians report that they often see infants with food allergy, whereas others state categorically that food allergy does not exist. It is crucial that an open-minded, yet critical, approach is adopted and that we listen carefully to what our patients and their parents tell us. After all, this is what most of us were supposedly taught to do as medical students.

GASTROINTESTINAL MANIFESTATIONS

Infantile Colic

The term *colic* means different things to different people. It has perhaps best been described as "intermittent abdominal pain assumed to be due to peristalsis" (1). In infancy it is associated with episodes of crying and restlessness, with drawing up of the legs, and it often occurs in the evening. It is a common problem and may affect up to one in eight babies (2). Several studies have suggested that cow's milk protein causes colic in some babies (3,4). It also appears that up to one-third of breast-fed babies with colic improve if their mothers avoid cow's milk (5), although other workers have found maternal cow's milk exclusion to be of no benefit (6). There is evidence that soya milk may also provoke colic (4).

There is no direct evidence that colic is mediated by an immune reaction, but it has been observed that many children subsequently shown to have cow's milk-sensitive enteropathy initially suffered from colic (7).

Cow's-Milk-Protein Enteropathy (CMPE)

This is largely a disease of infancy and is uncommon after the age of 3 years. Estimates of prevalence vary between 0.3% and 7%; this topic has been well reviewed by Bahna and Heiner (8), who suggest that the true prevalence may be between 1% and 3%. It occurs much more commonly in babies born into atopic families, and affected children often have other signs of allergic disease such as eczema, urticaria, or wheezing. It may be more common in children exposed to cow's milk in the neonatal period (9).

Affected infants sometimes present with an acute episode of vomiting and diarrhea that is indistinguishable from acute gastroenteritis, and such infection may precipitate the enteropathy (10). However, signs and symptoms persist and are shown to be cow's-milk-dependent. In other patients the onset of vomiting and diarrhea is more insidious, and failure to thrive is a more marked feature of the disease. The small bowel is mainly affected and an intestinal biopsy is usually abnormal, although the changes are more patchy and less severe than those seen in celiac disease (11,12).

The diagnosis is made by observing the response to the withdrawal of cow's milk and subsequent rechallenge, although this is rarely performed three times as was suggested by Goldman et al. (13).

There is usually a dramatic improvement on a cow's-milk-free diet, and a soya formula is often given as a substitute. However, soya milk is as antigenic as cow's milk (14), and probably about 24% of children with CMPE will develop soya-sensitive enteropathy (15). Not only soya, but also chicken, rice, fish, and egg, can provoke a similar condition (16).

Fortunately, CMPE almost always remits spontaneously, and the child will tolerate the food when given at a later date. It is usual to rechallenge every 6 months or so, but this needs to be done under medical supervision because anaphylaxis can occur (1).

Food Allergic Colitis

This rare condition is characterized by diarrhea mixed with blood and slime and, like CMPE, occurs almost exclusively in infancy. Unlike CMPE the large bowel is mainly involved. Colonoscopy reveals an inflamed, friable mucosa; biopsy shows a lamina propria infiltrated with eosinophils. In one series of cases, all were shown to remit when specific foods were excluded from the diet (17). In another series, however, only four of the 11 cases described proved to be food-related (18). Although uncommon, the florid nature of this disease, as well as the dramatic response to allergen avoidance, makes correct diagnosis and treatment important.

This condition may be triggered by very small amounts of antigen, as shown by the observation that the minute amounts of cow's milk protein that pass into breast milk can precipitate signs and symptoms in solely breast-fed infants (19,20).

Other Gastrointestinal Manifestations

Allergic reactions do not always fit neatly into clinical syndromes. Some infants with CMPE will be "colicky" and have a tendency to vomit without failing to thrive or without suffering from diarrhea. Only the trial of an alternative infant formula will reveal the diagnosis, and this may not be tried if the clinician is not disposed to considering the diagnosis. In others, cow's milk may cause an iron-deficiency anemia due to chronic low-grade blood loss (21), whereas in yet others it can provoke hypoproteinemia with edema and eosinophilia (22,23).

Sometimes a child will simply fail to thrive without there being any other gastrointestinal symptoms. In this situation a cow's-milk-free diet may be tried as a last resort after many negative investigations.

CUTANEOUS MANIFESTATIONS

Urticaria, Angioedema, and Anaphylaxis

These three conditions are all examples of immediate hypersensitivity and are IgE-mediated. Urticaria is characterized by wheals ("hives" or "nettle-rash"), which appear quite suddenly and usually disappear in a few hours. Such reactions are common in young children and often occur after direct contact with foods, particularly egg, cow's milk, and peanuts, although inhalant allergens such as dog, cat, and horse hair can also provoke urticaria. It is often forgotten that food additives such as azo dyes and benzoate preservatives are responsible for many cases of so-called "cryptogenic urticaria" (24). Urticarial reactions are especially common during weaning (25), and affected children are usually tolerant to the offending food by the second or third year of life, although sometimes serious hypersensitivity persists into adolescence and adult life. The condition is usually more alarming than serious, but the development of angioedema (subcutaneous swelling caused by an IgE-mediated reaction) can be much more dangerous, since involvement of the larynx and pharynx may lead to life-threatening upper-airways obstruction. More serious still, but fortunately much less common, is food-induced anaphylaxis (26). This, too, is mediated by IgE-triggered mast-cell degranulation, but the reaction is systemic and not purely local in nature. Anaphylactic reactions begin with sneezing and itching, followed by generalized urticaria, profound bronchospasm, and circulatory collapse. The time course is variable, but reactions occurring within minutes of ingesting the food allergen are potentially fatal. Fortunately, anaphylaxis responds very quickly to the administration of subcutaneous adrenalin and an intravenous injection of an antihistamine, although treatment may come too late. Patients known to develop anaphylaxis to foods should be given an oral antihistamine preparation to take immediately after inadvertent ingestion of the offending food, and some doctors give these patients an ampule of adrenalin to administer in emergency.

Eczema

This distressing condition usually starts in the first year of life. Itchy lesions appear on the face and then spread to the rest of the body. Involvement of the flexures is typical. The skin becomes thickened and rough and may exude serous fluid and blood. Itch is the hallmark of eczema, and the consequent scratching may account for much of the skin damage. It is probably becoming more common, with estimates that as many as 12% of preschool children in the United Kingdom suffer from it (27).

It is over 50 years since it was reported that dietary exclusion was a successful treatment for childhood eczema (28,29). More recently, Meara (30) reported improvement in 11 of 29 eczematous infants who had egg excluded from their diet, although only two deteriorated when egg was reintroduced. Freedman (31) studied 48 children with eczema, and he found that the parents of 12 of these children said that cow's milk aggravated their disease. However, cow's milk challenge, supervised by the author, did not appear to provoke eczema in any of the children studied. By contrast, Goldman et al. (13) studied 37 eczematous children said to be cow's-milk-sensitive; in 31 of these children there was convincing exacerbation following each of three separate challenges. Hammar (32) studied 81 unselected children with atopic eczema, all under 5 years of age. Cow's milk was thought to provoke eczema in seven cases, and the author confirmed this in six of the seven cases. Of the 73 children not thought to be sensitive to cow's milk, eight were considered to relapse when challenged with cow's milk. It is hard to draw conclusions from these studies because challenges were not given in a double-blind fashion, diagnostic criteria were very variable, and usually only single foods were studied.

Only in the last 10 years have double-blind studies been carried out. Atherton et al. (33) studied 20 eczematous children between the ages of 2 and 8 years. Each child was put on a diet that excluded cow's milk and egg for 12 weeks. For 4 weeks a milk substitute was taken daily, and after a "washout" period of an additional 4 weeks a second milk substitute was taken for the final 4-week period. One substitute contained egg and cow's milk, and the other contained soya milk. The substitutes were given double-blind, and the order in which they were taken was randomized. Overall the children's skin showed a highly significant improvement when they took the soya milk as opposed to the egg and cow's milk, and it was concluded that at least half the children enjoyed a worthwhile benefit from cow's milk and egg avoidance. Two other interesting findings emerged from this study: The first was that few of the parents whose children responded had previously thought that egg or cow's milk provoked their child's eczema, and the second was that there was no association between (a) a positive skin-prick test or IgE antibody test to egg or cow's milk and (b) benefit from cow's milk and egg avoidance. These two observations highlight food-allergic eczema as an example of a late, non-IgE-mediated reaction.

It is possible that some children's eczema was provoked by foods other than egg or cow's milk; thus further work has been carried out using an oligoantigenic diet consisting of only one meat, one carbohydrate, one vegetable, and one fruit, together with an oil or margarine and supplements to provide other essential nutrients. Nineteen children were placed on such a diet for 2 to 3 weeks, and 14 responded to whatever oligoantigenic diet they were given. Foods were reintroduced one at a time, and any that appeared to provoke eczema were noted. These foods were then given in a double-blind manner to nine children; in eight, challenge with an offending food provoked eczema, whereas in only one case did the challenge with the placebo provoke ecema (34).

Although Atherton's studies were performed in a painstaking and elegant manner, and the results were very striking, it must be remembered that the children he studied all attended a clinic at a tertiary referral center. Thus they may represent a very selected group. Although some children with eczema undoubtedly respond to dietary manipulations, it is not clear what proportion of the children seen at the District General Hospital would benefit from such treatment. Similar studies in this setting should answer this question.

RESPIRATORY MANIFESTATIONS

The association between food allergy and respiratory disease seems less well established, although nasal stuffiness, sneezing, and nasal discharge have been seen in children with cow's milk allergy (15). Lower-respiratory-tract diseases in infancy are poorly defined. There is little consensus concerning the use of terms such as bronchitis, wheezy bronchitis, and asthma. Inevitably the relationship between these disorders and food allergy is not clear. Nevertheless, in one series of 150 cow's-milk-sensitive children, 79 presented with "bronchitis" (i.e., cough and dyspnea) (35); in a further series, 10 of 59 did so (15). Wheezing has been noted in varying proportions of cow's-milk-sensitive children (15,16). Serious respiratory disease is probably less common, although Heiner and Sears (37) described a small group of affected children (mainly infants in whom cow's milk provoked a chronic cough accompanied by wheezing, vomiting, and failure to thrive). Their chest X-rays showed patchy consolidation, and they also had an iron-deficiency anemia and eosinophilia. Some developed hemoptysis and hemosiderosis (38).

So far, cow's milk has been the main offending allergen. This may be because cow's milk proteins are particularly allergenic or because they are usually the first "foreign" food protein encountered by the young infant's relatively immature mucosal immune system. Other food proteins, however, provoke allergic reactions in infancy and are probably more important than is generally recognized. Some authors consider soya formulas hypoallergenic, but they induce an antibody response similar to that induced by cow's milk (39). Not surprisingly, up to one-third of children with cow's milk allergy also react to soya milk (4,15). Even casein hydrolysate formulas may sometimes set off allergic reactions, possibly because of contamination with fragments of whey proteins (40). The relationship between weaning and allergy has rarely been studied, despite reports from many mothers that their child's allergic disease first developed at this time. Van Asperen et al. have confirmed this impression in a prospective study (41). Finally it should be remembered that breast-fed infants can react to food proteins ingested by their mothers (20,42).

FACTITIOUS FOOD ALLERGY

Food allergy has become one of the great preoccupations of our time, so it is not surprising that parents should sometimes present children with histories of food allergy, when in fact they are perfectly healthy. Warner and Hathaway (43) have reported 17 such cases and described them as suffering from "an allergic form of Meadow's syndrome (Münchhausen by proxy)" after Meadow's account (44) of factitious childhood illnesses that were elaborately fabricated by their mothers. Thirteen of Warner and Hathaway's cases were described in detail. All were put on a diet excluding at least four foods by their parents. None was shown to have diet-dependent disease; yet none of the mothers would accept this finding, and the children continued on their exclusion diets. The children all came from a poor social background and often came from disrupted families where there was an abnormal attachment between parent and child. Another feature of these cases was that the children had been seen by many different consultants and practitioners of alternative medicine. David (45) has described 15 similar cases and has given a lively account of the different "quack" remedies they had received.

Large numbers of patients were studied by Warner and Hathaway and by David, and those with factitious food allergy made up only a small proportion: 17 of 301 in Warner and Hathaway's series and 15 of 250 in David's series. Nevertheless the nutritional, psychological, and social problems experienced by these children are considerable, and the parental obsession is very difficult to eradicate. It is therefore important, if possible, to recognize this condition at an early stage, before abnormal behavior patterns are too rigidly set. It is probably also true that real food allergy and factitious food allergy are not mutually exclusive conditions. A child may have a genuine food allergy, which he outgrows, but his parents then persist in the belief that this is still present. Careful explanations and a good rapport with parents and child offer the best means of successfully normalizing the child's diet.

CONCLUSIONS

Food allergy in infancy has protean manifestations and is provoked by many different food proteins. The lack of really useful diagnostic tests, along with the difficulty of conducting double-blind challenges in general pediatric practice (46), means that the diagnosis is mainly a clinical one. This demands an open-minded, yet critical, approach in taking a careful history and observing the response to dietary challenge.

REFERENCES

1. Hutchins PJ, Walker-Smith JA. The gastrointestinal system. *Clin Immunol Allergy* 1982;2:43–76.
2. Hide DW, Guyer BM. Prevalence of infant colic. *Arch Dis Child* 1982;57:559–60.
3. Meuller HL, Weiss RJ, O'Leary D, Murray AB. The incidence of milk sensitivity and the development of allergy in infants. *N Engl J Med* 1963;268:1220–4.
4. Jakobsson I, Lindberg T. Prospective study of cow's milk protein intolerance in Swedish infants. *Acta Paediatr Scand* 1979;68:853–9.
5. Jakobsson I, Lindberg T. Cow's milk proteins cause infantile colic in breast-fed infants. *Pediatrics* 1983;1:268–71.
6. Evans RW, Fergusson DM, Allardyce RA, Taylor B. Maternal diet and infantile colic in breast-fed infants. *Lancet* 1983;i:1340–2.
7. Minford AMB, Macdonald A, Littlewood JM. Food intolerance and food allergy in children: a review of 68 cases. *Arch Dis Child* 1982;57:742–7.
8. Bahna SL, Heiner DC. *Allergies to milk.* New York: Grune & Stratton, 1980.
9. Stintzing G, Zetterstrom R. Cow's milk allergy: incidence and pathogenetic role of early exposure to cow's milk formula. *Acta Paediatr Scand* 1979;68:383–7.
10. Harrison M, Kilby A, Walker-Smith JA, France NE, Wood CBS. Cow's milk protein intolerance; a possible association with gastroenteritis, lactose intolerance and IgA deficiency. *Br Med J* 1976;1:1501–4.
11. Manuel PD, Walker-Smith JA, France NE. Patch enteropathy. *Gut* 1979;20:211–5.
12. Phillip AD, Rice SJ, France NE, Walker-Smith JA. Small intestinal lymphocyte levels in cow's milk protein intolerance. *Gut* 1979;20:509–12.
13. Goldman AS, Anderson DW, Sellars WA, Saperstein S, Knicker WT, Halpern SR. Milk allergy 1. Oral challenge with milk and isolated milk proteins in allergic children. *Pediatrics* 1963;32:425–43.
14. Eastham EJ, Lichauco T, Grady MI, Walker WA. Antigenicity of infant formulas: role of immature intestine on protein permeability. *J Pediatr* 1978;93:561–4.
15. Gerrard JW, MacKenzie JWA, Goluboff N, Garson JZ, Maningas CS. Cow's milk allergy: prevalence and manifestations in an unselected series of newborns. *Acta Paediatr Scand (Suppl)* 1973;234:1–21.
16. Vitoria JC, Camarero C, Sojo A, Ruiz A, Rodriguez-Soriano J. Enteropathy related to fish, rice and chicken. *Arch Dis Child* 1982;57:44–8.
17. Jenkins HR, Harries JT, Milla PJ, Pincott JR, Soothill JF. Food allergic colitis in childhood. *Arch Dis Child* 1984;59:326–9.
18. Chong SKF, Sanderson IR, Wright V, Walker-Smith JA. Food allergy and infantile colitis. *Arch Dis Child* 1984;59:690–1.
19. Lake AM, Whitington PF, Hamilton SR. Dietary induced colitis in breast-fed infants. *J Pediatr* 1982;101:906–10.
20. Cant AJ, Bailes JA, Marsden RA. Cow's milk, soya milk and goat's milk in a mother's diet causing eczema and diarrhoea in her breast fed infant. *Acta Pediatr Scand* 1985;74:467–8.
21. Wilson JF, Heiner DC, Lahey ME. Milk induced gastrointestinal bleeding in infants with hypochromic microcytic anemia. *JAMA* 1964;189:122–6.
22. Waldman TA, Wochner RD, Laster L, et al. Allergic gastroenteropathy: a cause of excessive gastrointestinal protein loss. *N Engl J Med* 1967;276:761–9.
23. Lebenthal E, Laor J, Lewitus Z, et al. Gastrointestinal protein loss in allergy to cow's milk lactoglobulin. *Isr J Med Sci* 1970;6:506–10.
24. Juhlin L. Recurrent urticaria: clinical investigation of 330 patients. *Br J Dermatol* 1981;104:369–81.
25. Van Asperen PP, Kemp AS, Mellis CM. Immediate food hypersensitivity reactions on first known exposure to food. *Arch Dis Child* 1983;58:253–6.

26. David TJ. Anaphylactic shock during elimination diets for severe atopic eczema. *Arch Dis Child* 1984;59:983–6.
27. Taylor B, Wadsworth M, Wadsworth J, Peckham C. Changes in the reported prevalence of childhood eczema since the 1939–45 war. *Lancet* 1984;ii:1255–7.
28. Talbot FB. Eczema in childhood. *Med Clin North Am* 1918;1:985–96.
29. O'Keefe ES. A dietary consideration of eczema in younger children. *JAMA* 1922;78:483–4.
30. Meara RH. Skin reactions in atopic eczema. *Br J Dermatol* 1955;67:60–4.
31. Freedman SS. Milk allergy in infantile eczema. *Am J Dis Child* 1961;102:106–11.
32. Hammar H. Provocation with cow's milk and cereals in atopic dermatitis. *Acta Dermatol Venereol* 1977;47:159–63.
33. Atherton DJ, Sewell M, Soothill JF, Wells RS, Chilvers CED. A double-blind controlled crossover trial of an antigen avoidance diet in atopic eczema. *Lancet* 1978;i:401–3.
34. Atherton DJ. Skin disorders and food allergy. *J R Soc Med* 1985;78(Suppl 5):7–10.
35. Gerrard JW, Lubos MC, Hardy LW, et al. Milk allergy: clinical picture and familial incidence. *Can Med Assoc J* 1967;97:780–5.
36. Buisseret PD. Common manifestations of cow's milk allergy in children. *Lancet* 1978;1:304–5.
37. Heiner DC, Sears JW. Chronic respiratory disease associated with multiple circulating precipitins to cow's milk. *Am J Dis Child* 1960;100:500–2.
38. Heiner DC. Pulmonary hemosiderosis. In: Gellis S, Kagan B, eds. *Current pediatric therapy*, 5th ed. Philadelphia: Saunders, 1971:139–41.
39. Eastham EJ, Lichauco T, Grady MI, Walker WA. Antigenicity of infant formulas: role of immature intestine on protein permeability. *J Pediatr* 1978;93:561–4.
40. Seban A, Konijn A, Freier S. Chemical and immunological properties of a protein hydrolysate formula. *Am J Clin Nutr* 1977;30:840–6.
41. Van Asperen PP, Kemp AS, Mellis CM. Immediate food hypersensitivity reactions on first known exposure to food. *Arch Dis Child* 1983;58:253–6.
42. Gerrard JW. Allergy in breast-fed babies to ingredients in breast milk. *Ann Allergy* 1979;42:69–72.
43. Warner JO, Hathaway MU. Allergic form of Meadow's syndrome (Münchhausen by proxy). *Arch Dis Child* 1984;59:151–6.
44. Meadow R. Münchhausen syndrome by proxy. *Arch Dis Child* 1982;57:92–8.
45. David TJ. The overworked or fraudulent diagnosis of food allergy and food intolerance in children. *J R Soc Med* 1985;78(Suppl 5):21–31.
46. Rossiter MA. Food intolerance—a general paediatrician's view. *J R Soc Med* 1985;78(Suppl 5):17–20.

DISCUSSION

Dr. Freier: I should first like to comment about Heiner's syndrome (1). I never understood why Heiner saw so many cases of his syndrome, with patchy infiltration of the lungs, hemoptysis, and so on, when I never saw a single case! However, from a subsequent article written by his group, of which he was a co-author, it appears that the symptoms which he originally attributed to respiratory food allergy are now thought to be the result of recurrent milk aspiration (2). I should also like to mention a condition which I call pseudo-obstruction due to cow's milk allergy. I have not seen this described in the literature, but I believe I have seen two cases, both of which presented with the classic symptoms of intestinal obstruction, with distension, vomiting, constipation, and fluid levels on X-ray. Both cases had features suggestive of cow's milk allergy and resolved with conservative management. One of them, who had been discharged on a soy bean formula, returned in anaphylactic shock when he was inadvertently put back on a cow's-milk-based formula. This child turned out to be allergic to beta-lactoglobulin. Finally, in relation to colitis and food allergy, I recall some work which suggests that children with enterocolitis form a special group who develop a proliferative response if their lymphocytes are stimulated with beta-lactoglobulin *in vitro*.

Dr. Cant: I believe that pseudo-obstruction is mentioned in an article by Professor Walker-Smith (3), though not, I think, in Heiner's book.

Dr. Rieger: I should like to add some information about Heiner's syndrome. We recently showed that recurrent milk aspiration in infants results in extremely high levels of antimilk antibodies, so this combination might explain the syndrome.

Dr. Frick: About 15 years ago there was great interest in milk precipitins. During the course of examining 1,000 patients with suspected food sensitivity for the presence of precipitins we only found one case, and this turned out to be a child with tracheoesophageal fistula. Within a couple of weeks we turned up another patient with positive milk precipitins, so we suggested a search for a tracheoesophageal fistula in this child as well, and they found it! In the last few weeks, after an interval of nearly 15 years, I saw a child with a history of incessant asthma which just did not seem like ordinary recurrent asthma. We looked for milk precipitins on the off chance, and found they were positive. This child also had a tracheoesophageal fistula. I should like to add to Dr. Cant's story of peanut allergy and aspirin. We have four patients with peanut allergy who only develop severe symptoms when they consume peanuts and alcohol at the same time.

Dr. Challacombe: I want to make a point about mood and behavior changes. I have, for many years, been studying the behavioral changes that occur in children with celiac disease when gluten is removed from the diet. An improvement in their mood occurs; and a similar change can also occur in some patients with a cow's-milk-protein enteropathy, when they are treated with a cow's-milk-protein-free diet. Whether or not the psychological changes in both are mediated through abnormalities of serotonin metabolism I do not know, but such abnormalities have been reported in celiac disease.

Dr. Kahn: In my clinical experience, I can confirm that changes in mood and even more so in behavior can be seen on modifying the diet in food allergy. Stress reactions to food allergy have been reported sporadically since the early part of the century but have usually been disregarded because of the lack of clinical observations based on objective data, which are of course difficult to obtain.

Dr. Cant: There is a tendency to see the immune system in isolation, which we must resist. There is sure to be more interplay between the immune system and the neuroendocrine system than we presently allow for.

Dr. Nusslé: I want to stress the changing symptoms of cow's-milk-protein intolerance with time in the same individual. Symptoms are often not reproducible, and the symptoms which are found at presentation may be quite different on subsequent provocation.

Dr. Cant: I quite agree. Without challenge tests we are facing a "moving target," and the symptoms a child has one month are absent or different the next. This is especially true in infancy.

DISCUSSION REFERENCES

1. Heiner D, Sears J, Knicker W. Multiple precipitating to cow's milk in chronic respiratory disease. *Am J Dis Child* 1962;103:634–54.
2. Lee S, Knicker W, Cook C, Heiner D. Cow's milk induced pulmonary disease in children. In: Barness L, ed., *Advances in pediatrics*. Chicago: Year Book Publishers, 1978:39–57.
3. Walker-Smith JA.

Food Allergy, edited by Eberhardt Schmidt.
Nestlé Nutrition Workshop Series, Vol. 17.
Nestec Ltd., Vevey/Raven Press, Ltd.,
New York © 1988.

Food Allergy and the Gut

J.K. Visakorpi

Department of Clinical Sciences, University of Tampere, 33101 Tampere 10, Finland

CLINICAL SYNDROMES

The clinical syndromes described in connection with cow's milk allergy and, more generally, food allergy are numerous. Symptoms coming from the gastrointestinal tract seem to be the most common (Table 1), which is quite understandable because the gastrointestinal tract is the first target of the food antigens.

Acute food-allergy-induced vomiting and diarrhea (without chronicity), as well as skin reactions, asthma, and rhinitis, usually seem to be mediated by an immediate reaginic-type allergic reaction.

Another type of syndrome is food (cow's milk)-induced enteropathy, which occurs with prolonged diarrhea and often with failure to thrive. The food sensitivity in these cases is of delayed onset. There is, however, a certain overlap in the sensitivity because about one-quarter to one-third of patients with this kind of delayed-onset enteropathy also show acute reactivity with reaginic activity and classic atopic symptoms in addition to the enteropathy.

The clinical picture of chronic enteropathy caused by cow's milk (Table 2) is usually a typical malabsorption syndrome where the gastrointestinal symptoms are combined with failure to thrive. The increased prevalence of atopic symptoms and Down's syndrome is noteworthy. The small-intestinal mucosal damage is, however, the most important finding in making the diagnosis.

In addition to this, food allergy (especially cow's milk allergy) has been connected with another chronic intestinal syndrome, namely, colitis (4,5). It is also known that patients with enteritis and small-intestinal damage often also have gastric mucosal lesions (6). Thus it seems that the gastrointestinal mucosa reacts more generally in food allergies than, for example, in celiac disease. It is not known, however, whether this reaction is always general or whether there are different target organs in different cases.

Two rare syndromes also have to be mentioned when we are speaking about food allergy and gastrointestinal diseases. These are eosinophilic gastroenteropathy and occult gastrointestinal blood and protein loss. The role of allergy in the pathogenesis of these syndromes has not, however, been very well documented.

137

TABLE 1. *Clinical symptoms of food allergies according to two clinical studies*

Symptoms	Percent of all reactions, Gerrard et al. (1)	Percent of all reactions, Jakobsson and Lindberg (2)
Gastrointestinal symptoms (vomiting, colic, diarrhea, failure to thrive)	44%	56%
Skin symptoms (eczema, urticaria)	24%	40%
Recurrent respiratory symptoms (rhinitis, bronchitis)	32%	4%

TABLE 2. *Symptoms in 54 patients with cow's-milk-induced enteropathy[a]*

Diarrhea	100%
Vomiting	67%
Severe dehydration	26%
Mean weight on admission	−3.3 SD
Eczema	22%
Recurrent respiratory infection	24%
Down's syndrome	7%

[a]Data are from ref. 3.

INTESTINAL MUCOSAL DAMAGE

Small-intestinal mucosal damage is, by definition, an essential finding in enteropathies caused by food. It has been clearly shown that this lesion of intestinal mucosa is really caused by cow's milk proteins (7).

There has been discussion from the practical, as well as the theoretical, point of view as to whether this damage is similar to that found in celiac disease and thus whether the final diagnosis can be made on the basis of the findings in the first biopsy.

The small-bowel mucosal damage in cow's-milk-induced enteropathy is very variable in severity, as can be seen in this series (Table 3). It shows that about half of the patients had a severe villous atrophy. But this percentage is not meaningful, because the result depends entirely on how you collect the material. If you study severely ill patients, as most of the patients in this series were, you get a high percentage of severe atrophy. Also, the so-called "patchy lesion," which has been said to be typical of cow's-milk-protein-induced enteropathy, is more common among milder cases (Fig. 1). The only really important point in these results is that cow's-milk-protein-induced enteropathy may cause a severe mucosal lesion indistinguishable from celiac disease.

TABLE 3. *Proximal jejunal biopsy findings in 48
infants with cow's-milk-induced enteropathy[a]*

Normal or slight villous changes	8%
Partial villous atrophy	36%
Subtotal villous atrophy	45%

[a]Data are from ref. 3.

What about the other histological parameters in cow's-milk-induced enteropathy? In the epithelium, changes can be found similar to those in celiac disease. After provocation the epithelium is flattened and the nuclei lose their elongated shape and perpendicular orientation to the surface (7). The number of intraepithelial lymphocytes increases. In the lamina propria there is heavy round-cell infiltration, mainly with IgA-producing cells like in celiac disease (8). Some researchers have suggested that a diagnosis of cow's-milk-protein-induced enteropathy can be made by quantifying the eosinophilic cells in the lamina propria (9). Kosnai et al. (10) found an increased count in only about half of their patients, but they made the same observation in celiac disease. Maluenda et al. (11) could

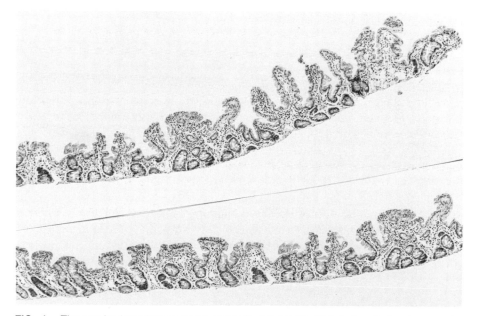

FIG. 1. The patchy intestinal mucosal lesion in a 3-month-old infant suffering from cow's-milk-induced enteropathy. In the upper part of the photograph, almost-normal finger-like villi are visible at one end of the biopsy specimen; in the lower part of the photograph, there are almost-flat mucosa from the other end of the specimen.

not verify an increased eosinophil count in the lamina propria, but they found an increased number of intraepithelial eosinophils, especially after provocation with cow's milk. There has been no comparison with celiac disease in this respect. There are two interesting observations among the morphometric studies showing some differences between the intestinal lesion in cow's-milk-induced enteropathy and celiac disease. Maluenda et al. (11) proved that the intestinal mucosa was thinner in cow's-milk-induced enteropathy regardless of whether the patients were on or off cow's milk. Kosnai et al. (12) again found that the cells in crypts and the mitotic indices were increased both in cow's-milk-induced enteropathy and in celiac disease. However, in cow's-milk-induced enteropathy the crypts were shorter than in celiac disease, but they showed a more vigorous mitotic activity, indicating a more rapid destruction of enterocytes.

In electron-microscopic studies, similar changes in celiac disease and cow's-milk-induced enteropathy have been found (7). After treatment the ultrastructure of epithelial cells is normal, but after challenge with cow's milk the microvilli are short and plump. A large collection of lysosomes can be seen. The nuclei are amoeba-like.

In summary, I should like to say that the severe lesion in cow's-milk-induced enteropathy is practically indistinguishable from the damage commonly found in celiac disease. Although certain differences between the lesions in the two diseases have been described, these cannot be used as a safe basis for differential diagnosis. I also have the feeling that the immune processes in the small-intestinal mucosa in both diseases must be rather similar, although the basic etiology is different.

FOOD SENSITIVITY

Although cow's milk is the best-known cause for allergic enteropathy, intolerance to other foods was also found in the first article [Lamy et al. (13)] in which the coexistence of the intestinal lesion and cow's milk allergy in one patient was described. Cow's milk is a rich source of allergens; it is also known that in cow's-milk-induced enteropathy (Table 4), several protein fractions may cause the reaction, and not only one. In addition, several patients (Table 5) had intolerances to foods they were receiving before the elimination of cow's milk, such as wheat, or during elimination, such as soy milk and Nutramigen. The intolerance to wheat is especially interesting because the clinical reaction is usually even stronger than the reaction against cow's milk and lasts longer, so that the patients still react to wheat when they have gained tolerance to cow's milk.

In spite of these observations of clinical sensitivity, only cow's milk was found to be a direct cause of intestinal mucosal damage. Recently, however, evidence of enteropathies caused by foods other than cow's milk has emerged. The type of intestinal mucosal injury observed has usually been very similar to that caused by cow's milk. In addition, most of these patients have either simultaneously had cow's milk allergy or they had it earlier. Table 6 summarizes the observations in-

TABLE 4. *Reactions to some cow's milk protein fractions in eight patients with cow's-milk-induced enteropathy*[a]

Case number	Casein	Lactalbumin	Lactoglobulin	Bovine serum albumin	Bovine globulin
1	+	−	+	−	−
2	+	−	−	−	−
3			+	−	
4	+		+	+	−
5					+
6	+	−	+	−	−
7	−	+	+	−	
8	+		+	−	
	5 of 6	1 of 4	6 of 7	1 of 7	1 of 5

[a]Data are from ref. 3.

TABLE 5. *Clinical intolerance to other foods in patients with cow's-milk-induced enteropathy*[a]

Soya	11%
Wheat	37%
Nutramigen	18%

9[a] Data from ref. 3.

TABLE 6. *Food-protein-induced enteropathies caused by foods other than cow's milk, according to literature*

Authors	Age of patient at challenge	Main intolerance	Additional intolerance
Walker-Smith (14)	19 months	Wheat	?
Ament and Rubin (15)	6 and 10 months	Soy milk and soy protein isolate	Cow's milk
Jyngkaran et al. (16)	9 months	Egg white	?
Vitoria et al. (17)	4 months	Fish	Cow's milk
	6 months	Rice	Cow's milk
	1 months	Chicken	Cow's milk

dicating intestinal damage caused by wheat, soy milk, egg white, chicken, and maize.

The most important diagnostic tool for verifying food allergy as a cause of enteropathy today is still provocation. However, challenging these young, and sometimes very sick, infants is difficult, and interpretation of the results is also sometimes problematic. The clinical sensitivity is transient and may disappear rather early (Table 7). Thus the absence of the clinical reaction does not exclude the diagnosis. The second difficulty is that the "time table" of reaction is variable. One would expect a rapid clinical reaction with a food allergy, but this is not the case in the food-induced enteropathies. In our series (3) about half of the patients reacted rapidly within 24 hr, but half reacted later. In some patients the mucosal damage reappeared slowly during several weeks on provocation, with very mild symptoms, thus simulating a reaction typical to that of gluten in celiac disease.

It has often been discussed that provocation tests with pre- and postchallenge small-bowel biopsies should be done in order to make the final diagnosis of cow's-milk-induced enteropathy (18,19). There is no single answer to this question because the circumstances vary greatly. My own view is that this kind of verification of the diagnosis is not necessary and not even reliable as described above. An intestinal biopsy at the beginning of the treatment is useful for verification of enteropathy. Thereafter the patients can be treated by the state of clinical intolerance. Thus, an allergen can be introduced into the diet when the patient tolerates it even if the intestinal mucosa is not yet completely normal. Table 8 shows that this is the case. In this series of patients with cow's-milk-induced enteropathy, cow's milk was introduced into the diet when patients tolerated it clinically in spite of

TABLE 7. *Age of the patients at the onset and at the disappearance of the symptoms in a series of 54 patients with cow's-milk-induced enteropathy*[a]

Number of patients	Mean age at onset of symptoms (range)	Mean age (and range) at time when patients no longer reacted to challenge
54	9 weeks (1 day to 22 weeks)	55 weeks (22–108 weeks)

[a]Data are from ref. 3.

TABLE 8. *Intestinal biopsy findings in cow's-milk-induced enteropathy at different stages of the elimination diet*[a]

	Age (mean)	Intestinal biopsy findings			
		Normal	Slight	PVA	SVA
Initial findings	15 weeks	1	3	17	27
At time of reintroduction of cow's milk	55 weeks	10	8	14	3
Follow-up at least 2 years on normal diet	4 years	33	4	0	5

[a]Data are from ref. 3.
SVA, subtotal villous atrophy; PVA, partial villous atrophy.

the fact that the intestinal mucosa was often still damaged. However, at the end-point the mucosa was normal except in five cases, where the patients were found to have additional celiac disease.

ETIOLOGY AND PATHOGENESIS

Not much is known about the etiology and pathogenesis of food-induced enteropathies. A lack of a good animal model makes it difficult to approach the problem.

There are, however, several clinical observations that might give some ideas for speculation (Table 9). First of all we know that cow's-milk-induced enteropathy is clearly confined to a certain age period, that is, to early childhood. This makes the whole discussion of maturation of the immune defense and immune tolerance relevant.

It is also quite obvious that the disease as such is not hereditary like celiac disease, and it is transient. In time the patient will be completely cured of the disease. Therefore we have to look for acquired factors. The reaction is not specific to one molecular structure, as it is in celiac disease, but is linked to antigenic material. This again favors the allergic type of immune reaction instead of an enzymatic defect.

The connection between food-induced enteropathy and the classic immediate type of allergy is interesting. It is well known that about one-third to one-half of the patients with an enteropathy also have signs of atopic hypersensitivity, namely, a typical atopy-like eczema, respiratory symptoms, eosinophilia, positive skin tests, RAST, etc. However, the other half of the patients do not have any signs of reaginic activity, and in these cases the development of severe intestinal damage is much more likely to be caused by a slower, nonreaginic immune reaction.

By studying the small-intestinal mucosa in atopic eczema caused by a food allergy without gastrointestinal symptoms or with only mild and immediate symptoms, it has been found that the overall appearance of the mucosa is normal (20,21). In a morphometric study, an increase of crypt depth and an increase of the IgA- and IgM-producing plasma cells in the lamina propria have been found.

TABLE 9. *Facts on food-protein-induced enteropathies based on clinical findings*

Age-bound
Nonhereditary and transient
Nonmolecule-specific
Bound to antigens
Connections with immediate food allergy (atopy)
Connection with acute gastroenteritis
Connections with other predisposing factors

This shows that in reaginic food allergy an activation of the immune reactivity exists in the gut, and perhaps a slightly increased epithelial-cell turnover exists. Thus it is possible that the reaginic reaction could be a predisposing factor for those more profound immune reactions which really cause the severe mucosal damage in enteropathies.

Acute gastroenteritis seems to be important as a triggering factor, especially in countries with endemic severe gastroenteritis (22). However, in other countries, such as Finland, this seems to be less common, as shown by Verkasalo et al. (23) (Table 10). In another Finnish study (24), two groups of infants and young children with acute gastroenteritis were treated either with early introduction of cow's milk and cow's milk products or elimination of these during treatment. No difference between the groups was found in terms of the number of clinical atopic symptoms, total and milk-specific IgE levels, and the levels of IgG and IgA antibodies to beta-lactoglobulin and casein. However, all 65 patients studied were older than 6 months of age, which might explain why the postgastroenteritis sensitization to cow's milk was not found. The decreasing incidence of acute gastroenteritis in young infants, coupled with an increasing number of breastfeeding mothers, obviously explains why the incidence of cow's-milk-induced enteropathy has greatly diminished in a country like Finland and why the connection between this disease and acute gastroenteritis is not so strong. The study of Verkasalo et al. (23) also shows some other interesting connections between cow's-milk-induced enteropathy and other conditions or diseases such as prematurity, Down's syndrome, and preceding intra-abdominal operations.

Thus several factors are obviously involved in the pathogenesis of food-protein-induced enteropathy (Table 11). The basic condition is established by feeding an infant with food containing strong antigens during early infancy, when antigen handling is physiologically immature and immune tolerance is not well developed. Prematurity, as well as 21-trisomy, may accentuate this immaturity. In addition, one or several triggering factors are needed. The hereditary background of atopic constitution could be one of these, and then there are local factors which may disturb the physiologic defense mechanisms in the gut. Acute gastroenteritis is certainly one of these, but there might also be others like celiac disease and intestinal disease, leading to surgery. The disease of food-induced enteropathy itself is thus

TABLE 10. *Some coexisting factors in a Finnish series*[a]

Atopy among first-degree relatives	30 of 144
21-Trisomy	5 of 65
Signs of atopy (e.g., eosinophilia)	19 of 54
Prematurity	6 of 65
Preceding intra-abdominal surgery	4 of 65
Infectious gastroenteritis	16 of 56

[a]Data are from ref. 23.

TABLE 11. *Hypothesis for pathogenesis of food-protein-induced enteropathy*

Basic factors	Triggering factors

Immaturity of antigen handling
Immaturity of development of oral tolerance
  Physiologic (age)
  21-Trisomy
  Prematurity
  Unknown
Feeding strong antigens
	Reaginic food allergy (heredity)
	Acute gastroenteritis
	Other gastrointestinal diseases and
	  surgery (e.g., celiac disease)
	Unknown factors (e.g., malnutrition)

a result of several triggering factors in favorable conditions, which induce the immunologic process in lamina propria, thus leading to the intestinal damage.

REFERENCES

1. Gerrard JW, Mackenzie JWA, Goluboff N, Garson JZ, Maningas CS. Cow's milk allergy: prevalence and manifestation in an unselected series of newborn. *Acta Paediatr Scand (Suppl)* 1973;234:1–21.
2. Jakobsson I, Lindberg T. Prospective study of cow's milk protein intolerance in Swedish infants. *Acta Paediatr Scand* 1979;86:853–9.
3. Kuitunen P, Visakorpi JK, Savilahti E, Pelkonen P. Malabsorption syndrome with cow's milk intolerance: clinical findings and course in the light of 54 cases. *Arch Dis Child* 1975;50:351–6.
4. Gryboski JD, Burkle F, Hillman R. Milk induced colitis in an infant. *Pediatrics* 1966;38:299–302.
5. Jenkins HR, Harries JT, Milla PJ, Pincott JR, Soothill JF. Food allergic colitis in childhood. *Arch Dis Child* 1984;59:326–9.
6. Kokkonen J, Similä S, Herva R. Impaired gastric function in children with cow's milk intolerance. *Eur J Pediatr* 1979;132:1–6.
7. Kuitunen P, Rapola J, Savilahti E, Visakorpi JK. Response of the jejunal mucosa to cow's milk in the malabsorption syndrome with cow's milk intolerance. *Acta Paediatr Scand* 1973;62:585–95.
8. Savilahti E. Immunochemical study of the malabsorption syndrome with cow's milk intolerance. *Gut* 1973;14:491–501.
9. Challacombe DN, Wheeler EE, Campbell PE. Morphometric studies and eosinophil cell counts in the duodenal mucosa of children with chronic nonspecific diarrhoea and cow's milk allergy. *J Pediatr Gastroenterol Nutr* 1986;5:887–91.
10. Kosnai I, Kuitunen P, Savilahti E, Sipponen P. Mast cells and eosinophils in the jejunal mucosa of patients with intestinal cow's milk allergy and celiac disease of childhood. *J Pediatr Gastroenterol Nutr* 1984;3:368–72.
11. Maluenda C, Phillips AD, Briddon A, Walker-Smith JA. Quantitative analysis of small intestinal mucosa in cow's milk-sensitive enteropathy. *J Pediatr Gastroenterol Nutr* 1984;3:349–56.
12. Kosnai J, Kuitunen P, Savilahti E, Rapola J, Kohegy J. Cell kinetic in the jejunal crypt epithelium in malabsorption syndrome with cow's milk protein intolerance and in coeliac disease in childhood. *Gut* 1980;21:1041–6.
13. Lamy M, Nezelof C, Jos J, Frézal J, Rey J. La biopsie de la muqueuse intestinale d'une des syndromes de malabsorption. *Presse Med* 1963;71:1267–70.
14. Walker-Smith J. Transient gluten intolerance. *Arch Dis Child* 1970;45:523–6.
15. Ament ME, Rubin CE. Soy protein—another cause of the flat intestinal lesion. *Gastroenterology* 1972;62:227–34.

16. Jyngkaran N, Abidin Z, Meng LL, Yadav M. Egg-protein-induced villous atrophy. *J Pediatr Gastroenterol Nutr* 1982;1:29–33.
17. Vitoria JC, Camarero C, Sojo A, Ruiz A, Rodriquez-Soriano J. Enteropathy related to fish, rice and chicken. *Arch Dis Child* 1982;57:44–8.
18. Berg NO, Jakobsson I, Lindberg T. Do pre- and postchallenge small intestinal biopsies help to diagnose cow's milk protein intolerance? *Acta Paediatr Scand* 1979;68:657–61.
19. Salazar de Sousa J, da Silva A, Pereira MV, Soares J, Magalhaes Ramalho P. Cow's milk protein-sensitive enteropathy: number and timing of biopsies for diagnosis. *J Pediatr Gastroenterol Nutr* 1986;5:207–9.
20. McCalla R, Savilahti E, Perkkiö M, Kuitunen P, Backman A. Morphology of the jejunum in children with eczema due to food allergy. *Allergy* 1980;35:563–71.
21. Perkkiö M. Immunohistochemical study of intestinal biopsies from children with atopic eczema due to food allergy. *Allergy* 1980;35:563–71.
22. Walker-Smith JA. Cow's milk intolerance as a cause of postenteritis diarrhoea. *J Pediatr Gastroenterol Nutr* 1982;1:163–73.
23. Verkasalo M, Kuitunen P, Savilahti E, Tiilikainen A. Changing pattern of cow's milk intolerance. *Acta Paediatr Scand* 1981;70:289–95.
24. Isolauri E, Vesikari T, Saha P, Viander M. Milk versus non-milk in rapid refeeding after acute gastroenteritis. *J Pediatr Gastroenterol Nutr* 1986;5:254–61.

DISCUSSION

Dr. Challacombe: First a comment: If you examine sections of the small-intestinal mucosa in cow's-milk-induced enteropathy, you will find that clusters of eosinophils are present in various parts of the tissue, and these clusters appear to be associated with mast cells. Initially, there appears to be a patchy reaction occurring in the lamina propria in some patients; and as the reaction spreads, so the biopsy appearances become indistinguishable from those of celiac disease. Total eosinophil counts in the lamina propria are increased in cow's-milk-protein intolerance and also in a small number of children with toddler's diarrhea (chronic nonspecific diarrhea). It is therefore important to examine small-gut biopsies from suspected cases of food allergy very carefully and to quantify the eosinophils present, much as one does in the blood. I should like now to pose a more general question: Professor Visakorpi talks about wheat intolerance, and we know that an IgE-mediated reaction to wheat can develop after introducing wheat into the diet in infancy. Can any member of the audience tell me what component of wheat causes this reaction?

Dr. Visakorpi: I do not know.

Dr. Aas: I have seen a number of patients with true immunologic wheat allergy. About 50% will tolerate small amounts of gluten-free flour, but the other 50% do not. Some of these seem to react to the same components as the celiac disease patients, but with a true immunologic type of reaction. The problem is that there is a kind of "Münchhausen syndrome by physicians" which plays an important role in both wheat allergy and cow's milk intolerance. A large number of patients show positive reactions to skin tests and RASTs which have nothing to do with food allergy, but the reactions are interpreted as being specific. These patients should not be put on elimination diets, but they often are. Luckily for them there are plenty of ignorant physicians who allow them to have rye flour in the belief that wheat allergy will not interfere with rye tolerance, whereas in fact the majority of people with genuine wheat allergy will also react to rye flour.

Dr. Rossipal: I would like to comment on some aspects of the group of infants who develop cow's-milk-induced enteropathy. In the last 12 years I have not seen a single case occurring in a child whose first introduction of cow's milk with the diet was later than the third month of life. My experience also showed me that prematurity is not a factor which increases the likelihood of this condition developing.

Dr. Visakorpi: I agree that very early exposure to cow's milk seems to be essential, perhaps even during the first few weeks.

Dr. Wahn: I still have a problem with nomenclature. My impression is that the patients you describe with "food-protein-induced enteropathy" are rather a heterogeneous group. Is it not possible to devise a more precise definition of this condition or conditions, assuming that there are subgroups?

Dr. Visakorpi: The difficulty is that my patients were all sick babies from a gastroenterology clinic. When I first started to collect such patients and describe the syndrome, it was on the basis of a clinical syndrome of failure-to-thrive with gastrointestinal symptoms, which I called, for safety, "cow's milk intolerance" because I did not know what was behind it. After a while, many people started to use this name, or perhaps "cow's-milk-protein intolerance," meaning the same thing. When it later became apparent that there was an immunologic basis to the condition and that immune reactions caused the damage to the intestine, the name was changed to "cow's-milk-induced enteropathy" or "cow's-milk-protein enteropathy."

Dr. Müller: I don't want to rake up the discussions that have been going on for over 80 years about the value of antibody determinations in cow's milk allergy, but I think we all know that there are at least two types: the immediate-type reaction, mainly with urticaria, and the other type of reaction which you have demonstrated. In addition to the data which you showed, these young infants with enteropathy usually show (a) high IgG- and IgA-specific antibody titers to milk proteins and (b) nearly normal levels of IgE-specific isotypes. On the other hand, the immediate reactors usually have no IgG-specific antibodies to milk proteins, and they commonly show high IgE titers measured by RAST or ELISA. So I think we can say that there are two different types of reactors, though maybe these are just the two different sides of the same medal.

Dr. Visakorpi: I agree with that. I do not think we can say that there are two different diseases. They are linked in some way because you often see patients with changing type of reaction, perhaps initially an anaphylactic response, becoming later an enteropathy without other symptoms. I do not like to divide this condition into two separate diseases because there are so many things in common, and in the gastrointestinal tract you see only one disease.

Dr. Shmerling: I have some doubts about the uniformity of the population of children with predominantly gastrointestinal forms of cow's milk intolerance, the reason being that, from the results of prospective studies, the patients who present early with a very severe syndrome of malabsorption with IgG and IgA antibodies usually do not have associated symptoms of allergy. They do not come from atopic families, they are cured within a year or two, and even by the age of 20 (my longest follow-up so far) they do not have any other allergic manifestations. I accept that this is a disease which is initiated and maintained in the gut by immunologic mechanisms, but it is different from the other types of cases where there are generalized symptoms including enteropathy but where the enteropathy is not the initial or only manifestation. These patients go on later to get eczema and asthma, they tend to remain atopic, they come from allergic families, and they have IgE-mediated symptoms. It is possible that the picture has become confused in the literature by the inclusion of these atopic patients in the group of children with purely gastrointestinal symptoms, probably because a good family history has not been obtained or because the child was too young at diagnosis to have developed atopic manifestations.

Dr. Visakorpi: I recognize the two types of patients you are describing, but I meant that the histological appearance of the small-gut mucosa in the two forms are very similar. I agree that the most severe forms, where there is a flat mucosa, are perhaps found predominantly in children with no family history of atopy.

Dr. Bellanti: The differences may reflect different immunologic mechanisms. Returning to the basic pathophysiology of these diseases, we see that the first event seems to be a structural break in the mucosa. Whether caused by acute gastroenteritis, medications, or other toxic causes, that seems to initiate the disorder; and following it there is absorption of macromolecular substances which leads, in one group of children, to IgE-mediated immediate hypersensitivity and, in another, to the production of a cell-mediated immune disorder. Thus we must keep in mind the different immunologic mechanisms. We have used an animal model to demonstrate how injury may initiate an immunologic disorder. When guinea pigs are fed methotrexate, there is injury to the gut mucosa; and after a period of ingestion of food proteins, intestinal reactions very similar to those found in celiac disease occur, with a flat mucosa and lymphocytic infiltration. These effects are transient, and healing occurs. I think the basic problem in the human model is to discover what factors favor transience and what factors favor chronicity.

Dr. Mittal: You have highlighted the question of differentiating cow's-milk-induced enteropathy from celiac disease, but what about the child who presents with persistent diarrhea, malnutrition, and an enteropathy? How do you decide whether he or she has malnutrition alone, or contaminated bowel syndrome, or tropical enteropathy, or cow's-milk-induced enteropathy, or all of them?

Dr. Visakorpi: This is a very difficult problem. There may well be a connection between cow's milk allergy and these other enteropathies; for example, in some of the postdiarrheal cases a flat mucosa may be caused by sensitization to cow's milk. Of course you can study it by excluding cow's milk proteins from the diet.

Dr. Nusslé: Using formula with chicken meat or lactalbumin hydrolysate we have had the opportunity, with the help of the Nestlé Nutrition Research Fund, to study prospectively about 60 patients with chronic diarrhea and malnutrition in Bolivia. We were unable to find any cases of cow's-milk-protein intolerance with the usual diagnostic criteria in this very poor population. All the children were older than 9 months (mean 16 months) and were breast-fed until that age. Lactose and milk challenges were done separately, and only lactose intolerance could be demonstrated.

Dr. Frick: It was shown in Australia a few years ago that some of these cases of cow's-milk-induced gastroenteropathy were preceded by rotavirus infections. Have you had a chance to look at virus antibody titers in your cases?

Dr. Visakorpi: We have not looked at this specifically, but the incidence of gastroenteritis is now very low in young infants, so I do not think it is likely to be important in the etiology of cow's milk enteropathy.

Dr. Rieger: I think we should stay open-minded about all the possible mechanisms for the production of intestinal allergy, but I should like to ask whether there is such a thing as protein intolerance leading to chronic gastrointestinal disease which is *not* mediated by immunologic mechanisms. It has already been said that protein intolerance is not the same as allergy, but are we seeing the same situation as in asthma, where there is extrinsic allergic asthma and intrinsic nonallergic asthma, i.e., an undefined entity?

Dr. Visakorpi: I do not know, but I believe that where there is an enteropathy of this kind there is always an immunologic reaction.

Dr. Müller: I think there *is* a similar picture in respiratory disease, where you have immediate-type reactions in asthma and type-3 reactions in allergic alveolitis. The former has an IgE response mainly, and the latter goes on to very high titers of precipitating antibodies. In the gut we may well be seeing the same thing in cow's milk allergy, or whatever you want to call it. On the one hand you have a type-1 response with immediate symptoms, and on the other hand you have a type-3 response confined to a chronic enteropathy. This is at least some sort of working concept.

Food Allergy, edited by Eberhardt Schmidt.
Nestlé Nutrition Workshop Series, Vol. 17.
Nestec Ltd., Vevey/Raven Press, Ltd.,
New York © 1988.

Food Intolerance in Respiratory Tract Disease

Oscar L. Frick

Department of Pediatrics, School of Medicine, University of California, San Francisco, California 94143

An asthma attack precipitated by wine was noted in 1679 by Thomas Willis (33). Salter (1) observed sneezing, rhinorrhea, nasal congestion, coughing, and wheezing after ingestion of certain foods; he suggested avoiding old cheese, preserved foods, nuts, and malt liquor. Salter also observed milk-precipitated wheezing in a child.

For many years Rowe (2) made a strong case for foods causing coughing and wheezing in about half of his asthmatic patients. In his 1948 survey of 1,491 asthmatic patients, 40% of children <5 years old, 25% of children 5 to 15 years old, 20% of adults 15 to 55 years old, and 40% of adults >55 years old had asthmatic reactions only with foods. These results were based upon history, skin tests, and response to the Rowe 1-2-3 elimination diets. He felt that if physicians actually took the trouble to look, they would find that half the cases of intrinsic asthma and psychogenic asthma in adults were really caused by allergy to foods. Most of his professional colleagues dismissed Rowe's studies as those of an uncritical enthusiast, but today's interest in adverse reactions to foods, as evidenced by these recent Nestlé symposia, would please Dr. Rowe greatly.

Van Metre et al. (3) evaluated the Rowe's cereal-free diet 1,2,3 along with a second high-allergenic-foods diet in double-blind crossover fashion on 18 randomly selected adult asthmatics, in whom a role for foods as relevant allergens had not been established. After 3 weeks on each diet, there was no difference in frequency or severity of asthmatic symptoms or in medication scores. In rebuttal, Rowe (4) pointed out that Van Metre's patients were only on the Rowe diet for 3 weeks and that it takes 2 to 3 weeks to clear the body of antigenic food, so that the diet trial period was insufficiently long to expect to see a change in the patients' respiratory symptoms.

Dr. Rowe's enthusiasm to look into foods as a possible cause of respiratory allergy rubbed off on several of his California colleagues, namely Dr. William Deamer and myself. Deamer became convinced that allergy in children was caused by inhalants in 60% of cases; inhalants and foods together in 30% of cases, and foods alone in 10% of cases (5). We have tried to document, with newly developed immunologic tests, *in vitro* reactions to foods that correlated with clinical sensitivity (6). On the basis of two elimination diet trials and exacerbation of symptoms upon reintroduction of suspected foods (modified Goldman criteria) (7), 40 patients were classified as having either immediate or delayed reactions to foods; 30% of these had upper or lower respiratory symptoms upon open food challenge. Immunologic tests, such as skin tests, IgE precipitation, and leukocyte histamine release, were performed. Patients with immediate reactions had (80%) positive test results with suspected food. However, in those with delayed-onset symptoms, these immunologic tests were mostly negative.

DIAGNOSIS

Blinded food challenges have become the "gold standard" for the diagnosis of food sensitivity; these were introduced by Loveless (8). Of eight milk-sensitive patients with positive skin tests, two had positive reactions, one with wheezing; two were inconclusive; and four were negative. May and Bock (9) established a systematic double-blind food challenge protocol. In a recent summary (10), Bock evoked symptoms in 81 of 209 (39%) older (>3 years of age) children, with 96 of 431 (22%) positive challenges. All had positive skin-prick tests. Symptoms involved gastrointestinal >skin>respiratory systems and occurred within 2 hr of challenge. In 131 younger children (<3 years of age), symptoms occurred in 51 of 131 (39%) cases, with 69 of 110 (63%) positive challenges. Immediate reaction (<2 hr) occurred in 84% with 80% positive skin-prick tests, whereas 15% had late-onset (>4 hr) diarrhea and one had a rash reaction; in the latter group, only 10% had positive skin-prick tests. Respiratory symptoms occurred in 10% with wheezing usually associated with sneezing, rhinorrhea, or otitis with effusion.

Of 57 children with reported cow's-milk-induced symptoms, Hill et al. (11) found only 17 children with positive cow's milk open challenges. Before and after challenge, duodenal biopsies were done in eight children. In subsequent blinded challenges, two of 17 had wheezing, both had positive skin-prick tests, and one had mild intestinal mucosal damage. Skin symptoms occurred in seven of 17; all had positive skin-prick tests; mucosal damage occurred in one. Gastrointestinal symptoms occurred in eight of 17; only three were immediate; none had positive skin-prick tests or RAST; and mucosal damage occurred in four. IgA deficiency was present in one-third of the children. The parents observed milk-induced severe symptoms in 57 children, although only 17 actually had symptoms induced by milk challenges; this marked discrepancy was attributed to small volumes in challenge which were not increased beyond onset of first symptoms. This was a major drawback in demonstrating respiratory symptoms for such blinded challenges; often much larger challenge doses over a longer period of time may be needed to elicit respiratory symptoms. Another potential problem is desensitization (exhausting mast cells' mediators) with first small challenge doses, so that insufficient mediators remain to give a positive challenge with larger doses of food antigen. Hill concluded that "there is no single laboratory test on which to base the diagnosis for cow's milk hypersensitivity and that diagnosis still rests on a reproducible response to challenge under controlled conditions."

Adults ($n = 22$) with food-induced multisystem allergic symptoms were given double-blind food challenges by Bernstein et al. (12). They found that nine of 22 (41%) had 13 of 46 (28%) positive challenges with suspected food, whereas two of 10 (20%) patients had a positive placebo challenge. Respiratory symptoms (rhinorrhea and/or shortness of breath with antigen) occurred in three patients and stomatitis and sore throat occurred in an additional three. Six patients with negative challenges also complained of similar respiratory symptoms. Positive skin tests occurred in only 30% with positive challenges. With almost identical results in 25 adults, Atkins et al. (13) found 10 of 24 (42%) patients with 12 of 75 (16%) positive double-blind food challenges and *no* positive placebo challenges. Of these, six had upper respiratory symptoms (sneezing, rhinorrhea, and nasal congestion) and four had hoarseness and dysphagia indicative of laryngeal edema; one required ephinephrine. Skin tests were positive in 90% of positive challenge reactors and were positive in 21% of the negative challenge group. These studies in adults confirmed the value of the double-blind food test, with a significant number of subjects having respiratory symptoms from foods.

In a large asthma clinic, Onorato et al. (14) screened 300 consecutive asthmatic patients for foods that could contribute to their asthmatic symptoms. Only 25 had a strongly suggestive history and/or positive food skin-prick tests of IgE RAST. Of these patients, 20 had double-blind food challenges performed that were interpretable. In Table 1, a summary of data from Onorato et al. (14), showed that blinded food ingestion caused asthmatic symptoms in six patients and nonrespiratory symptoms in five, such as atopic dermatitis flare and gastrointestinal upset. The patients with positive food challenges had significantly elevated total serum IgE as compared to that of nonatopic patients, but these values were similar to atopic subjects with negative food challenges. The onset of asthma occurred significantly in younger patients with positive food challenges as compared to nonallergic asthmatics. There was a highly significant association of current atopic dermatitis in subjects with asthma with positive food challenges. On blind rechallenge with food after ingesting 300 mg of cromolyn sodium, the asthmatic response was blocked in four of five patients with positive food challenges. These investigators concluded that foods can induce asthmatic symptoms but that its incidence was low and that such symptoms might be blocked with oral cromolyn treatment.

Serial twice-a-day peak-flow monitoring while off suspected foods in an elimination diet or on an oligoallergonic (few foods) diet and open or blinded challenge with food were successful in many patients who charted decreases in PEFR over hours or days after food challenge (15). Immediate reactions, mostly gastroenteritis and itching (and three with wheezing), occurred in 20 patients with positive RAST. Late reactions, mostly asthma, occurred in 36 patients; 18 of which had positive RASTs, many with cereal flour; the other 18 with negative RAST had

TABLE 1. *Double-blind food challenges in subjects with asthma[a]*

Parameter	Nonallergic subjects	p	Positive food challenge	Negative food challenge	Pollen allergy	Perennial allergy
Number of subjects	102	< 0.01	11	9	102	74
Asthma-causing foods			6[b]			
Age (years), mean	1–80		12.5	16.2	25.7	34.3
Age at onset of asthma	24.1	< 0.05	6.5	8.5	16.4	15.1
Total serum IgE (kU/L)	84	< 0.01	1908	2236	605	698
Nonasthma symptoms % Current atopic dermatitis	5.3	< 0.001	45.4	11.1	21.1	10.8
Previous atopic dermatitis	2.5		36.4	44.1	7.0	6.8
Acute urticaria	13.5		9.0	11.1	15.4	15.7
Gastrointestinal symptoms	22.1		36.3	22.2	28.2	23.5

[a]Data are from ref. 14.
[b]Egg, 4; wheat, 2; corn, 1.

eczema flareup along with asthma, most commonly in response to egg and milk, in 1 to 6 hr. Therefore, serial peak flow measurements may be useful in following delayed reactions to foods.

As a further assessment of such delayed food-induced asthmatic reactions and recognition of late-phase inflammatory reactions after food antigen ingestion, Silverman and Wilson (16) found increased bronchial hyperreactivity to histamine inhalation after food challenges. Increased histamine reactivity was maximal in 90 min and was wearing off by 120 to 150 min. For logistic reasons, they could not measure reactivity after 2 to 3 hr, but such measurements should be made in the future.

Along this line, May (17) reported high spontaneous baseline leukocyte histamine release in patients with food sensitivity. Podleski (18) has described a spontaneous autocytotoxicity with $16.6\% \pm 1.3$ SE trypan-blue-stained leukocytes in six food-sensitive asthmatics as compared to $3.8\% \pm 0.4$ in 18 nonallergic controls ($p<0.001$). Addition of the relevant food antigens *in vivo* increased the direct allergic autocytotoxicity in all six patients' cells significantly ($p<0.001$); increases ranged from 5% to 13% over baseline specific autocytotoxicity with antigen. It had been suggested that circulating immune complexes consisting of IgG, IgM, IgA, or IgE antibodies and antigens from constantly absorbed food antigens increased spontaneous releasibility of granules from leukocytes. Podleski et al. showed earlier (19) that eosinophils from a milk-allergic subject degranulated *in vitro* in the presence of cow's milk and this was inhibited in the presence of ketotifen.

NON-IgE-MEDIATED HYPERSENSITIVITIES TO FOODS

Immune complexes in Type-III serum-sickness-like mechanism has been proposed to explain some food reactions. Complement activation after milk feeding in children with cow's milk allergy was reported by Matthews and Soothill (20). Cow's-milk-induced nephrotic attacks occurred in six children with steroid-dependent nephrosis (21).

Recurrent pneumonia or Heiner's syndrome (22) was described in children with hypersensitivity to cow's milk. Additional components of the syndrome were: (a) allergic rhinitis, otitis media, cough, wheezing, or hemoptysis; (b) anorexia, vomiting, colic, or diarrhea; (c) failure to thrive; (d) iron-deficiency anemia; (e) recurrent or persistent eosinophilia; (f) serum precipitating antibodies to multiple (five or more) constituents of cow's milk. A positive 4-hr intradermal test to milk antigen was frequent. It was felt that this was a Type-III Arthus-like reaction to cow's milk that, if severe, resulted in necrosis of pulmonary vessels, hemorrhage, and deposition of hemosiderin in the lung. Iron-laden macrophages were commonly observed in gastric washings from such children. Wilson et al. (23) also reported milk-induced gross or occult intestinal bleeding in milk-sensitive infants that led to severe microcytic iron-deficiency anemia. Elimination of cow's milk from the diet of children with either syndrome resulted usually in marked improvement.

Circulating immune complexes containing IgE antibodies were described in two egg-sensitive eczematous asthmatic adults whose reactions resulted from egg ingestion challenge (24). Paganelli et al. (25) subsequently demonstrated that both IgA and IgG antibodies complexed with foods in asthmatic subjects. Cunningham-Rundles et al. (26) observed 13 children and 17 adults with selective IgA deficiency who had both circulating immune complexes shown by Raji cell test and milk precipitins in close association. Both IgG and casein complexes in serum rose dramatically within 30 to 60 min following milk ingestion in two such IgA-deficient patients (27). In our own study (28), increased levels of circulating immune complexes in sera were demonstrated in 20 of 25 food-sensitive, but normal, IgA children by both Raji cell and C1q-binding studies. The levels of such immune complexes in sera varied with compliance with the elimination diet. Twelve of the 25 children had perennial rhinitis, eight of whom also had wheezing worsened by ingestion of the suspected food allergen.

Finally, a Type-IV cellular immunity in food allergy has been proposed. In our study (29), 34 children and 7 adults had delayed-onset (>2 hr to 2 days) food intolerance as evidenced by two or more open challenges after 2 weeks of being on the elimination diet; 11 had asthma; and 18 had chronic rhinitis. Leukocyte inhibition factor (LIF) assays were positive ($>20\%$ inhibition of migration) with corn in five of 41 patients, all with a positive history and positive open challenges with corn. With cow's milk or its fractions, 21 of 34 children and four of seven adults had positive LIF; differences in LIF in patients versus nonallergic controls were significant with $p<0.001$.

Concomitant with our publication, Ashkenazi et al. (30) reported that 24 patients with cow's milk allergy had positive LIF to beta-lactoglobulin

(23.5% ± 6.4). LIF was negative in three control groups—10 newborn infants, 10 infants with acute gastroenteritis, and 24 nonallergic children ($p<0.0005$). Months later, when five children had recovered from milk allergy symptoms, LIF became negative. Ashkenazi et al. (31) had significantly positive LIF tests with gluten in active celiac disease patients. LIF test became negative upon a gluten-free diet and became positive again upon oral gluten challenge; therefore, the LIF can be used to monitor the progress of a celiac patient's course as well as to monitor his or her compliance with the gluten-free diet.

Subsequently, in India, Khoshoo et al. (32) tested for LIF activity in 98 infants with protracted diarrhea and failure to thrive; 12 of these fulfilled Goldman's criteria for cow's-milk-protein intolerance. Controls were 12 healthy children, 12 malnourished children, and 16 children with acute gastroenteritis. LIF test was positive in all 12 infants with cow's milk allergy (58.83% ± 11.98) as compared with healthy controls (8.25% ± 3.9) ($p<0.05$). LIF was positive in four others with protracted diarrhea and in two with lactose malabsorption but was negative in acute gastroenteritis and malnutrition. In five cow's-milk-allergic infants who improved on milk-free diet, LIF returned toward normal (24.74% ± 4.87). These investigators concluded that LIF was a sensitive test for monitoring cow's milk allergy in infants. We have adopted the LIF test routinely in our clinic to monitor many food intolerances, including those in a group of patients with intrinisic asthma that appear to have food intolerance as part of their problem.

In conclusion, hypersensitivity to foods causes typical upper and lower respiratory allergic symptoms such as sneezing, rhinorrhea, and nasal congestion (upper respiratory tract) and cough and wheezing (lower respiratory tract). Immediate (>1 hr) respiratory reaction can usually be documented with double-blind food challenges, skin-prick tests, and RAST. Delayed food-induced respiratory symptoms may sometimes be reproduced by double-blind food challenges, but because of the large food amounts needed for challenge and repeated administration of these, such patients often must be confirmed by elimination diet and blind challenge and monitoring changes in pulmonary function tests such as PEF. Many delayed-onset food-intolerant patients exhibit positive tests for circulating immune complexes and LIF that suggest non-IgE-mediated hypersensitivity of Types III and IV.

REFERENCES

1. Salter HH. *On asthma: Its pathology and treatment*. London: J. & A, Churchill, 1860.
2. Rowe AH, Rowe A Jr. *Bronchial asthma*. Springfield, Ill.: Charles C Thomas, 1963.
3. Van Metre TE, Anderson AS, Barnard JH, et al. A controlled study of the effects on manifestations of chronic asthma of a rigid elimination diet based on Rowe's cereal-free diet 1,2,3. *J Allergy* 1968;41:195–208.
4. Rowe AH, Rowe A Jr. Letter on "cereal-free diet 1,2,3." *J Allergy* 1968;42:243–6.
5. Deamer WC. In: Breneman JC, ed. *Basics of food allergy* Springfield, Ill.: Charles C Thomas, 1978:48.
6. Galant SP, Bullock JD, Frick OL. An immunological approach to the diagnosis of food sensitivity. *Clin Allergy* 1973;3:363–72.

7. Goldman AS, Anderson DW Jr, Sellers WA, et al. Milk allergy. I. Oral challenge with milk and isolated milk proteins in allergic children. *Pediatrics* 1963;32:425–43.
8. Loveless MH. Milk allergy: a survey of its incidence; experiences with a masked ingestion test. *J Allergy* 1950;21:489–99.
9. May CD, Bock SA. A modern clinical approach to food hypersensitivity. *Allergy* 1978;33:166–88.
10. Bock AS. A critical evaluation of clinical trials in adverse reactions to foods in children. *J Allergy Clin Immunol* 1985;78:165–74.
11. Hill DJ, Davidson GP, Cameron DJS, Barnes GL. The spectrum of cow's milk allergy in childhood. *Acta Paediatr Scand* 1979;68:847–52.
12. Bernstein M, Day JH, Welsh A. Double-blind food challenge in the diagnosis of food sensitivity in the adult. *J Allergy Clin Immunol* 1982;70:205–10.
13. Atkins FM, Steinberg SS, Metcalfe DD. Evaluation of immediate adverse reactions to foods in adult patients. I. Correlation of demographic, laboratory, and prick skin test data with response to controlled oral food challenge. II. A detailed analysis of reaction patterns during oral food challenge. *J Allergy Clin Immunol* 1985;75:348–55, 356–63.
14. Onorato J, Merland N, Terral C, Michel FB, Bousquet J. Placebo-controlled double-blind food challenge in asthma. *J Allergy Clin Immunol* 1986;78:1139–46.
15. Wraith DG. Diagnostic methods and criteria: respiratory diseases. In: Coombs RRA, chairman. *Proceedings of the 1st food allergy workshop*. Oxford: Medical Education Services, 1980:64.
16. Silverman M, Wilson N. Clinical physiology of food intolerance in asthma. In: Read CE, ed. *Proceedings of the XII international congress of allergology and clinical immunology*. St. Louis: C. V. Mosby, 1986:457–62.
17. May CD. High spontaneous histamine release *in vitro* from leukocytes of persons hypersensitive to food. *J Allergy Clin Immunol* 1976;58:432–7.
18. Podleski WK. Spontaneous allergic autocytotoxicity in bronchial asthma associated with food allergy. *Am J Med* 1986;81:437–42.
19. Podleski WK, Panaszek BA, Schmidt JL, Burns RB. Inhibition of eosinophils degranulation by Ketotifen in a patient with milk allergy, manifested as bronchial asthma—an electron microscope study. *Agents Actions* 1984;15:177–81.
20. Matthews TS, Soothill JF. Complement activation after milk feeding in children with cow's milk allergy. *Lancet* 1970;2:893–5.
21. Sandberg DH, McIntosh RM, Bernstein CW, et al. Severe steroid-responsive nephrosis associated with hypersensitivity. *Lancet* 1977;1:388–90.
22. Heiner DC, Sears JW, Kniker WT. Multiple precipitins to cow's milk in chronic respiratory disease. *Am J Dis Child* 1962;103:634–54.
23. Wilson JF, Heiner DC, Lahey ME. Milk-induced gastrointestinal bleeding in infants with hypochromic microcytic anemia. *JAMA* 1964;189:122–6.
24. Brostoff J, Carini C. Production of IgE complexes by allergen challenge in atopic patients and the effect of sodium cromoglycate. *Lancet* 1979;1:1268–70.
25. Paganelli R, Levinsky RI, Brostoff J, Wraith DG. Immune complexes containing food proteins in normal and atopic subjects after oral challenge and effects of sodium cromoglycate on antigen absorption. *Lancet* 1979;1:1270–2.
26. Cunningham-Rundles C, Brandeis WE, Pudifin DJ, et al. Autoimmunity in selective IgA deficiency: relationship to anti-bovine antibodies, circulating immune complexes, and clinical disease. *Clin Exp Immunol* 1981;45:299–304.
27. Cunningham-Rundles C. The identification of specific antigens in circulating immune complexes by an enzyme-linked immunosorbent assay: detection of bovine x-casein IgG complexes in human sera. *Eur J Immunol* 1981;11:504–509.
28. Chang TT, Char D, Frick OL. Immune complexes in sera of delayed onset food allergy patients demonstrated by Raji cell and C1q-binding assays [Abstract 13]. *J Allergy Clin Immunol* 1981;68:4.
29. Minor JD, Tolber SG, Frick OL. Leukocyte inhibition factor in delayed-onset food allergy. *J Allergy Clin Immunol* 1980; 66:314–21.
30. Ashkenazi A, Levin S, Idar D, et al. *In vitro* cell-mediated immunologic assay for cow's milk allergy. *Pediatrics* 1980;66:399–402.
31. Ashkenazi A, Idar D, Handzel ZT, et al. An *in vitro* immunological assay for the diagnosis of coeliac disease. *Lancet* 1978;1:627–30.
32. Khoshoo V, Bhan MK, Arora NK, et al. Leucocyte migration inhibition in cow's milk protein intolerance. *Acta Paediatr Scand* 1986;75:308–12.

33. Willis T. *Pharmacentrices rationalis,* second part. 1697, London, Dring, Harper & Leigh, p 82, cited in Major RH. *Classic descriptions of disease.* Springfield, Ill.: Charles C Thomas, 1945:578.

DISCUSSION

Dr. Müller: Do you have any idea what it is that makes a food cause symptoms away from the gut, in the lung for instance? And are you aware of any reliable studies showing *specific* immune complexes to foods?

Dr. Frick: I don't think anyone really knows why the lung should be a target organ for food allergy, but I suppose that incompletely digested proteins get through the gut into the circulation and then end up anywhere in the body where they may be capable of initiating a reaction. As to the specificity of immune complexes, we have studied this using a double-labeling technique. We used the C_{1q}-binding test that we described before (1), labeling with *staph*-A protein and using ELISA to detect immune complexes (or C_{1q}-binding at least, which we presume indicates immune complexes). In the same plate we also used a rapid anti-beta-lactoglobulin [121]I label, i.e., a radiolabeling assay. We then studied a group of nonallergic children and another group of children from our previous study with cow's milk allergy, and we showed that there was increased lactoglobulin demonstrable in the allergic children's sera, in the same samples that also had C_{1q}-binding. We feel this is indirect evidence that there are immune complexes and that the immune complexes, or at least the sera, contained beta-lactoglobulin in these milk-sensitive individuals.

Dr. Rieger: I don't think anyone knows why food allergy may lead to wheezing, but one thing we should remember is that an asthmatic may tolerate a lot of inhaled allergen for a long time without symptoms, but when he gets a respiratory infection he will develop airway hyperreactivity and will respond with wheezing to the same allergens which he has tolerated before. I think we tend to forget this phenomenon when we test for pulmonary reactions to food allergens. We should be taking care to test such patients during a period of airways hyperreactivity, or we should try to create such a situation for the tests. Another point is that people tend to have a fixation on wheezing; but before somebody starts to wheeze, a lot of other things happen—peripheral airway obstruction, bronchitis, subtle changes in pulmonary function tests, and so on. We should be thinking of these features when trying to establish the incidence of airways disease due to food allergy.

Dr. Frick: This is exactly why I think that those studies which have looked at pulmonary function tests after food challenge are particularly interesting (2,3). For instance, I think it is important that Silverman's study showed increased histamine sensitivity of the bronchi after food challenge, so one may expect to see a late-phase asthmatic response even if there is no immediate reaction to the food.

Food Allergy, edited by Eberhardt Schmidt.
Nestlé Nutrition Workshop Series, Vol. 17.
Nestec Ltd., Vevey/Raven Press, Ltd.,
New York © 1988.

Food Allergy and the Central Nervous System

Joseph Egger

University Children's Hospital, 8000 Munich 2, West Germany

The idea that what one eats influences how one feels and behaves is not new. More than two thousand years ago, Titus Lucretius Carus (55 B.C.) coined the saying "One man's meat is another man's poison." In the seventeenth century, Richard Burton proclaimed in the "Anatomy of Melancholy" that milk, as well as everything that is derived from milk, increases melancholy. The anaphylactic nature of some responses to foods was only recognized at the beginning of this century (38). Almost 30 years later, a comprehensive monograph was published on associations between food allergy and different symptoms of the central nervous system (68), to which little can be added to date.

Interactions between psyche and soma are complex, and nowhere is this better demonstrated than in patients with multiple allergies. In these patients, psychosomatic and somatopsychic influences sometimes interact to such an extent that without systematic controlled provocation studies it would be impossible to accept a causative role for food-allergic disease.

IS IT ALLERGY?

Most clinical immunologists prefer to restrict the term "allergy" to immunologically mediated intolerances, and some prefer to restrict it to IgE-mediated reactions only. Others, applying a more historical perspective (86), use it as a more general term for adverse reactions. Food allergy provoking symptoms of the central nervous system is not IgE-mediated, and no known immunological mechanisms have been identified to explain this association. Moreover, the interval between eating an allergy-provoking food and appearance of symptoms may last several days, which, from an immunological point of view, is not easily explained. However, several features suggest allergy rather than other types of intolerance: (a) a wide variety of foods with, as far as we know, nothing in common can provoke symptoms; (b) a food-allergic reaction can be outgrown, which would not be expected from other types of intolerance; and (c) foods provoking symptoms of the central nervous system sometimes also provoke eczema and/or wheezing and/or rhinitis. For these reasons the term "allergy" is used in this chapter. Excluded are symptoms of the central nervous system caused by known metabolic, pharmacological, or toxic mechanisms.

FOOD ALLERGY AND NEUROLOGICAL DISORDERS

Migraine

The cause of migraine is not known. Perhaps migraine is best regarded as a neurovascular syndrome with a generalized vasomotor instability and vulnerability to multiple factors. The apparent precipitating factors (Table 1) may be the final event leading to decompensation of the system. Whether food intolerance is but one of the precipitating factors or whether it is causing the neurovascular instability cannot be answered at present.

Publications concerning the relationship between migraine and dietary factors can be separated into two groups according to whether they support the tyramine hypothesis or the food allergy hypothesis.

Tyramine Hypothesis

Hannington (44) reported that foods containing tyramine or other vasoactive amines may precipitate headaches, particularly in patients who are treated with monoamino-oxidase inhibitors. A defect in the conjugation of tyramine and phenylethylamine was incriminated by some authors (71), whereas others proposed a deficiency of platelet phenolsulfotransferase (51), but double-blind administration of tyramine to patients who seemed to be affected in this way did not provoke migraine (15).

TABLE 1. *Precipitating factors*

Emotions
Food
Trauma
Exertion
Upper-respiratory-tract infection
Hypoglycemia
Lactose intolerance
Irregular sleep
Weather changes
Travel
Bright light
Noise
Hormones

Food Allergy Hypothesis

There are multiple case reports in the older literature of migraine attacks which have been associated with severe generalized allergic reactions to foods (8,42,52,58,59,61,68,74,77,85). Although most were purely anecdotal and are now regarded as impressionistic and unscientific, there is good evidence to incriminate food allergy in children with severe migraine (33). However, it does not appear that this is due to central involvement of allergic mechanisms but rather to an influence on the permeability of the gut allowing increased ingress of vasoactive substances.

The Oligoantigenic Approach

All foods are potential allergens, and an oligoantigenic diet should contain as few foods as possible (Table 2). Sometimes the foods chosen may be provoking ones, and if there is no improvement or deterioration, an alternative oligoantigenic diet avoiding foods included in the first diet should be tried. If recovery or definite improvement occurs during 3 or 4 weeks of oligoantigenic diet treatment, other foods are reintroduced one by one at weekly intervals. If symptoms occur reproducibly with a certain food, it is withdrawn and eventually tested in a double-blind placebo-controlled crossover study (12).

The value of an oligoantigenic diet was demonstrated by a double-blind, placebo-controlled crossover trial (35), during which 93% of children with severe and frequent migraine ($>$1 per week) were shown to benefit.

During the sequential reintroduction of foods at weekly intervals, 90% of the responders relapsed with one or more foods (Table 3) but recovered by avoiding them. The interval between eating a provoking food and migraine varied from minutes to more than a week but was usually 2 to 3 days.

Forty-six children, in whom a provoking food was identified, entered a double-blind placebo-controlled crossover trial of the provoking food, and significantly more patients had headaches with active material ($p<0.001$) than with placebo (Table 4).

TABLE 2. *Example of an oligoantigenic diet*

Lamb, turkey
Potatoes, rice
Pears, bananas
Brassicas
Sunflower oil
Water, mineral water
Calcium, vitamins

TABLE 3. *Provocative foods in migraine (76 patients)*

Food	Number tested	Number reacted	Percent
Cow's milk	75	29	39
Chocolate	64	24	37
Benzoic acid	46	17	37
Eggs	71	26	36
Tartrazine	45	15	33
Wheat	71	22	31
Cheese	48	15	31
Citrus	72	22	30
Coffee	21	5	24
Fish	51	11	22
Maize	53	9	17
Grapes	23	4	17
Goat's milk	44	7	16
Tea	44	7	16
Pork	60	8	13
Beef	64	8	12
Beans	42	9	12
Malt	33	3	9
Lentils	21	2	9
Apples	74	6	8
Yeast	54	4	7
Pears	69	4	6
Apricots	48	3	6
Sugar	56	3	5
Potatoes	76	4	5
Peas	37	2	5
Bananas	78	4	5
Carrots	76	3	4
Chicken	73	3	4
Peaches	51	2	4
Lamb	75	2	3
Rice	75	9	1
Brassica	76	1	1

TABLE 4. *Double-blind placebo-controlled crossover trial[a,b]*

Occurrence of headaches on:	AP	PA	Both
Neither food	2	6	8
Active food	14	12	26
Placebo	0	2	2
Both foods	1	3	4
Total:	17	23	40

[a]AP versus PA = NS; A versus P = S ($p < 0.001$).
[b]A, active material; P, placebo; NS, not significant; S, significant.

Epilepsy

Throughout this century, a possible provocation of seizures by foods or other allergens has variously been reported (9,19,23,33,35,77,83). Some other clinical studies of epileptics reported an unusually high prevalence of allergic disorders (1,11,22,24,25,76,87,89), whereas an increased prevalence of electroencephalographic abnormalities, often with occipital dysrhythmias, was present in patients with allergic disorders (5,10,14,24–26,41,78,82). However, others have not found an association between allergy and epilepsy (36), and the majority of reports on foods and seizures are anecdotal and open to alternative hypotheses. An exception is the study with double-blind placebo-controlled provocations in only one patient by Crayton et al. (19) and the double-blind placebo-controlled provocation studies on 16 children with epilepsy who had undergone oligoantigenic diet treatment for migraine and/or hyperkinetic behavior (33,35). The results of these studies clearly show that some patients with epilepsy recover by avoiding certain foods. However, a subsequent study on 63 patients (34) indicated that patients with epilepsy who also suffer from migraine and/or the hyperkinetic syndrome respond to dietary treatment, whereas patients with epilepsy alone do not. It is possible that these patients suffer from an otherwise latent form of epilepsy which is activated by migraine-induced disturbances of cerebral perfusion (50). Similarly, focal cerebral hypoperfusion was shown to occur in children with the hyperkinetic syndrome (53). Although there was marked clinical improvement of the epilepsy and of migraine in these patients, there was little change on the EEG (34). This, along with the fact that epilepsy did not improve as long as the patients continued to have headaches, would support the hypothesis that migraine was the trigger of an otherwise latent epilepsy. Both epileptic seizures and migraine and/or hyperkinetic behavior recurred reproducibly when allergy-provoking foods were eaten. In patients who responded to dietary treatment, it was possible to phase out anticonvulsants without relapse of seizures. Although it seems that only the minority of epileptic patients who suffer from both epilepsy and migraine respond to dietary treatment, this is an important step because some might recover by just avoiding certain foods.

FOOD ALLERGY AND PSYCHIATRIC DISORDERS

The Hyperkinetic Syndrome

Hyperkinetic behavior is defined by overactivity, impulsivity, distractability, and excitability. There is no standard of what is a normal level of activity on which to base comparisons, and the threshold for viewing such behavior as pathological or as a specific syndrome varies very markedly between countries, between parents, and between different physicians.

So far, reliable and valid tests of overactivity are not available. For practical purposes, behavior rating scales are used such as that of Conners (16) (Table 5), and classification is by the criteria of the Diagnostic and Statistical Manual III (3).

Etiology

Many causes of overactivity have been proposed (Table 6), and more than 92 terms have been used to describe hyperactive children; the most common of these terms are "attention-deficit disorder," "minimal brain dysfunction," and "hyperkinetic syndrome."

Therapy

A number of treatments have been used, the most common of which are psychostimulant drugs (40), behavioral approaches (64), and diets.

Concern about the undesirable effects of drug treatment, as well as the mounting evidence for the lack of long-term efficacy of both drug treatment and behavioral methods, has led to a focus on diets. The diets tested in double-blind controlled trials were Feingold's diet (17,45,81,84,90,92), Hafer's phosphate-reduced diet (88), and oligoantigenic diets (33).

The Feingold Hypothesis

In June 1975 a preliminary report was presented by Feingold (37), in which it was proposed that hyperkinesis in childhood is associated with the ingestion of

TABLE 5. *Conners' abbreviated rating scales*

	Degree of activity			
Observation	Not at all	Just a little	Pretty much	Very much
Restless or overactive				
Excitable, impulsive				
Disturbs other children				
Fails to finish things				
Short attention span				
Constantly fidgeting				
Inattentive, easily distracted				
Demands must be met immediately				
Easily frustrated				
Cries often and easily				
Mood changes quickly and drastically				
Temper outbursts				
Explosive and unpredictable behavior				
Scoring:	0	1	2	3

TABLE 6. *Suspected causes of overactivity*

Inherited hyperkinetic syndrome
Adverse psychosocial situations
Perinatal problems
Brain damage
Brain dysfunction
Epilepsy
Anticonvulsants
Lead poisoning
Maternal smoking during pregnancy
Maternal alcohol intake during pregnancy
Maternal drug abuse or drug intake during pregnancy
Atopy
Hypersensitivity to salicylates and synthetic food additives
Food allergy
Malnutrition
Metabolic disorders
Syndromes
Chromosomal abnormalities

salicylates, food additives, and colors. Feingold treated hyperactive children with diets that eliminated all food additives as well as natural salicylates, and he claimed success in 70% of these cases. His findings were impressionistic, anecdotal, and lacking in objective evidence. Subsequently, a number of double-blind trials involving control diets and diets eliminating artificial colors, flavors, and salicylates were conducted on children with well-defined hyperkinetic syndrome (17,45,81,84,90,92). The results of these controlled studies of Feingold's hypothesis are all somewhat equivocal, but the broad conclusions were that Feingold's claims had probably been exaggerated. The reason for the uncertainty is the lack of comparability between studies because of (a) the heterogeneity of patients studied and (b) differences in dietary manipulations. Moreover, research designs were inadequate; control diets were used whose effects on behavior had not been studied (17,45); no washout periods were inserted in between the test periods, which were probably disturbed by carry-over effects (45,81,84,90,92); both active and placebo material were disguised in chocolate and sugar-containing materials (81,84,92), although it is known that these substances are likely to have adverse effects on behavior (33); and the challenges were administered only for 1 or 2 days (81,90), thus not allowing the symptoms to develop. However, all studies showed that some hyperactive children, or certain subgroups of them, may benefit from an additive-free diet.

The Phosphate Hypothesis

According to Hafer (13), phosphate is thought to play a major role in causing the hyperkinetic syndrome. Again, her evidence was purely anecdotal, and a controlled study on 35 children did not show a reproducible effect of the phosphate (88). However, children on a phosphate-reduced diet would avoid many foods, including cow's milk, chocolate, and foods containing artificial colors and preservatives, and it is not unlikely that occasionally children improve with this diet.

The Food Allergy Hypothesis

A role for food allergy in the hyperkinetic syndrome has been postulated since early this century (18,21,47,65,67,69,77). Because of the lack of scientific documentation, this hypothesis was rejected until the highly significant results of a double-blind placebo-controlled crossover trial were published (33). Seventy-six children took part in this experiment. All were socially handicapped by their behavior, and overactivity and inattention were prominent features. The children were selected for severe overactivity and may not be representative of hyperkinetic children in the general population. A surprisingly high proportion had associated symptoms such as recurrent headaches, abdominal pains, limb pains, and epileptic seizures, and ony 10 did not have any associated symptoms. Of all the children, 82% responded to an oligoantigenic diet. However, only 27% recovered completely. Most of the associated symptoms also improved with diet. During the subsequent reintroduction, the substances that most commonly caused problems were tartrazine and benzoic acid, but no child reacted to these alone. Forty-six other provocative foods were also identified (Table 7), and most patients reacted to several of these (Table 8) reproducibly. The interval between eating an allergy-provoking food and reaction was usually 2 to 3 days, but it varied from a few minutes to more than 7 days. Comparison between synthetic additives and foods showed that there was no difference in type of reaction and length of the interval between eating the allergy-provoking item and appearance of symptoms.

Twenty-eight patients completed the double-blind placebo-controlled crossover trial of the effect of reintroduction of an allergy-provoking food. The parents kept daily Conners' scores, and a pediatrician and a child psychologist independently made an assessment of the children's behavior for each arm of the double-blind trial. The psychologist also employed actometer readings, "matching familiar figures" tests, and the Forteus maze test. Parents, the pediatrician, and the psychologist assessed the period in which the placebo material was administered as being linked significantly more often with better behavior (Table 9).

Prognosis

Some of the patients don't react to the allergy-provoking food when they are tested again after avoiding it for about 1 year. On the other hand, sometimes foods previously shown not to cause problems (usually after viral infections) start to provoke symptoms and have to be avoided.

TABLE 7. *Provocative foods in 62 patients with hyperkinetic syndrome*

Food	Number tested	Symptoms	Percent
Colorant and preservatives	34	27	79
Soya	15	11	73
Cow's milk	55	35	64
Chocolate	34	20	59
Grapes	18	9	50
Wheat	53	25	49
Oranges	49	22	45
Cow's-milk cheese	15	6	40
Hen's eggs	50	20	39
Peanuts	19	6	32
Maize	38	11	29
Fish	48	11	23
Oats	43	10	23
Melons	29	6	21
Tomatoes	35	7	20
Ham/bacon	20	4	20
Pineapple	31	6	19
Sugar	55	9	16
Beef	49	8	16
Beans	34	5	15
Peas	33	5	15
Malt	20	3	15
Apples	53	7	13
Pork	38	5	13
Pears	47	5	12
Chicken	56	6	11
Potatoes	54	6	11
Tea	19	2	10
Coffee	10	1	10
Other nuts	71	1	10
Cucumbers	32	3	9
Bananas	52	4	8
Carrots	55	4	7
Peaches	47	3	7
Lamb	55	3	5
Turkey	22	1	5
Rice	51	2	4
Yeast	28	1	4
Apricots	34	1	3
Onions	49	1	2

Early investigators thought that the hyperkinetic syndrome was a time-limited condition that disappeared after adolescence. Although hyperactivity may diminish with age, it is now recognized that antisocial behavior, educational retardation, depression, and psychosis are prevalent in adolescents and adults who were hyperkinetic children (56,57,91). It is too early to speculate whether dietary management will influence the prognosis of hyperkinetic children. However, there are reports suggesting that antisocial behavior in young delinquents was often related

TABLE 8. *Number of patients reacting to different numbers of food*

Number of foods	Number of patients
1	5
2	4
3	4
4	8
5	4
6	9
7	3
8	4
9	3
10	3
11	2
12	2
18	1
21	1
27	1
30	2

TABLE 9. *Double-blind placebo-controlled crossover trial[a,b]*

Behavior better on:	Pediatrician			Parents			Psychologist		
	PA	AP	Both	PA	AP	Both	AP	PA	Both
Neither	3	4	7	2	2	4	5	4	9
Placebo	12	8	20	13	10	23	7	6	13
Active	0	1	1	0	1	1	0	2	2
Total:	15	13	28	15	13	28	12	12	24

[a]PA versus AP = NS; A versus P < 0.001.
[b]A, Active material; P, placebo; NS, not significant; S, significant.

to certain foods and food additives (73) and that schizophrenics on a milk-free and cereal-free diet were released from the hospital twice as fast as those given the regular hospital diet (30).

Schizophrenia

Variously, an association between foods and schizophrenia has been reported (30,31,54,75). Dohan observed that a cereal-free and milk-free diet lessens psychiatric symptoms in hospitalized patients, and he was able to discharge patients on this diet twice as fast as those on usual hospital diets. His approach was based

TABLE 10. *Schizophrenia: avoidance of wheat*

Study	Sample size	Improvement	Statistically significant
Dohan et al. (30)	115	Yes	Yes
Dohan et al. (31)	102	Yes	Yes
Storms et al. (79)	26	No	No
Singh and Kay (75)	14	Yes	Yes
Potkin et al. (63)	8	No	No
Osborne et al. (60)	5	No	No

on epidemiological evidence for an association between celiac disease, wheat consumption, and schizophrenia (28). Singh and Kay (75) studied the effects of blind administration of wheat on hospitalized schizophrenics and found worsening of multiple psychopathological symptoms during the 4 weeks on wheat. An increased rate of antibodies to wheat and rye, detected by indirect immunofluorescence (46), and the finding that 17% to 20% of schizophrenics have antibodies to wheat gliadin, detected by enzyme-linked and latex agglutination techniques (32,46), seem to support the hypothesis of a wheat intolerance in patients with schizophrenia. However, other researchers were unable to confirm these observations (60,63,79) (Table 10).

Subsequently, alternative hypotheses were proposed, for example that of peptide effects of specific foods. Dohen (29) suggested that the basic biological defect in schizophrenia was a genetic impairment of the gut and other barriers of the body which permits the passage of food-derived neuroactive peptides from the gut to the brain. Other researchers discovered that digestion of wheat generates exorphins (49), which could act as neuromodulators and thereby alter behavior.

Direct evidence for any of these hypotheses is still needed, and the role of foods in schizophrenia has to be confirmed by double-blind controlled trials.

Affective Disorders

Several publications on food allergy contain statements that mania, depression, and other neurotic and psychotic changes can be induced by food (7,39,66,68,77). Surprisingly few systematic studies are available on this issue. Although the double-blind study by King (48) showed a definite deterioration of cognitive-emotional symptoms after allergen challenges, it cannot be accepted as evidence, since both active and placebo material were not disguised properly and it is likely that the patients were able to taste the difference. In another double-blind placebo-controlled study of capsule food challenges in 40 depressed patients and 20 control subjects, a subgroup of patients experienced provocation of their psychiatric symptoms with specific food challenges (20) as well as activation of the early components of complement. However, Pearson et al. (62), using double-blind placebo-controlled challenges of dried foods in capsules, were unable to confirm true reactions to foods in a significant number of patients who believed that they were sensitive to certain foods. Moreover, they found that patients in whom food allergy was not confirmed had neurotic depressive disorders.

Studies of immunological tests in patients with depression showed positive allergen-specific IgE antibodies to a wide range of inhalant substances and foods in a greater percentage of depressive patients than in controls (80), and in a similar study it appeared that unipolar depressed women had the highest frequency of allergic disorders (55). A number of other immunological abnormalities has been reported in association with depression (2,4,72). At present, however, immunological abnormalities in patients with psychiatric disorders are poorly understood, and it is not clear whether (a) a depressed mood per se induces immune dysfunction (2,4,72), (b) adverse food reactions trigger both the depression and the immunological abnormality, or (c) an immunological abnormality induces food allergy and depression. Further research on the biopsychosocial dimensions may elucidate the complex interactions between these variables.

CONCLUSION

Taken together, the available research suggests that particular types of adverse food reactions sometimes correlate with neurological, psychiatric, and psychophysiological symptoms.

The diversity of foods involved, which apparently have nothing in common, is suggestive of allergy, and the adverse food effects may correlate with immunological abnormalities. However, diets may affect brain function in different ways.

Research into affective disorders and into Parkinson's disease has highlighted the importance of amino-acid-derived neurotransmitters in the regulation of brain function and has shown that brain levels can be affected by dietary precursors (93).

On the other hand, it has variously been reported that these patients may suffer specific food cravings, addiction, and withdrawal symptoms (66). The discovery of opiate-like peptides in milk (6) and wheat (49), as well as a possible induction of mast-cell degranulation by opiates (13), makes a relationship between food addiction and food allergy in some patients a possibility.

A similar relationship might exist between food-allergic reactions and presently unknown enzyme defects which might lead to abnormal metabolism of chemical compounds and other substances.

In humans and experimental animals, allergic changes may become a conditioned reflex after repeated allergen exposure (27,70). These data suggest a two-way communication between mind and body as well as between the central nervous system and the immune system (2); it's not all in the mind, but some of it might be.

REFERENCES

1. Adamson WD, Sellers ED. Observations on the incidence of a hypersensitive state in 100 cases of epilepsy. *J Allergy* 1932;4:315–23.
2. Ader R. *Psychoneuroimmunology*. New York: Academic Press, 1981.
3. American Psychiatric Association. *Diagnostic and statistical manual of mental disorders*, 3rd edition. Washington, DC: American Psychiatric Association, 1980:42–4.
4. Bartrop RW, Luckhurst E, Lazarus L, et al. Depressed lymphocyte function after bereavement. *Lancet* 1977;1:834–6.
5. Beauchemin JA. Allergic reactions in mental diseases. *Am J Psychiatry* 1935;92:1190.
6. Brantl V, Teschenmacher HA. A material with opioid activity in bovine milk and milk products. *Naunyn-Schmiedebergs Arch Pharmacol* 1979;306:301–4.
7. Brown M, Gibney M, Husband PR, Radcliffe M. Food allergy in polysymptomatic patients. *Practitioner* 1981;225:1651–4.
8. Brown RC. The protein of foodsuffs as a factor in the cause of headache. *Wisconsin Med J* 1920;19:337.
9. Campbell MB. Allergy and epilepsy. In: Speer F, ed. *Allergy of the nervous system*. Springfield, Illinois: Charles C Thomas, 1970:59–78.
10. Campbell MB. Neurologic manifestations of allergic disease. *Ann Allergy* 1973;31:485–98.
11. Campbell MB. Neurological and psychiatric aspects of allergy. *Otolaryngol Clin North Am* 1974;7:805.
12. Carter CM, Egger J, Soothill JF. A dietary management of severe childhood migraine. *Hum Nutr Appl Nutr* 1985;39A:294–303.
13. Casale TB, Bowman S, Kaliner M. Induction of human cutaneous mast cell degranulation by opiates and endogenous opioid peptides: evidence for opiate and non-opiate receptor participation. *J Allergy Clin Immunol* 1984;73:775.
14. Chobot R, Dundy HD, Pacella BL. The incidence of abnormal electroencephalographic patterns in allergic children. *J Allergy* 1950;21:334–8.
15. Congdon PJ, Forsythe WI. Migraine in childhood: a study of 300 children. *Dev Med Child Neurol* 1979;21:209–16.
16. Conners CK. Rating scales for use in drug studies with children. *Psychopharmacol Bull* (Special Issue: Pharmacotherapy with children) 1973;24–48.
17. Conners CK, Goyette CH, Southwick DA, et al. Food additives and hyperkinesis: a controlled double-blind experiment. *Pediatrics* 1976;58:154–66.
18. Cooke RA. Studies in specific hypersensitiveness. On the phenomenon of hyposensitization (the clinically lessened sensitiveness of allergy). *J Immunol* 1922;7:219.
19. Crayton JW, Stone T, Stein G. Epilepsy precipitated by food sensitivity: report of a case with double-blind placebo-controlled assessment. *Clin Electroencephalogr* 1981;12:192–8.
20. Crayton JW. Effects of food challenges on complement components in food-sensitive psychiatric patients and controls. *J Allergy Clin Immunol* (Suppl) 1984;73:134.
21. Crook WG, Harrison WW, Cawford SE, Emmerson BS. Systemic manifestations due to allergy. *Pediatrics* 1961;27:790–9.
22. Cunningham AS, Allergy, immunodeficiency and epilepsy. *Lancet* 1975;II:975.
23. Davison HM. Allergy of the nervous system. *Q Rev Allergy Immunol* 1952;6:157–88.
24. Dees SC. Electroencephalography in allergic epilepsy. *South Med J* 1953;46:618–20.
25. Dees SC. Neurologic allergy in childhood. *Pediatr Clin North Am* 1954;1:1017–27.
26. Dees SC, Loewenbach H. Allergic epilepsy. *Ann Allergy* 1951;9:446–58.
27. Dekker E, Pelser HE, Grosen J. Conditioning as a cause of asthmatic attacks: a laboratory study. *J Psychosom Res* 1957;2:97–108.
28. Dohan FC. The possible pathogenetic effect of cereal grains in schizophrenia. Celiac disease as a model. *Acta Neurol (Napoli)* 1976;31:195–205.

29. Dohan FC. Schizophrenia and neuroactive peptides from food. *Lancet* 1979;1:1031.
30. Dohan FC, Grasberger JC. Relapsed schizophrenics: earlier discharge from the hospital after cereal-free milk-free diet. *Am J Psychiatry* 1973;130:685–8.
31. Dohan FC, Grasberger JC, Lowell FM, et al. Relapsed schizophrenics: more rapid improvement on a milk- and cereal-free diet. *Br J Psychiatr* 1969;115:595–6.
32. Dohan FC, Martin L, Grasberger JC, et al. Antibodies to wheat gliadin in blood of psychiatric patients: possible role of emotional factors. *Biol Psychiatry* 1972;5:127–37.
33. Egger J, Carter CM, Graham PJ, Gamley D, Soothill JF. Controlled trial of oligoantigenic diet treatment in the hyperkinetic syndrome. *Lancet* 1985;1:540–5.
34. Egger J, Carter CM, Soothill JF, Wilson J. Oligoantigenic diet treatment in children with epilepsy and migraine. *In press*.
35. Egger J, Carter CM, Wilson J, et al. Is migraine food allergy? A double-blind controlled trial of oligoantigenic diet treatment. *Lancet* 1983,II:865–9.
36. Fein BT, Kamin PB. Allergy, convulsive disorders, and epilepsy. *Ann Allergy* 1968;26:241–7.
37. Feingold BF. Hyperkinesis and learning disabilities linked to artificial food flavours and colors. *Am J Nurs* 1975;75:797–803.
38. Finkelstein H. Kuhmilch als Ursache akuter Ernährungsstörungen bei Säuglingen. *Monatsschr Kinderheilk* 1905;4:65.
39. Finn R, Cohen NH. Food allergy: fact or fiction? *Lancet* 1978;1:426–8.
40. Flintoff MM, Barron RW, Swanson JM, et al. Methylphenidate increases selectivity of visual scanning in children referred for hyperactivity. *J Abnorm Child Psychol* 1982;10:145–63.
41. Fowler WM, Heimlich EM, Walter RD, et al. Electroencephalographic patterns in children with allergic convulsive and behaviour disorders. *Ann Allergy* 1962;20:1–14.
42. Grant HEC. Food allergies and migraine. *Lancet* 1977;I:966–9.
43. Hafer H. Nahrungsphosphat—Die heimliche Droge. *Ursache für Verhaltensstörungen, Schulversagen und Jugendkriminalität.* Heidelberg: Kriminalistik Verlag, 1984.
44. Hannington E. Preliminary report on tyramine headache. *Br Med J* 1967;II:550–1.
45. Harley PJ, Ray RS, Tomasi L, et al. Hyperkinesis and food additives: testing the Feingold hypothesis. *Pediatrics* 1978;61:818–28.
46. Hekkens, WThJM, Schipperijn AJM, Freed DLJ. Antibodies to wheat proteins in schizophrenia: relationship or coincidence? In: Hemmings G, ed. *Biochemistry in schizophrenia and addiction.* Lancaster: MTP Press. 1980:125–33.
47. Hoobler BR. Some early symptoms suggesting protein sensitization in infancy. *Am J Dis Child* 1916;12:129.
48. King DS. Can allergic exposure provoke psychological symptoms? A double-blind test. *Biol Psychiatry* 1981;16:3–19.
49. Klee WA, Zioudrou, Streaty RA. Exorphins: peptides with opioid activity isolated from wheat gluten, and their possible role in the etiology of schizophrenia. In: Usdin E, Bunney WE, Kline NS, eds. *Endorphins in mental health research.* New York: Oxford University Press, 1979:209–18.
50. Lauritzen M, Olessen J. Regional cerebral blood flow during migraine attacks by Xenon-133 inhalation and emission tomography. *Brain* 1984;107:447–461.
51. Littlewood J, Glover V, Sandler M. Platelet phenolsulfotransferase deficiency in dietary migraine. *Lancet* 1982;II:983–6.
52. Liveing E. *On megrim, sick headaches and some allied disorders.* London: J & A Churchill, 1873.
53. Lou HC, Henriksen L, Bruhn P. Focal cerebral hypoperʼusion in children with dysphasia and/or attention deficit disorder. *Arch Neurol* 1984;41:825–8.
54. Macharness R. *Not all in the mind.* London: PanBooks, 1976.
55. Matussek P, Agerer D, Seibt G. Allergic disorders in depressive patients. *Compr Psychiatry* 1983;24:25–34.
56. Mendelson W, Johnson N, Stewart M. Hyperactive children as teenagers: a follow up study. *J Nerv Ment Dis* 1971;153:237–9.
57. Menkes MM, Rowe JS, Menkes JH. A twenty-five year follow-up study on the hyperkinetic child with minimal brain dysfunction. *Pediatrics* 1967;39:393–9.
58. Minot GR. The role of low carbohydrate diet in the treatment of migraine and headache. *Med Clin North Am* 1923;7:715.

59. Monro J, Brostoff J, Carini C, Zilkha KJ. Food allergy in migraine. *Lancet* 1980;II:1–4.
60. Osborne M, Crayton JW, Javaid J, Davis JM. Lack of effect of a gluten-free diet on neuroleptic blood levels in schizophrenic patients. *Biol Psychiatry* 1982;17:627–9.
61. Pagniez P, Vallery-Raddt P, Nast A. Therapeutique preventative de certaines migraine. *Presse Med* 1919;27:172.
62. Pearson, DJ, Rix KJ, Bentley SJ. Food allergy: how much in the mind? A clinical and psychiatric study of suspected food hypersensitivity. *Lancet* 1983;1:1259–61.
63. Potkin SG, Weinberger D, Kleinman J, et al. Wheat-gluten challenge in schizophrenic patients. *Am J Psychiatry* 1981;138:1208–11.
64. Prior M, Griffin M. *Hyperactivity. Diagnosis and management.* London: William Heinemann Medical Books, 1985.
65. Randolph TG. Allergy as a causative factor for fatigue, irritability, and behaviour problems of children. *J Pediatr* 1947;31:560–72.
66. Randolph TG. Specific adaptation. *Ann Allergy* 1978;40:333–45.
67. Rapp DJ. *Allergies and the hyperactive child.* New York: Cornerstone Library, 1979.
68. Rowe AH. *Food allergy, its manifestations, diagnosis and treatment.* Philadelphia: Lea & Febiger, 1931.
69. Rowe AH. Allergic toxemia and fatigue. *Ann Allergy* 1950;8:22.
70. Russel M, Dark KA, Cummins RW, et al. Learned histamine release. *Science* 1984;225:733–4.
71. Sandler MMBH, Hannington E. A phenyl-aethylamine oxidizing defect in migraine. *Nature* 1974;250–335.
72. Schleifer SJ, Keller SE, Meyerson AT, et al. Lymphocyte function in major depressive disorder. *Arch Gen Psychiatry* 1984;41:484–6.
73. Schoenthaler SJ. Diet and delinquency: a multi-state replication. *Int J Biosoc Res* 1983; 5:70–117.
74. Sheldon JM, Randolph TG. Allergy in migraine-like headaches. *Am J Med Sci* 1935;190–232.
75. Singh MM, Kay SR. Wheat gluten as a pathogenic factor in schizophrenia. *Science* 1976;191:401–2.
76. Spangler RH. Allergy and epilepsy *J Lab Clin Med* 1927;12:41–58.
77. Speer F. *Allergy of the nervous system.* Springfield, Illinois: Charles C Thomas, 1970.
78. Sternberg TH, Baldridge GD. Electroencephalographic abnormalities in patients with generalized neurodermatitis. *J Invest Dermatol* 1948;11:401–3.
79. Storms LH, Clopton JM, Wright C. Effects on gluten on schizophrenics. *Arch Gen Psychiatry* 1982;39:323–7.
80. Sugerman AA, Southern DL, Curran JF. A study of antibody levels in alcoholic, depressive and schizophrenic patients. *Ann Allergy* 1982;48:166–71.
81. Swanson JM, Kinsbourne M. Food dyes impair performance of hyperactive children on a laboratory learning test. *Science* 1980;207:1485–7.
82. Terrel CO, Stephens WE, Morris R. Eosinophilia and neurological dysfunction—a preliminary report. *Ann Allergy* 1967;25:673–7.
83. Thompson J. Clinical types of convulsive seizures in very young babies with a special consideration of so-called idiopathic convulsions of early infancy and their treatment. *Br Med J* 1921;II:679–83.
84. Thorley G. Pilot study to assess behavioural and cognitive effects of artificial food colours in a group of retarded children. *Dev Med Child Neurol* 1984;26:56–61.
85. Unger AH, Unger L. Migraine is an allergic disease. *J Allergy* 1952;23:429–40.
86. van Pirquet CE. Allergie. *Klin Wochenschr* 1906;53:1457.
87. Wallis RM, Nicol WD, Craig M. The importance of protein hypersensitivity in the diagnosis and treatment of a special group of epileptics. *Lancet* 1923;i:741–3.
88. Walther B. Nahrungsphosphat und Verhaltensstörung im Kindesalter. Ergebnisse einer kontrollierten Diätstudie. In: Steinhausen HC, ed. *Das Konzentrationsgestörte und hyperaktive Kind.* Berlin: Kohlhammer Verlag Stuttgart, 1984.
89. Ward JF, Peterson HA. Protein sensitization in epilepsy. *Arch Neurol Psychiatry* 1927;17:427–43.
90. Weiss B, Williams JH, Margen S, et al. Behavioral response to artificial food colors. *Science* 1980;207:1487–9.
91. Weiss G, Minde K, Werry JS, et al. Studies on the hyperactive child. VIII 5 year follow-up. *Arch Gen Psychiatry* 1971;24:409–14.

92. Williams JJ, Cram DM, Tausig FT, Webster E. Relative effects of drugs and diet on hyperactive behaviors: an experimental study. *Pediatrics* 1978;61:811–7.
93. Wurtman RJ. Behavioural effects of nutrients. *Lancet* 1983;i:1145–7.

DISCUSSION

Dr. Bellanti: In the patients with epilepsy who improved under diet, what happened to their antiepilepsy treatment? Were the drugs discontinued or reduced, or did they stay the same?

Dr. Egger: All the patients had been on anticonvulsants, and we made no changes to the treatment until we had done the double-blind provocations or completed the reintroduction phase, at least in the case of the most obviously offending foods, because we did not know what was going to happen. After this we were, in many cases, able to reduce and discontinue the drugs.

Dr. Bellanti: Had the patients been monitored with plasma anticonvulsant levels?

Dr. Egger: Yes. All patients were being treated in the Hospital for Sick Children, Great Ormond St., London, and their drug levels were monitored closely.

Dr. Challacombe: What effect did the diet have on the EEG in these patients?

Dr. Egger: We were not able to study EEG changes consistently, since this was not part of the original study design and we felt it was not justifiable to subject the children to yet more investigations when they had already had so much done. In the few cases where we were able to get EEG data, there was no consistent change. It seems to me to be probable that these children all, or mostly, have latent epilepsy, which is activated by the perfusion changes which occur in the brain during migraine but is otherwise not evident.

Dr. Frick: Would you comment on the possibility that food allergy induces confusion in these patients, in addition to seizures? The reason I ask is that there is a professor on our staff who is extremely sensitive to wheat, and when he is not on strict wheat elimination he is unable to respond to students' questions appropriately, although he is still able to give his lectures. When he is off wheat his performance is normal.

Dr. Egger: This could be part of the migraine complex. The "Alice in Wonderland" syndrome, or confusional states, are very well known in migraine patients, even in migraine without headache. They probably result from changes in perfusion in the brain. Recent studies have shown that children with hyperkinesis have abnormal perfusion patterns as well, though in these cases it is mainly the frontal lobe which is affected, whereas in migraine it is the occipital lobe initially.

Dr. Guesry: You speculate that ketogenic diets may work in epilepsy because such a diet is usually hypoallergenic. However, there is a recent report showing that medium-chain triglycerides (MCT) given in a diet which is not specifically hypoallergenic alleviate epilepsy through ketogenesis.

Dr. Egger: I think that if you consume a large amount of MCT you are bound to eat less of other foods. To become ketotic the patients will certainly have to cut down their carbohydrate intake. I have tried ketogenic diets on occasions, and it is very difficult to get children to be consistently ketotic.

Dr. Boelacher: I have some experience with ketogenic diets, and I think there are certain definite indications for it. However, they are mainly for those groups of epilepsies like the Lennox Syndrome in which you had no effect with the diet, or only partial effects. Therefore I think that ketogenic diets do not work because they are oligoallergenic.

Dr. Egger: I can only say that in my experience it is very difficult to keep a child on a ketogenic diet. Therefore, children with types of epilepsy which are more responsive to drug treatment than the myoclonic epilepsies are only rarely given ketogenic diets. However, I have found such diets to be effective on occasion in patients with other forms of epilepsy, so I would not rule out the possibility that the effect is mediated through a reduction in the allergenicity of the diet rather than ketosis per se.

Dr. Bakken: Do you have any idea of the molecular basis for the dietary effects you have shown?

Dr. Egger: No, we have no evidence about the mechanism, which remains to be elucidated. We believe that gut hormones and neurotransmitters probably play a role because many of the children have abdominal symptoms, and abdominal symptoms are the first ones to improve on diet. There were no patients with headache or other symptoms who responded to diet without gastrointestinal symptoms which responded too. During the reintroduction phase, gastrointestinal symptoms were always the first to appear when a provoking food was given, usually bloating, abdominal discomfort, loose stools, with an interval of up to 1 to 2 days before the onset of cerebral symptoms.

Dr. Lenard: Some of your patients with migraine were as young as 2 to 3 years of age. How do you define migraine in this age group?

Dr. Egger: We attached the label "abdominal migraine" to children in this age range who had abdominal symptoms with other signs of migraine such as pallor and vomiting.

Food Allergy, edited by Eberhardt Schmidt.
Nestlé Nutrition Workshop Series, Vol. 17.
Nestec Ltd., Vevey/Raven Press, Ltd.,
New York © 1988.

Immunologic Diagnostic Tests in Food Allergy

Alain L. de Weck

Institute for Clinical Immunology, Inselspital, University of Bern, 3010 Bern, Switzerland

Both for the clinician and the laboratory immunologist, the diagnosis of food allergies is a frustrating exercise, due to the pathophysiological complexity of food-induced adverse reactions on the one hand, and to the difficult interpretation of single immunologic tests or techniques on the other. A complete review of diagnostic tests of possible use in food allergy falls far beyond the scope of this chapter. Such reviews have been recently presented (1,2). We shall here restrict ourselves to food allergies as observed in infants and children, in particular to adverse reactions due to cow's milk (CMA).

GENERAL DIAGNOSTIC FEATURES OF COW'S MILK ALLERGY

In infants, adverse reactions to cow's milk take many clinical forms, a number of which are not due to allergy in a classic sense; that is, these reactions are not based on some form of immune response to cow's-milk antigens. Indeed, a number of adverse reactions are due to other causes, such as enzymatic defects (e.g., lactose intolerance), and are generally covered under the category of cow's milk intolerance. The various clinical aspects of adverse reactions to cow's milk in infants have been recently reviewed (3–5).

Even when considering only those reactions that appear to be based on immunologic mechanisms and to come under the general heading of CMA, one is impressed by the diversity of symptoms and symptom associations, as well as by marked differences in the kinetics of the reactions, in the doses of allergen required for challenge and in the persistence of symptoms over the years. An analysis of CMA case histories makes it clear that several immunopathological mechanisms (e.g., IgE, IgG, immune complexes, cellular immunity) may be involved, either singly or concomitantly. Exposure to the CM allergens may occur in various hidden ways (e.g., *in utero*, breast-feeding), and several other food allergens (e.g., egg, fish, nuts) are frequently involved as well. For all these reasons, it is not astonishing that according to a general consensus, "there is no

177

single and reliable laboratory test that can distinguish individuals allergic to cow milk from normal people'' (3,5,6).

Nevertheless, a subclassification of patients according to the nature and kinetics of their symptoms following ingestion of CM, as based on history and provocation challenge, throws some light on the immunologic mechanisms probably involved and reflected by various immunologic diagnostic tests (Table 1). The diagnosis is difficult in many individual cases because, in numerous instances, overlaps in symptomatology and poor correlation between clinical history and immunologic tests prevail.

The arsenal of diagnostic measures at our disposal for ascertaining the diagnosis of CMA is listed in Table 2. In the following, only problems related to immunologic tests will be discussed.

IMMUNOLOGIC TESTS IN CMA

As indicated in Table 1, CMA patients may be roughly classified as immediate, protracted, and late reactors, on the basis of CM challenge and history. It is assumed that most immediate reactions are related to the presence of IgE antibodies to CM proteins, whereas late reactors may primarily manifest a specific cellular hypersensitivity to CM. This interpretation, to some extent, dominates the current literature on CMA immunologic tests. As will be discussed below, the effective situation is probably much more complex.

TABLE 1. *Classification of clinical allergic reactions to cow's milk*

Type	Skin-prick test for CM	Total IgE	CM IgE	Lymphokine tests
Immediate reactors (45 min post-CM challenge) Acute perioral or generalized skin eruption; vomiting; wheezing; coughing; rhinitis	+ + +	+ + +	+ + +	+ or −
Protracted reactors (45 min to 20 hr post-CM challenge) Pallor; vomiting; diarrhea; irritation; failure to thrive; collapse (high CM amounts)	−	Normal	−	+ or −
Late reactors (> 20 hr post-CM challenge) Diarrhea (no vomiting); respiratory symptoms; eczema (AD)	+ or − (AD)	Normal or + + + (AD)	− or + + + (AD)	+ + +

AD, atopic dermatitis.

TABLE 2. *Diagnostic measures in cow's milk*
allergy/intolerance

Intolerance:	Xylose absorption test
	Lactose and sucrose tolerance test
	Stool fecal leukocyte test, fecal fat
	Small or large intestine biopsy
	X-ray examination
Allergy:	Skin-prick test with CM proteins
	Total IgE
	Specific IgE to CM
	IgG, IgA, IgG subclasses to CM
	Lymphocyte transformation test
	Leukocyte migration inhibition test (LIF)
	Elimination diet
	Placebo-controlled CM challenge

Skin Tests

Immediate wheal-and-erythema scratch or skin-prick tests for CM and/or for isolated CM proteins—in particular, beta-lactoglobulin—are positive in a high proportion (80–100%) of infants with immediate clinical reactions to CM, espe cially when affected also with atopic dermatitis (4). However, some infants with positive history of immediate reaction and positive CM challenge may have negative skin tests. Furthermore, 5% of healthy children (7) and 12% of atopic children without CMA symptoms show positive scratch tests to CM (8). Intradermal tests for CM are of little practical interest, since they are as often (if not more often) positive in atopic children without clinical CMA (68%) than in children with CMA (59%) (9).

Total IgE Determination

Infants with CMA frequently show abnormally elevated IgE levels, but this may be due primarily to the frequently associated atopic hereditary condition rather than to CMA itself. By itself, therefore, a high total IgE cannot be diagnostic of CMA. The early determination of total IgE in newborns and infants may, however, become of great practical importance in prevention of atopic diseases in general and of CMA in particular. As shown by numerous groups, newborns showing IgE levels higher than 1 IU/ml are at considerable risk of developing CMA, atopic dermatitis, and upper-airway allergies to inhalation allergens within the first 5 to 7 years of life. Early detection of such children, while still in the nursery, would enable us to take preventive measures, such as breast-feeding and/or hypoallergenic formulas.

The recent development (by our group) of a quick and simple total IgE assay

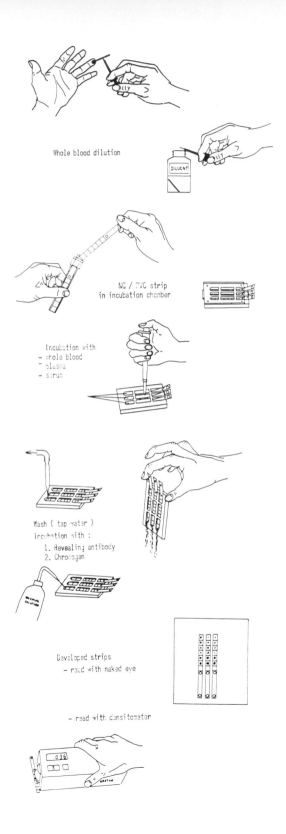

Whole blood dilution

NC / PVC strip
in incubation chamber

Incubation with
— whole blood
— plasma
— serum

Wash (tap water)
Incubation with :
　　1. Revealing antibody
　　2. Chromogen

Developed strips
　　— read with naked eye

　　— read with densitometer

FIG. 1. Total IgE assay.

(10,11) which discriminates cord bloods possessing IgE levels >1 IU/ml and which can be performed by nonlaboratory personnel (Fig. 1) should make the proper indication and use of these preventive measures easier.

Specific IgE Tests (RAST and Analogues)

According to several studies (reviewed in refs. 4 and 5), specific IgE antibodies to CM proteins are to be found in the majority of children with atopic dermatitis and immediate CMA. However, in children where CMA manifestations are protracted or delayed, especially in those where the symptoms remain strictly intestinal, the CM RAST tests are mostly negative. A positive RAST test for CM is relatively frequent in children who are not clinically sensitive to CM: 13% of children with atopic dermatitis and 3.5% of normal children. A positive RAST test is therefore no evidence of CMA (4).

It may be questioned as to whether technical problems with the usual RAST test with CM proteins may not interfere with the results. It is evident that most infants fed with CM develop rather high levels of IgG antibodies to CM proteins—hence the possibility that competition between IgE and IgG antibodies for the CM allergens bound to the solid phase might lead to false-negative results. We have obtained evidence that such competition phenomena do indeed occur in some categories of RAST tests, where high levels of IgG of the same specificity have to be expected.

For the screening of IgE specific to various CM proteins, an immunodot procedure similar to that described above for determination of total IgE may also be used (12). The advantages of this technique are: (a) a high sensitivity (~0.05 IU IgE/ml) and a quantitative discrimination over a high range of IgE levels; and (b) the possibility of screening IgE against a large variety of CM proteins in a single manipulation, thus enabling us to identify those allergens that are clinically relevant for individual patients.

The use of this technique makes it easy, for example, to check whether CM-allergic patients possibly possess IgE or IgG antibodies against milk proteins or against hypoallergenic formulas (Fig. 2) (M. Bättig, *personal communication*).

Specific IgG Antibodies Against CM Proteins

The presence of IgG antibodies against CM proteins is a normal finding in healthy individuals. In cord blood, about 50% of newborns show IgG anti-CM antibodies, presumably transferred from the mother, although they are usually in lower titer (4). Feeding with CM is followed by a rise in IgG anti-CM antibodies, especially in infants receiving CM in the first days after birth. In infants given CM soon after birth, the peak of IgG antibodies is reached at the age of 3 months, after which it remains stable or slowly declines over years.

Several tests have been used to detect IgG or IgA anti-CM antibodies: passive

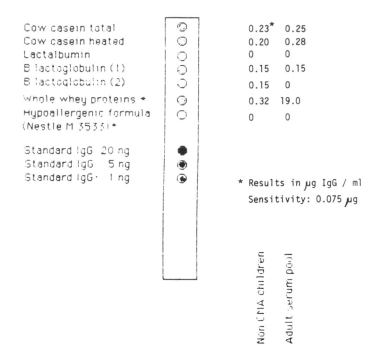

Cow casein total   0.23*   0.25
Cow casein heated   0.20   0.28
Lactalbumin   0   0
B lactoglobulin (1)   0.15   0.15
B lactoglobulin (2)   0.15   0
Whole whey proteins *   0.32   19.0
Hypoallergenic formula   0   0
(Nestle M 3533) *

Standard IgG 20 ng
Standard IgG   5 ng
Standard IgG· 1 ng

* Results in μg IgG / ml
Sensitivity: 0.075 μg

Non CMA children   Adult serum pool

FIG. 2. Detection of anti-CM IgG by immunodot.

hemagglutination, double diffusion in agar, and radioimmunoassays (4). According to the sensitivity of the test used, the percentage of positive healthy controls or of patients varies widely. In general, IgA deficiency and various intestinal diseases with mucosal damage (e.g., celiac disease, ulcerative colitis) are accompanied by rather high titers of anti-CM IgG antibodies; these seem also to be elevated in CMA.

Not yet fully clarified is the possible role in the pathogenesis or protection against the development of CMA of various anti-CM IgG subclasses (especially IgG_4) and of anti-CM IgA and IgM. Systematic follow-up studies of this kind are still relatively few, mostly because the RIA technology required for such studies is relatively cumbersome. In this respect also, the availability of the immunodot technique and of monoclonals against Ig subclasses could facilitate in-depth studies.

Other Serologic Tests

Among the other serologic tests that may be relevant for the diagnosis of CMA, we should include the determination of complement activation and of CM-containing immune complexes.

Although some positive results have been reported, the majority of controlled studies where complement components were followed during positive CM challenge revealed no sizable complement activation *in vivo* (4). This aspect, however, would deserve to be revisited with the help of the more sensitive and specific techniques which have become available during recent years.

The occurrence of immune complexes containing CM proteins following challenge has been reported (13). However, this finding alone does not mean that such complexes should exert pathogenic effects. To what extent more systematic investigations of CM-IgE and CM-IgG complexes would help in resolving the mechanism of the protracted intestinal manifestations of CMA remains unresolved.

Cellular Tests in Immediate-Type CMA

As in other IgE-mediated allergies, it is theoretically to be expected that peripheral blood basophils from CMA patients should undergo degranulation and histamine release when challenged *in vitro* with CM or CM proteins. Indeed, a few reports (14,15) along these lines have appeared, but studies have not been sufficiently extended and comparative between CMA patients and healthy individuals or atopics without CMA to evaluate the potential diagnostic interest of such tests.

Cellular Tests in Delayed-Type CMA

It can be postulated that reactions occurring more than 20 hr after CM challenge are primarily manifestations of interaction of CM allergens with sensitized T lymphocytes, with the release of inflammatory lymphokines.

Lymphocyte stimulation tests for CM proteins in patients with CMA are positive in 35% to 60% of the cases (4), to an equal extent whether the *in vivo* reaction upon CM challenge had been immediate or delayed. The lymphocyte stimulation appears not to be affected by the length of the CM-free diet or by recent feeding by CM. In controls without CMA, the incidence of positive lymphocyte stimulation to CM proteins is 9.3%.

Several groups have reported the interest of the leukocyte migration inhibition test (LIF), a lymphokine-detecting assay, in the evaluation of CMA patients with protracted or delayed onset (16–18). Although the LIF test has been used in clinical allergy in a wide range of indications in the 1970s, its popularity has considerably diminished in recent years, essentially because the test is relatively cumbersome and difficult to standardize. However, some more modern versions have recently been proposed (19).

A major drawback of most cellular tests performed on peripheral blood cells in infants is the fact that the number of cells which can be made available is relatively limited, while correct interpretation of the results would require the use of several CM antigens, dose-response curves, and appropriate controls. Although not yet applied to the problem of food allergy, a new technology which we have developed (quantitative kinetic microfluorometry, QKM) might, in the future, permit a

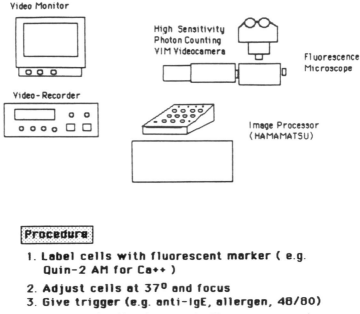

FIG. 3.   Quantitative kinetic microfluorometry (QKM).

whole new array of cellular investigations in infant allergy. This technique, the principle of which is shown in Fig. 3, enables us to assess kinetically and quantitatively the stimulation of single cells by allergens, in a mixed-cell population. This technique has only been applied to peripheral blood cells, bronchial lavage cells, and nasal scrapings, but it could probably be applied to intestinal biopsies and/or lavages.

INTERPRETATION OF IMMUNOLOGIC DIAGNOSTIC TESTS IN CMA: A LOOK INTO THE FUTURE

One of the major problems in the interpretation of immunologic tests in CMA is their imperfect correlation with clinical history of disease and provocation challenges. Patients with positive challenges may show negative immunologic tests, and healthy infants without clinical signs of CMA may exhibit positive immunologic tests. Although similar situations are also occasionally encountered in other types of allergic diseases—for example, in allergy to inhalation allergens—the case of CMA, particularly in its protracted and delayed forms, is often difficult. The reason for this is probably not so much the imperfection or poor sensitivity of the immunologic tests but rather the uncertainty and hesitations generated by provocation tests that are difficult to perform and that frequently yield somewhat subjective results.

Another difficulty in the interpretation of immunologic tests is the fact that none of the elements of an immune response occurs alone and/or exhibits a specific and exclusive correlation to a clinical type of response. For example, the presence of CM-specific IgE and immediate-type skin reactivity may not necessarily be associated with clinical symptoms following challenge. Several factors may be responsible for this, such as (a) the competition between CM-specific IgE, IgG, and IgA for CM reaching IgE-sensitized submucosal mast cells or (b) the relative ratio between CM-specific and other IgE bound to reactive mast cells. Indeed, recent studies have pointed out that the ratio between allergen-specific and total IgE is decisive for the size of the allergen-induced immediate skin reaction (C.S. Hong, *personal communication*). Similar competitive effects may be visualized between various IgG subclasses.

In terms of cellular reactivity, the obvious candidates as effector cells of reactions to CM proteins are specifically sensitized T-lymphocytes. However, it will soon have to be clarified as to whether helper and or suppressor lymphocytes are equally involved. It should also be investigated as to whether other cell types coated with CM-specific antibodies—for example, macrophages, eosinophils, and platelets, which have all been shown to become cytotoxic when armed with IgE antibodies—may also be involved in protracted or delayed CMA reactions.

In conclusion, it has become obvious that a correct and predictive immunologic diagnosis of CMA requires the simultaneous use of a battery of tests, which have to become more practical and standardized. Even then, the development of investigational techniques at the local (gut) level will increasingly become required for understanding the pathogenic factors involved.

SUMMARY

The various serologic and cellular immunologic tests that have been used in the diagnosis of CMA reactions have been briefly described. The relative value of serologic tests such as total IgE determination, evaluation of specific IgE and IgG antibodies against CM proteins, and other tests (complement activation, histamine release) for the detection and prediction of immediate-type CMA has also been discussed. The development of new immunodot techniques based on multiple assays should permit better assessment of the reaction patterns to be observed. For evaluation of cellular immunity to CM proteins, the development of new cytofluorometric assays at the single-cell level should enable us to perform tests on a very limited number of cells, as usually required in infants.

ACKNOWLEDGMENT

This work was supported, in part, by grants of the Swiss National Foundation for Scientific Research (No. 3,882,083).

REFERENCES

1. Brostoff J, Challacombe SJ. *Food allergy and intolerance*. London: Baillière Tindall, 1987.
2. Businco L. *Advances in pediatric allergy*. Amsterdam: Excerpta Medica, 1983.
3. Hill DJ. Cow's milk allergy in infants: some clinical and immunologic features. *Ann Allergy* 1986;57:225–8.
4. Savilahti E. Cow's milk allergy. *Allergy* 1981;36:73–88.
5. Businco L, Benincori N, Cantani A. The spectrum of food allergy in infancy and childhood. *Ann Allergy* 1986;57:213–8.
6. Jakobsson I, Lindberg T. A prospective study of cow's milk protein intolerance in Swedish infants. *Acta Paediatr Scand* 1979;68:853–9.
7. Buckley RH, Dees SC. Nutritional and antigenic effects of two bovine milk preparations in infants. *J Pediatr* 1966;69:238–45.
8. Bachman KD, Dees SC. Milk allergy II. Observations on incidence and symptoms of allergy to milk in allergic infants. *J Pediatr* 1957;20:400–7.
9. Goldman AS, Anderson DW, Sellers WA, et al. Milk allergy II. Skin testing of allergic and normal children with purified milk proteins, *Pediatrics* 1963;32:572–9.
10. Hong CS, Stadler BM, Wälti M, de Weck AL. Dot-immunobinding assay with monoclonal anti-IgE antibodies for the detection and quantitation of human IgE. *J Immunol Methods* 1986;95:195–202.
11. Derer M, De Weck AL, Stadler B, Guérin B. Dipstick for quick screening of total IgE in adults and infants blood. 1987, *submitted for publication*.
12. Hong CS, Wälti M, Stadler BM, de Weck AL. Dot-Immunobinding assay for the detection and quantitation of allergen specific human IgE. *J Immunol Methods (in press)*.
13. Cunningham-Rundles C. The identification of specific antigens in circulating immune complexes by an enzyme-linked immunosorbent assay: detection of bovine x-casein IgG complexes in human sera. *Eur J Immunol* 1981;11:504–9.
14. McLaughlan P, Coombs RRA. Latent anaphylactic sensitivity of infants to cow's milk proteins. Histamine release from blood basophils. *Clin Allergy* 1983;13:1–9.
15. Hartleib H, Heine W, Kusak H. Der Wert des Histaminliberationstestes für die Diagnostik der intestinalen Eiweissunverträglichkeit. *Monatschr Kinderheikd* 1983;131:451–4.
16. Minor JD, Tolber SG, Frick OL. Leukocyte inhibition factor in delayed-onset food allergy. *J Allergy Clin Immunol* 1980;66:314–21.
17. Ashkenazi A, Levin S, Idar D, et al. *In vitro* cell-mediated immunologic assay for cow's milk allergy. *Pediatrics* 1980;66:399–402.
18. Khoshoo V, Bhan MK, Arora NK, et al. Leukocyte migration inhibition in cow's milk intolerance. *Acta Paediatr Scand* 1986;75:308–12.
19. Sandru G. A method using ^{3}H-leucine-labeled granulocytes and macrophages for migration inhibition assay. *J Immunol Methods* 1984;69:23–32.

DISCUSSION

Dr. Strobel: I was very impressed with the immunodot technique you described. Maybe I missed the point, but I understood you were looking at antibodies against the "hypoallergenic" formulas. What was your positive control, and did you make sure that the peptides actually bound to the nitrocellulose? How did you obtain and measure antibodies against your so-called "hypoallergenic" feeds?

Dr. Weck: The question we tried to answer was whether these preparations still react with the natural IgG antibodies produced by cow's milk. What we can say is that, using the hypoallergenic formula, the capacity of reacting with human anti-milk IgG has been reduced to the point where you no longer detect it under these conditions.

Dr. Leroy: This last technique has enormous potential. Did I understand you correctly that it can be used in *in vivo* situations? How would you do that?

Dr. de Weck: It can be used *ex vivo*—in other words, on cells obtained from washings or scrapings (e.g., bronchial lavage).

Food Allergy, edited by Eberhardt Schmidt.
Nestlé Nutrition Workshop Series, Vol. 17.
Nestec Ltd., Vevey/Raven Press, Ltd.,
New York © 1988.

Physicochemical Treatment of Food Allergens: Application to Cow's Milk Proteins

R. Jost

Nestlé Research Department, Nestec Ltd., 1000 Lausanne 26, Switzerland

The scope of the present chapter is to discuss technologic treatments leading to a substantial reduction in the allergenicity of food proteins. In the case of cow's milk, general dairy technology comes into application. Thus, concerns about bacteriological safety and minimum heat damage to proteins obviously limit the operational range. In the particular field of infant formulas, CODEX principles have to be considered. With a relatively limited freedom of operation, we must consider in great detail the physicochemical properties of the proteins involved, in order to direct our treatments toward products of low allergenicity.

PHYSICAL PROPERTIES OF MILK PROTEINS RELATED TO THEIR ALLERGENIC POTENTIAL

According to mass balance in milk, caseins (CNs) might be considered as the major antigens of cow's milk for humans. However, because of "adaptation" of the casein/whey-protein (CN/WP) ratio, the situation is changed in industrial formulas. It is therefore not surprising to find some WPs frequently cited as allergens in hypersensitive infants (1,2). Basically all cow's milk proteins are potential allergens in view of a greater or lesser degree of sequence nonhomology (Table 1) between bovine and human proteins. Besides differences in primary structure, some physical properties affecting solubility, acid stability, or digestibility may be important factors. Thus beta-lactoglobulin (β-LG) is the most acid stable WP and will not be coagulated at the stomach pH. However, if heated in the presence of CNs (e.g., in UHT milks or condensed milks), it will be associated with the micelle and will consequently be co-precipitated with the CNs (3). Such a situation may be important in the low β-LG-related antigenicity of strongly heated milk.

TABLE 1. *Properties of the major cow's milk proteins related to their allergenic potential*

Property	Caseins				Whey proteins			
	αs₁-CN	αs₂-CN	β-CN	κ-CN	β-LG	α-LA	BSA	IgG
Concentration (g/liter) in milk	12–15	3–4	9–11	2–4	3–4	0.6–1.5	~ 0.4	0.4–0.8
Calculated molecular weight[a]	23,600	25,200	24,000	19,000[b]	18,300	14,200	66,300	150,000[c]
Association with casein micelle	+	+	+(−)[d]	+	−(+)[e]	−(+)[e]	−	+
Solubility at pH < 4, > 2	−	−	−		+		+	+
Sequence homology (%) bovine vs. human	nd[f]	nd[f]	47[g]	Low[h]	25[i]	72[i]	80[k]	nd[f]

[a]Calculated from sequence data and rounded to next 100.
[b]Carbohydrate neglected.
[c]Composed of two H chains (each ~ 53,000 molecular weight) and two L chains (each 22,000 molecular weight).
[d]Partial dissociation from micelle to serum at low temperature.
[e]Heat-induced complex with micelle in severely heated milk.
[f]nd, not determined.
[g]β-CN is the major casein of human milk (27).
[h]For the glycomacropeptide part only (28).
[i]No equivalent in human milk. Human serum retinol binding protein is homologous to some extent with β-LG (29,30).
[j]Refs. 18 and 31.
[k]Main immunoglobulin of human milk is secretory IgA.

HEAT STABILITY OF MILK PROTEINS AND EFFECT OF HEAT PROCESSING ON ANTIGENICITY

Caseins possess ordered structure to a relatively low extent (Table 2). They resist heating at very high temperature for prolonged time. In contrast, the globular WPs are easily heat coagulated in the absence of the CN micelle, such as in whey. Their transition temperatures, as measured by differential scanning calorimetry, are within a range of 60°C to 80°C (4). The corresponding transitions lead to irreversible denaturation in the case of β-LG, bovine serum albumin (BSA), and IgG. In contrast, alpha-lactalbumin (α-LA) renatures after cooling and in the presence of Ca ions (5). Despite its relatively low transition temperature, α-LA is the most heat-stable WP from a practical point of view (2).

Denaturation of BSA starts above 50°C with partial helix disruption. At 60°C, heat-induced aggregation takes place (6). BSA, which is partially or fully saturated with fatty acids, shows an increased heat stability (7). Biologic activity of immunoglobulins is very heat-labile and is rapidly destroyed above 70°C, but we have little information as to whether its antigenicity as a bovine protein is likewise heat-labile.

The thermal denaturation of β-LG appears to follow either a second-order process (8) or, at least in milk, a reaction of the order 1.5 (9). The lesson from these data is that heat processing of milk will mainly reduce WP-related antigenicity, but it is unlikely that CN-dependent antigenicity will be greatly affected.

Early studies on the allergenicity of heated milks in guinea pigs demonstrated an inverse relationship between antigenicity and the intensity of heat treatment (10–12). While CN-dependent allergenicity could not be satisfactorily abolished, WP antigenicity was decreased to a very large extent or even completely. Accordingly, if one wants to rely on heat processing alone, the ideal substrates are the WPs in the form of whey or whey protein concentrate (WPC). This option was indeed adopted (13,14); and it was shown that heating at 100°C, or under steam pressure at 120°C, drastically reduced the oral sensitization capacity of whey in guinea pigs, whereas the reduction in eliciting capacity was not entirely satisfactory (14).

Simplicity and low costs seem to be attractive features of such an ''all-whey hypoallergenic formula''; on the other hand, however, one can foresee some problems related to the low protein solubility in heated whey both during processing and in the final application of the product. It is not yet clear to what extent the achieved level of hypoallergenicity will provide sufficient safety for infants predisposed to hypersensitivity.

SENSITIVITY OF MILK PROTEINS TO PROTEOLYTIC CLEAVAGE

Limited cleavage of the polypeptide chains of milk proteins by specific endopeptidases such as trypsin, chymotrypsin, papain, pepsin, and others leads to a

TABLE 2. Properties of cow's milk caseins and whey protein related to their heat stability

Property	Caseins				Whey proteins			
	α_{s1}-CN	α_{s2}-CN	β-CN	κ-CN	β-LG	α-LA	BSA	IgG
Number of S-S bridges/mole	—	1	—	1	2	4	17	4
Number of SH groups/mole	—	—	—	—	1	—	1	1
Secondary structure content (% of total chain)	Low[a]	nd[b]	Low[c]	Medium[d]	High[e]	Medium[f]	High[g]	High
α-helix	4–15	—	1–10	14	15	25	50	nd
β-sheet			16	31	40	15	15	nd
Transition temperature (°C) by DSC[h]	—	—	—	—	78	63	68(74)	78
Heat coagulability in serum at 80–100°C	+	—	—	—	+	±	+	+
Holding time (sec) for > 90% denaturation in skim milk[i]								
at 90°C					200	900	< 200	< 200
at 130°C					20	100		

[a]Ref. 32.
[b]nd, not determined.
[c]Ref. 33.
[d]Ref. 34.
[e]Ref. 35.
[f]Refs. 36 and 37.
[g]Ref. 38.
[h]Ref. 4.
[i]Ref. 9.

drastic reduction in antigenicity (15). Because of the exposing of new ionized terminal amino and carboxyl groups, conformation-dependent antigenic sites collapse. Progressive hydrolysis gradually eliminates sequential (conformation-independent) determinants, more recently recognized as protein regions inducing antipeptide responses (15). It is quite impossible to specify general and precise limits of molecular weights for peptide immunogenicity, but polypeptides of less than 5,000 molecular weight tend to be weakly immunogenic, and oligopeptides are considered nonimmunogenic (16,17).

If we analyze CNs and WPs for their number of trypsin-sensitive sites in the chain, we find between 7 and 14 sites per 100 total residues (Table 3). If these sites were all attacked and cleaved in an *in vitro* process, the mean tryptic peptide would be about 10 residues long and would range between 800 and 1600 molecular weight. In terms of immunogenicity, such peptides would already be at or below the limit. Few of them would be expected to be plurivalent antigens capable of triggering anaphylactic reactions.

In practice, the number of cleaved sites is lower than the total number of theoretical sites. Such resistance to endopeptidase attack may result from disulfide bridges shielding segments of the chain. This is clearly the case for BSA. Trypsin and other proteases were shown to produce large antigenic fragments (18). Cleavage of bovine immunoglobulins leads to formation of Fab-type fragments with antigen-combining capacity (19).

Both α-LA and β-LG are extensively hydrolyzed by trypsin, chymotrypsin, or pancreatin. Antigenic properties of tryptic fragments of β-LG were recently studied (20). Hydrolysis of undenatured β-LG by tosyl-phenylalanine chloromethyl ketone (TPCK)-treated trypsin led to the fragmentation pattern shown in Fig. 1.

Of 18 T-sites, 11 sites were cleaved as theoretically expected, whereas seven were cleaved at a very low rate or were not attacked at all. Some of the fragments were active in binding anti-β-LG rabbit antibody, but a single fragment gave a precipitation line in agar gel diffusion with anti-β-LG serum (Table 4). This disulfide-linked two-chain fragment (molecular weight 2,700) did not trigger passive cutaneous anaphylaxis (PCA) at a maximum concentration of 2 mg/ml in passively sensitized guinea pigs in which 10 μg/ml of β-LG repeatedly gave a positive response. The total digest was active at 20 mg/ml but was inactive at 2 mg/ml. The triggering activity of the unfractionated digest might be to residual β-LG or, alternatively, to cooperation between nontriggering peptides.

Caseins, because of their open and strongly hydrated structure, should *a priori* be easier substrates than WPs. This is what is also observed in practice, with the limitation that the highly acidic regions containing the phosphoserine clusters are rather protease-resistant.

Cyanogen bromide cleavage of β-CN (which contains six methionine residues) yielded large fragments which, in mixture, reconstituted close to 100% of the total antibody-precipitating activity of β-CN (21). This observation is of interest because it presents an experimental possibility of determining the chain-length limit for precipitating antigenic peptides. Punctual hydrolysis of αs₁-CN with TPCK-

TABLE 3. *Properties of the cow's milk casein and whey proteins related to their sensitivity to proteolytic cleavage*

Property	Caseins				Whey proteins			
	αS₁-CN	αS₂-CN	β-CN	κ-CN	β-LG	α-LA	BSA	IgG
Σ residues/mole	199	207	209	169	162	123	582	470/200
Mean residue weight[a]	119	122	115	112	113	115	114	~115
Σ lysine, arginine/mole	20	30	15	4	18	12–13	82	nd[b]
Mean molecular weight, tryptic peptide[c]	1,184	842	1,602	4,732	1,017	1,132	809	
Mean molecular weight, tryptic/chymotryptic peptide[d]	592	505	829	1,051	654	577	510	
Hydration (g H₂O/g protein)	> 3	nd	> 6		< 1	< 1	< 0.5	nd
Observed *in vitro* digestibility[e]	High	nd	High	Limited	High	High	Limited	Limited
Formation of plurivalent antigens during tryptic *in vitro* digestion	+[f]	nd	+[f]	nd	+[g]	–[h]	+ + +[i]	+ + +[j]

[a] Molecular weight/residue per mole.
[b] nd, not determined.
[c] [Σ residual per mole/Σ (Lys, Arg)] × mean residue weight.
[d] [Σ residual per mole/Σ (Lys, Arg, Trp, Tyr, Phe)] × mean residue weight.
[e] Trypsin pH 8, 40°C, 4 hr.
[f] Precipitating antiprotein antibodies in a quantitative immunoprecipitation test (21,22).
[g] Precipitation arc in agar gel; see also Table 4.
[h] Pancreatin instead of trypsin (39).
[i] High-molecular-weight antigenic fragments obtained (40).
[j] Fragments corresponding to Fab, Fab', and Fc (19).

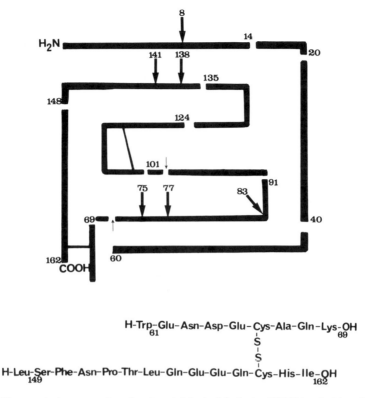

FIG. 1. Observed cleavage of undenatured β-lactoglobulin by TPCK-treated trypsin at 1% E/S ratio, pH 7.8, 4 hr at 40°C (20). ↑, Lys-Lys sequences giving rise to free lysine; ➤, sites which were not cleaved or at a very low rate only. (**Bottom**) Disulfide-bridged tryptic fragment which represents a major antigen of the total tryptic digest.

trypsin led to a variety of fragments, some of which retained rather limited precipitating capacity (22). Extended hydrolysis of total CN with pancreatin and fungal proteases led to hydrolysates devoid of sensitizing or eliciting capacity (23). Casein hydrolysates (such as those present in therapeutic formulas) have been shown to be safe in hypersensitive infants. Their major disadvantages are a low palatability and bitterness or off-flavors. Bitterness is the result of bitter peptide formation during proteolysis of CN (24). Debittering procedures exist, but they lead to even higher costs and disequilibration of the amino acid composition of the hydrolysate (25).

ANTIGENICITY OF WHEY PROTEIN HYDROLYSATES

WPCs such as those produced by ultrafiltration of whey are very potent allergens to guinea pigs (oral route). Such protein concentrates contain close to 30%

TABLE 4. *Immunoreactivity of tryptic fragments of β-LG in vitro and in vivo*[a]

Peptides	Calculated molecular weight	Concentration		Activity RIA[b]	Precipitation arc[c]	Eliciting capacity[d]
		mg/ml	Molar			
β-LG 15–20	696	2.0	2.9×10^{-3}	$\ll$	–	–
β-LG 21–40	2,030					
β-LG 41–60	2,314	~2	$\sim 10^{-3}$	6×10^{-6}	–	–
β-LG 61⌐ 69s̄	2,761	2.0	0.7×10^{-3}	4×10^{-4}	+	–
140⌐162s						
β-LG 92–101	1,065	2.0	1.9×10^{-3}	1.7×10^{-6}	–	–
β-LG 125–135	1,245	2.0	1.6×10^{-3}	0.8×10^{-6}	–	–
Total digest[e]		2.0		0.8×10^{-3}	–	–
Total digest		20.0			+	+
β-LG		2×10^{-3}			–	–
β-LG		2×10^{-2}			+	+

[a]Data are from ref. 20.
[b]Solid-phase RIA with rabbit anti-LG serum. Relative reactivity of pure β-LG is 1.
[c]Ouchterlony double-diffusion test.
[d]PCA: donor sera from whey protein sensitized animals.
[e]TPCK-treated trypsin (2% weight/weight), pH 7.8, 4 hr at 40°C. The digest was separated by reverse-phase LC on C-18 column (20).

of immunoreactive β-LG, estimated by RIA. Table 5 shows that trypsin-hydro-lyzed WP was nonsensitizing (oral route) and had no eliciting capacity (intrave-nous route) in guinea pigs sensitized to either WP or milk (26). The hydrolysate showed about a 300-fold decrease in β-LG specific antigenicity and gave (at 50 mg/ml) a weak precipitation line in the Ouchterlony diffusion test. It also showed (at an antigen dilution up to 1:8) a precipitation arc with anti-BSA serum. Accord-ingly, tryptic hydrolysis had reduced this antigen by not more than a factor of about 8 (titer in WPC 1:64). Electrophoresis (SDS-PAGE) revealed that the anti-gen(s) consisted of intact BSA. In addition, BSA fragments of 20,000 to 24,000 had accumulated. Heating of the hydrolysate at 80°C or higher led to the inactiva-tion of these antigens (Table 5).

Hydrolysates fractionated by ultrafiltration and diafiltration gave permeates, es-sentially composed of peptides. The permeate fraction, obtained in yields ranging from 50% to 60% of the parent hydrolysates, showed no precipitation lines in im-munodiffusion with anti-β-LG, anti-α-LA, or anti-BSA sera. Their β-LG-specific binding activity was about one order of magnitude lower than that of the original hydrolysates (Table 5). The same observations were made with pancreatic hydro-lysates, fractionated by heat coagulation and desludging of insolubles.

Despite clear-cut differences in residual antigenicity *in vitro*, the lower level of antigenicity of fractionated hydrolysates was not reflected in the guinea pig tests because the unfractionated hydrolysates were already unreactive. It is possible that such a difference in allergenicity becomes manifest if, instead of oral sensitization, another route would be used to sensitize the animals.

TABLE 5. *Immunoreactivity of whey protein hydrolysates* in vitro *and* in vivo

Preparation	Activity RIA[a] (μg β-LG/mg)	Precipitation arc (Ouchterlony)[b] anti-β-LG	anti-α-LA	anti-BSA	Allergenicity (guinea pigs)[c] Oral sensitization (positive/total)	Eliciting capacity (PCA) A	B
Whey protein concentrate[d]	280 ± 50	+ (1/1,024)	+ (1/256)	+ (1/64)	+ (9/9)	+	+
Trypsin-hydrolyzed WPC[e]	~ 1.0	± (1/1)	−	+ (1/8)	− (0/11)	−	−
Heated (20 min/80°C) hydrolysate[f]	0.4−1.0	−	−	−	nd[g]	−	−
Heated (120 sec/125°C) hydrolysate[h]	0.4−1.0	−	−	−	(0/8)	−	−
Ultrafiltrated hydrolysate (permeate[i])	0.03−0.15	−	−	−	− (0/8)	−	−
Pancreatic hydrolysate (soluble fraction[j])	0.02−0.10	−	−	−	− (0/8)	−	−
For comparison: human milk whey[k]	0.06−0.10	−	−	+	nd[g]	nd[g]	nd[g]

[a]Solid-phase RIA (26).
[b]Initial antigen concentration 50 mg/ml.
[c]Guinea pig model described in ref. 26. Donor sera from whey-sensitized animals (A) and from skim-milk-sensitized animals (B).
[d]Essentially undenatured WP produced by ultrafiltration of sweet whey. Protein content 84% total dry solids.
[e]Porcine trypsin (2% weight/weight), pH 7.5, 55°C, 4 hr.
[f]Hydrolysates heated batchwise.
[g]nd, not determined.
[h]Hydrolysate heated continuously.
[i]Hydrolysate ultrafiltrated and diafiltrated on membranes with nominal cut-off 10,000; permeate fraction recovered.
[j]Pancreatin (5% weight/weight), pH 7.5, 55°C, 4 hr. Heat coagulation (20 min/80°C), separation of insolubles by desludger and filtration.
[k]Pool of several wheys dialyzed to remove lactose and salts. Protein: 75% on total dry solids.

CONCLUSIONS

Limited or extensive hydrolysis with proteases followed by heat treatment, as well as hydrolysis followed by fractionation, is a practical way of reducing milk protein antigenicity. Purified CN hydrolysates, as well as hydrolysates of WP, are on the market and were found to be extremely well tolerated in allergic infants.

Technologically, the route from a heat-modified whey formula to the purified hydrolysates used in therapeutic oligopeptide diets is long. En route we lose palatability and functionality and we increase costs.

In the near future we hope, by an appropriate combination of enzyme and heat treatments, to achieve more palatable and less expensive hypoallergenic formulas. Their more general availability and better organoleptic properties could make an important contribution to preventing hypersensitivity to cow's milk proteins in infants.

REFERENCES

1. Freier S, Kletter B, Gery I, Lebenthal E, Griefman, M. Intolerance to milk proteins. *J Pediatr* 1969;75:623–31.
2. Savilahti E. Cow's milk allergy. *Allergy* 1981;36:73–88.
3. Sawyer WH. Complex between β-lactoglobulin and k-casein. A review. *J Dairy Sci* 1969;52:1347–55.
4. de Witt JN, Klaarenbeek G. Effects of various heat treatments of structure and solubility of whey proteins. *J Dairy Sci* 184;67:2701–10.
5. Bernal V, Jelen P. Effect of calcium binding on thermal denaturation of bovine α-lactalbumin. *J Dairy Sci* 1986;67:2452–4.
6. Lin VJC, Koenig JL. Raman studies on bovine serum albumin. *Biopolymers* 1976;15:203–18.
7. Gumpen S, Hegg PO, Martens H. Thermal stability of fatty acid serum albumin complexes studied by DSC. *Biochem Biophys Acta* 1979;574:189–96.
8. Lyster RL. The denaturation of α-lactalbumin and β-lactoglobulin in heated milk. *J Dairy Res* 1970;37:233–43.
9. Dannenberg F. Ph.D. thesis 1986. Technische Universität München.
10. Ratner B, Dworetzky M, Oguri S, Ascheim L. Studies on the allergenicity of cow's milk. *Pediatrics* 1959;23:648–57.
11. Anderson KJ, McLaughlan P, Devey, ME, Coombs RRA. Anaphylactic sensitivity of guinea pigs drinking different preparations of cow's milk and infant formulas. *Clin Exp Immunol* 1979;35:454–61.
12. McLaughlan P, Anderson KJ, Widdowson EM, Coombs RRA. Effect of heat on the anaphylactic-sensitizing capacity of cow's milk, goat's milk, and various infant formulae fed to guinea pigs. *Arch Dis Child* 1981;56:165–71.
13. Kilshaw PJ, Heppell LM, Ford JE. Effects of heat treatment of cow's milk and whey on nutritional quality and antigenic properties. *Arch Dis Child* 1982;57:842–7.
14. Heppell LM, Cant AJ, Kilshaw PJ. Reduction in the antigenicity of whey proteins by heat treatment: a possible strategy for producing a hypoallergenic infant milk formula. *Br J Nutr* 1984;51:29–36.
15. Lerner RA. Antibodies of predetermined specificity in biology and medicine. *Adv Immunol* 1984;36:1–45.
16. de Weck AL. Low molecular weight antigens. In: *The Antigens, Vol II*. New York: Academic Press, 1974:141–248.
17. Adda G, Skehel JJ. Are peptides good antigens? *Nature* 1985;316:764–5.
18. Peters, Th. Serum albumin. *Adv Protein Chem* 1985;37:161–245.
19. Fang WD, Mukkur TKJ. Physicochemical characterization of proteolytic cleavage fragments of bovine colostrial immunoglobulin G1. *Biochem J* 1976;155:25–30.
20. Monti JC, Jost R, Pahud JJ, Hughes G. Antigenic sites in bovine lactoglobulin. *Abstr Experientia* 1986;42:670.
21. Otani H, Higashiyama S, Tokita F. Studies on the antigenic structure of bovine β-casein. *Milchwissenschaft* 1984;39:469–72.
22. Otani H, Takayama K, Tokita F. Studies on the antigenicity of bovine α-sl-casein. *Milchwissenschaft* 1986;41:565–8.
23. Takase M, Fukuwatari Y, Kiyosawa I, Ogasa K, Suzuki S, Kuroume T. Antigenicity of casein hydrolysate. *J Dairy Sci* 1979;62:1570–6.

PHYSICOCHEMICAL TREATMENT OF FOOD ALLERGENS

24. Guigoz Y, Solms J. Bitter peptides, occurrence and structure. *Chemi Senses Flavor* 1976;2:71–84.
25. Cogan U, Moshe M, Mokady S. Debittering and nutritional upgrading of enzymatic casein hydrolysates. *J Sci Food Agric* 1981;23:459–66.
26. Pahud JJ, Monti JC, Jost R. Allergenicity of whey protein: its modification by tryptic *in vitro* hydrolysis of the protein. *J Pediatr Gastroenterol Nutr* 1985;4:408–13.
27. Greenberg R, Groves ML, Dover HJ. Human β-casein. *J Biol Chem* 1984;259:5132–8.
28. Chobert JM, Mercier JC, Bahy Ch, Haze G. Structure primaire du caseinomacropeptide des caseines k porcine et humaine. *FEBS Lett* 1976;72:173–7.
29. Brew K, Pervaiz S. Homology of β-lactoglobulin, serum retinol binding protein, and protein HC. *Science* 1985;228:335–7.
30. Godovac-Zimmerman J, Conti A, Liberatori J, Braunitzer G. Homology between the primary structures of β-lactoglobulin and human retinol binding protein; evidence for similar biological function. *Biol Chem Hoppe-Seyler* 1985;366:431–4.
31. Findlay JBC, Brew K. The complete amino-acid sequence of human α-lactalbumin. *Eur J Biochem* 1972;27:65–86.
32. Herskovits TT. On the conformation of caseins. Optical rotatory properties. *Biochemistry* 1966;5:1018–25.
33. Andrews AL, Atkinson D, Evans MTA, Finger EG, Green JP, Phillips MC, Robertson RN. The conformation and aggregation of bovine β-casein A. *Biopolymers* 1979;18:1105–21.
34. Loucheux-Lefebvre MH, Aubert JP, Jolles P. Prediction of the conformation of the cow and sheep d-caseins. *Biophys J* 1978;23:323–36.
35. Townsend R, Kumosinski TF, Timasheff SN. The circular dichroism of variants of β-lactoglobulins. *J Biol Chem* 1967;242:4538–45.
36. Robbins FM, Holmes LG. Circular dichroism spectra of α-lactalbumin. *Biochem Biophys Acta* 1970;221:234–40.
37. Barel AO, Prieels JP, Maes E, Looze Y, Leonis F. Comparative physicochemical studies of human α-lactalbumin and human lysozyme. *Biochem Biophys Acta* 1972;257:288–96.
38. Shechter E, Blout ER. An analysis of the optical rotatory dispersion of polypeptides and proteins. *Proc Natl Acad Sci USA* 1964;51:665–70.
39. Fushiki T, Yamamoto N, Naeshiro I, Iwai K. Digestion of α-lactalbumin in rat gastrointestinal tracts. *Agric Biol Chem* 1986;50:95–100.
40. Wahn U, Peters Th, Siraganian R. Allergenic and antigenic properties of bovine serum albumin. *Mol Immunol* 1981;18:19–28.

Food Allergy, edited by Eberhardt Schmidt.
Nestlé Nutrition Workshop Series, Vol. 17.
Nestec Ltd., Vevey/Raven Press, Ltd.,
New York © 1988.

Control of Hypoallergenicity by Animal Models

J.J. Pahud, K. Schwarz, and D. Granato

Nestlé Research Department, Nestec Ltd., 1000 Lausanne 26, Switzerland

The normal immune response of experimental animals to ingested antigens is usually an increased mucosal immunity associated with an active suppression of the systemic response (1–3). Orally induced tolerance through the persistent feeding of antigens should prevent the hypersensitivity phenomenon. However, the wide use of formulae most frequently based on modified cow's milk is linked to the frequent incidence of cow's milk allergy in infants (4). The pathogenesis of food allergies may be governed by various immunologic mechanisms: immediate manifestations mediated by reagins, inflammatory reactions caused by immune complexes, or delayed hypersensitivity associated with specific T-lymphocytes. One major component of the pathomechanism involved in food allergy is a deficient or immature immune regulation. Children with cow's milk allergy have a decreased immune suppressor T-cell activity, and the immaturity of this control system is suggested by the usually transient character of the disease. The global allergenicity of cow's milk is contributed, to some degree, by the different protein fractions, which are all potential allergens. Among the most likely candidates, we should mention caseins, beta-lactoglobulin (β-LG), alpha-lactalbumin, serum albumin, and immunoglobulins. The large number of milk proteins, in addition to the different immunologic mechanisms possibly involved, are all contributing factors of complexity in the pathogenesis of the disease. This is reflected by a multiplicity of symptoms in various intestinal, respiratory, dermatologic, and hematologic disorders (5).

GENERAL CONCEPTS FOR HYPOALLERGENIC FORMULAE

The ability of mother's milk to prevent the development of atopic diseases in childhood has been suggested by a number of well-documented clinical studies. Exclusive breast-feeding during the first few months of life appears to be the best measure to prevent, or to delay the onset and to attenuate, the symptoms of early food allergy (6,7). However, the excellent prognosis of breast-feeding is highly dependent on an appropriate maternal diet during late pregnancy and lactation (e.g., complete avoidance of the most offending foods such as milk and eggs) (8,9). When high-risk newborns cannot be breast-fed, a formula with reduced allergenic properties is the major alternative that can be recommended. Modulating the immune system of the neonate by other dietetic manipulations remains premature and debatable. Protein chemists and immunologists of the food industry have considered several concepts in the development of hypoallergenic infant formulae. The most reasonable proposals until now involve technological procedures such as heat denaturation and enzymatic proteolysis. Protein sources other than cow's milk have also been frequently substituted in a number of modern formulae. Soya preparations, for instance, have been considered to be less sensitizing than bovine milk, but their wider application has, in turn, increased the occurrence of allergies to soya (10).

Reduction in allergenicity of infant formulae must remain compatible with impeccable nutritional qualities and industrial feasibility. Currently, application of enzymatic *in vitro* hydrolysis to the milk casein or the whey protein fraction appears to be the most successful technique employed to guarantee a hypoallergenic source of nitrogen (11). Our contribution in product development has been to provide *in vivo* procedures for evaluating the sensitizing capacity of different food products as well as the potential influence of industrial treatments on subsequent immunologic reactivity. Two independent animal models have been developed in order to follow up the effect of enzymatic hydrolysis on reducing whey protein allergenicity. The hybridoma technology was applied to a mouse model with the production and experimental use of monoclonal IgE antibodies in a test of passive intestinal anaphylaxis (12). Independently, an oral screening procedure in the guinea pig was adapted to evaluate the sensitizing capacity of whey protein hydrolysates (13,14). Both model systems essentially diagnose Type-I hypersensitivity with the implication of reaginic antibodies in immediate systemic or local manifestations.

INTESTINAL ANAPHYLAXIS EXPLORED WITH A MOUSE MONOCLONAL IgE ANTIBODY AGAINST BOVINE MILK BETA-LACTOGLOBULIN

In most cases of cow's milk allergy, children exhibit gastrointestinal disorders such as vomiting and diarrhea. These funtional abnormalities are usually associated with alterations of the intestinal mucosa, mostly in the proximal jejunum, which are characterized by villous atrophy, hyperplasia of the crypts, and inflammation. Several animal models of intestinal anaphylaxis have previously been proposed to reproduce human symptoms (15,16). The manifestations of gastrointestinal hypersensitivity observed in rats and guinea pigs were mainly of the immediate type. However, reaginic antibodies involved in these reactions have not been fully characterized and might have been superimposed on other factors. The synthesis and use of a monoclonal IgE antibody against bovine beta-lactoglobulin enabled us to select for an authentic IgE mediation in testing milk allergy. The IgE-secreting hybridoma was produced in our laboratory by fusion of NS1 myeloma cells with spleen cells of Balb/c mice immunized specifically against the pure milk protein. The secreted antibody was fully characterized and identified as an IgE. On radioimmunoassay, this antibody was found to react with both native and aggregated β-LG. However, positive *in vivo* reactions such as passive cutaneous anaphylaxis (PCA) were obtained with aggregated β-LG only. Approximately 1 ng of purified antibody was capable of passively sensitizing mast cells of local skin sites in the PCA test.

The monoclonal IgE was examined for its capacity as a mediator of intestinal anaphylaxis in a mouse model. Mice (immunologically virgin hosts) were systemically sensitized with the amount of IgE antibodies giving a positive reverse PCA reaction (about 500 μg of monoclonal IgE per mouse). After 24 hr of fasting, the animals were challenged with aggregated β-LG (8 mg in 0.4 ml) by gastric intubation. Gut manifestations were evaluated after 1 hr following intravenous injection of colloidal carbon black (0.5 ml of Pelikan biological ink diluted 1:10 in saline) in order to demonstrate increased vascular permeability (17). Thirty minutes later, the gut was removed and flushed with ice-cold Carnoy's fixative for histological studies. Carbon leakage was most pronounced in the jejunum and was of decreasing intensity along the small intestine. Histology showed edema of the villi but showed no detectable modifications of the epithelial cells. The vessels of the submucosa were heavily labeled with carbon, mainly along the bottom of the crypts but to a lesser extent along the villous axis. Intestinal anaphylaxis following passive sensitization of mice occurred without any obvious morphologic alterations of the mucosae or cellular infiltration. Vascular leakage in the submucosae was a transient phenomenon observable within 2 to 3 hr post-challenge. It seems likely that more chronic anaphylactic reactions of this type within the gastrointestinal tract would also result in mucosal damage. This model system helps to demonstrate that certain gastrointestinal manifestations of food allergy could be mediated by reaginic antibodies alone. However, at this point of our investigation, it does not provide a routine procedure for the control of hypoallergenicity in modified milk formulae. One major problem would be to produce, for instance, a battery of monoclonal reagins against the most significant epitopes of the different milk proteins.

ORAL SENSITIZATION TO FOOD PROTEINS IN A GUINEA PIG MODEL

A convenient *in vivo* model was necessary to determine orally the global allergenicity contributed to all protein fractions of cow's milk also present in infant formulae. The oral screening procedure worked out in our laboratory was a modification of the guinea pig model proposed by Coombs and co-workers in Cambridge (18,19). Guinea pigs and humans may both become anaphylactically sensitized to dietary proteins. Oral sensitization can be assessed by hypersensitivity reactions of the immediate type upon systemic challenge with these proteins. The complex symptoms of food allergy in humans, such as distinctive respiratory and cutaneous manifestations, may be partially reproduced in this model.

Weaned Dunkin-Harley guinea pigs (Madörin AG, CH-4414 Füllingsdorf) were used in the model (13). The animals originated from a breed that was maintained on a cow's-milk-free and soya-free diet (Kliba Sodi 3000, Klingentalmühle AG, CH-4303 Kaiseraugst) for a minimum of three generations. Test diets were given in liquid form instead of water over 2 weeks. The occurrence of hypersensitivity was then tested by intravenous challenge for systemic anaphylaxis (16–18 mg protein/0.5 ml) and passive cutaneous anaphylaxis (PCA) (1–2 mg/0.5 ml), after an additional week on Sodi 3000 and water.

Optimal sensitization was achieved by oral presentation of food proteins in solution as mentioned by the Coombs protocol. In these conditions, protein intake was at least twice as high as that from a pelleted diet. Also, natural bacterial contaminants could proliferate (up to 10^9 total germs and 10^7 enterobacteria per milliliter) and possibly enhance the reaginic response. The immunostimulating properties of their amphipathic products (LPS, peptidoglycans) have been established (20). Food allergies have often been seen as a sequel to acute gastroenteritis (21). However, feeding did not by itself trigger any local or systemic reactions and caused no apparent damage in the intestinal mucosa, although sensitization had been induced by the same route. These observations indicate that other factors in addition to infection might be leading to oral sensitization.

Feeding spray-dried milk initially failed to induce oral sensitization to milk proteins. Guinea pigs are usually raised on commercial feeds containing 1% to 2% milk whey complement (roughly 0.1% of the diet in terms of milk proteins). This unforeseen complication was probably not encountered by the Cambridge scientists, who never mentioned this factor in their own development of this model system. Diet supplementation with small amounts of milk proteins appeared to be sufficient in suppressing subsequent sensitization to these allergens. Pregnant females were transferred to a milk-free diet at midgestation, and further breeding was resumed under these conditions. Their F1 offspring could only be partially sensitized by feeding, and anaphylactic manifestations were transient and weak. The F2 and later generations became fully responsive to oral exposure to cow's milk or moderately processed whey proteins.

Consequently, oral sensitization proved to be dependent on the absence of an anamnestic response caused by previous maternal exposure to the food antigens. Maternal factors transferred either *in utero* or in milk appeared to be responsible for a suppression of reaginic responsiveness in the offspring. In the young rat, suppression of the IgE response was linked to specific IgG antibodies (22,23) and maybe also to secretory IgA and other factors transferred in milk from immunized mothers. Though responsiveness in guinea pigs or rats may be suppressed by maternal immunity, clinicians usually doubt that human beings may acquire reaginic tolerance in the same manner (6–9,24,25). However, the amounts of bovine milk proteins (0.1%) contained in standard guinea pig feed are minute in comparison with Western human diets, where these proteins are usually present in many hidden forms as well as in dairy products. Maternal control over the reaginic responsiveness of the infant might be overtaken by an excessive load of food antigens. Transmucosal transfer of intact macromolecules or antigenic fragments from the intestinal lumen to the mammary secretions is well documented (26,27). These conditions would then favor sensitization to these antigens and would probably lead to a decreased transfer of maternal suppressive factors, either transplacental or from breast milk.

The systemic and local allergic reactions observed in this system (bronchospasm, cutaneous anaphylaxis) can be associated with antibodies differing from the IgE reagin. Previous work by Coombs et al. on a similar model suggested that the sensitizing antibodies belonged to the IgG1a isotypes but not to the IgE class (28). Our own findings support this statement, although no formal identification of the isotype by serology has been performed. The reaginic activity can be fully recovered from guinea pig serum by two types of affinity gels, with the immobilized ligand being either Protein A or specific antigens (ovalbumin, β-LG). The affinity-purified antibodies against ovalbumin were characterized by heavy chains with a molecular weight of approximately 55,000 to 60,000 on SDS polyacrylamide. However, cytophilic activity cannot be attributed to the whole population of isolated IgG antibodies on this sole basis. Trace amounts of specific IgE undetectable by electrophoresis cannot be ruled out. When testing for circulating reagins, skin reactions are optimal after a sensitization phase of 4 to 18 hr prior to intravenous challenge in the PCA test. The skin reactions remain faint or undetectable after 72 hr. The conformational stability and the biological activity of the reagins seemed unaffected by thermal treatment at 56°C for 4 hr or by acid elution in affinity chromatography.

The animal model was expected to provide a sensitive *in vivo* evaluation of dietary proteins and technologies aiming at the prevention of food allergies. Oral screening was initially applied to milk products. The specificity of the systemic immune response induced orally was determined by a screening of the circulating reaginic antibodies. Thus, serum from animals orally sensitized against whey proteins was tested with pure fractions in the PCA test. The reaginic antibodies produced by orally exposed guinea pigs demonstrated a specific activity associated with β-LG, α-lactalbumin, and IgG_1 but demonstrated no detectable allergenicity that could be attributed to bovine serum albumin. However, the brunt of the *in vivo* reactivity was carried by β-LG in this animal model (Table 1).

The sensitivity of the animal model was evaluated by oral sensitization and systemic challenge. The lowest protein concentration range for a detectable oral induction of the reaginic response was of the order of 200 to 500 μg protein per milliliter for whole milk but only 10 to 20 μg/ml for whey proteins. The minimal allergen concentration in the provocation phase was roughly 20 to 50 μg/ml for whey proteins and 5 to 10 μg/ml for pure β-LG. By comparison, radioimmunoassays could detect 0.01 to 0.1 μg β-LG per milliliter in processed whey, which is

TABLE 1. *Anaphylactic sensitization to milk whey proteins and to the hypoallergenic formula based on its tryptic hydrolysate*

Challenge with specific milk proteins	PCA titers in recipient animals following:	
	Oral sensitization to untreated whey proteins[b]	Parenteral sensitization to hypoallergenic formula[c]
Beta-lactoglobulin	500–1,250	500–1,000
Alpha-lactalbumin	1–15	0
Colostral IgG₁	1–10	0–10
Serum albumin (BSA)	0	0–10
Sodium caseinate	0	0–5

[a]Intravenous injection of 1 mg of specific protein in 0.5 ml of physiological saline including 2% Evans Blue.
[b]No detectable oral sensitization to trypsin-hydrolyzed whey protein and to the hypoallergenic formula.
[c]Three weekly injections (~ 10 mg of hydrolyzed protein or 10–30 μg of immunoreactive peptides) in 0.15 ml of physiologic saline, ± 0.15 ml complete Freund intracutaneously (injection 1) and in 0.15 ml of physiologic saline ± 0.15 ml 2% AL(OH)₃ intraperitoneally (injections 2 and 3). Parenteral sensitization with the tryptic hydrolysate alone gives similar titers.

at least 100 times more sensitive than the *in vivo* model. The relatively low response to whole milk suggests a rather minor contribution of caseins to the global allergenicity of milk in the guinea pig.

It was assumed that lactic bacteria might reduce the allergenicity of milk proteins by acidification, partial proteolysis, improved protein digestibility, and a barrier effect against pathogenic microorganisms (29). Microbial acidification by different lactic strains (effect due to *S. lactis*) had a negligible effect on cow's milk allergenicity. The reaginic antibodies produced in these animals had a specially high affinity for bronchiolar mast cells. This characteristic was demonstrated indirectly during PCA testing (titers 1:25–1:50), because intradermal injection of the test sera produced anaphylactic shock in the recipient animals, associated mainly with bronchospasm. Reagin diffusion out of the skin site and into the blood stream was sufficient to cause passive systemic anaphylaxis. Heat treatment of milk proteins usually leads to a reduction of their antigenicity (30). It was suggested that a well-adapted heat process could produce a nonsensitizing cow's milk formula (31). Knowing the heat stability of casein, a similar treatment applied to whey proteins looked more promising (32). A significant reduction of *in vivo* reactivity affecting both the sensitization and the provocation steps could be achieved by heat treatment of whey proteins. However, this effect did not reach a level acceptable for clinical applications.

In modern infant nutrition, hypoallergenicity refers to a strict avoidance of intact protein determinants from the diet. Hypoallergenic formulae based on this concept usually include hydrolyzed proteins (casein, whey) or crystallized amino acids as a nitrogen source. Pancreatic and tryptic hydrolysis of whey proteins completely abolished their capacity to sensitize orally and to trigger systemic or cutaneous anaphylaxis (PCA). A 1,000-fold reduction of immunoreactivity in radioimmuno-assays seemed sufficient to avoid oral sensitization and allergic manifestations in the guinea pig (13,14).

Without any detectable oral sensitization to trypsin-hydrolyzed whey, the potential allergenicity of the peptide pool was then evaluated by parenteral sensitization. In these conditions, the tryptic peptides of β-LG are responsible for most of the residual immunoreactivity in the hydrolysate. Minor or no observable reactivity was linked to peptides from other milk proteins (Table 1).

The experimental conditions established for oral sensitization to cow's milk proteins were also applied for the evaluation of protein allergenicity from soya, carob germ, and egg white. According to reagin titration by PCA, egg white was comparatively the most sensitizing protein source, followed by milk, soya, then carob germ (Table 2). By administration of egg albumin, lethal systemic anaphylaxis was shown to affect all test animals, with a very quick onset of shock manifestations. The sensitizing capacity of soya was dependent upon the different alternatives involved in technological processing: milling, solvent extraction, and heat treatment. The highest level of sensitization concerned 60% to 80% of the animals, including 30% to 40% lethal shock. Carob germ flour was the least sensitizing product by the oral route, with two weakly positive responses out of 12 animals tested.

Animal models provide comparative indications on the allergenicity of proteins from various sources and on the impact of different technologies affecting their immunoreactivity in vivo. The validity of these model systems is restricted by the limited information concerning the prevailing epitopes in humans and animals (33). The introduction of new conformational determinants by enzymic proteolysis (34) appears to be considerably less significant than the elimination of native epitopes in food proteins. The role of other epitopes and control mechanisms in delayed-type hypersensitivity equally deserves to be closely examined in the future.

TABLE 2. Oral sensitization to food proteins

Proteins[a]	PCA titers[b]
Egg albumin	1,000–2,000
Whey proteins	100–500
Soya cold extract	20–50
Carob germ	0–5

[a]Oral sensitization by ad libitum feeding of protein solutions (~ 20 mg/ml). Challenge: intravenous injection of 5 mg of protein in 0.5 ml of saline + 2% Evans Blue.
[b]PCA titrations in immunologically virgin hosts with crude unfractionated food proteins.

REFERENCES

1. Challacombe SJ, Tomasi TB. Systemic tolerance and secretory immunity after oral immunization. *J Exp Med* 1980;152:1459–72.
2. Tomasi TB. Oral tolerance. *Transplantation* 1980;29:353–6.
3. Stokes CR. In: Newby TJ, Stokes CR, eds. *Local immune response of the gut.* Boca Raton, Fla.: CRC Press, 1984:97–142.
4. Bahna SL, Heiner DC. *Allergies to milk.* New York: Grune and Stratton, 1980.
5. Walker-Smith JA, Ford RPK, Phillips AD. The spectrum of gastrointestinal allergies to food. *Ann Allergy* 1984;53:629–36.
6. Saarinen UM, Kajosaari M, Backman A, Siimes M. Prolonged breast feeding as prophylaxis for atopic disease. *Lancet* 1979;ii:163–6.
7. Sarfati M, Vanderbeeken Y, Rubio-Trujillo M, Duncan D, Delespesse G. Presence of IgE suppressor factors in human colostrum. *Eur J Immunol* 1986;16:1005–8.
8. Businco L, Beninconi N, Cantani A. Epidemiology. Incidence and clinical aspects of food allergy. *Ann Allergy.* 1984;53:615–22.
9. Bellanti JA. Prevention of food allergies. *Ann Allergy* 1984;53:683–8.
10. Gerrard JW, Mackenzie JWA, Goluboff N, Garson JZ, Maningas CS. Cow's milk allergy: prevalence and manifestations in an unselected series of newborns. *Acta Paediatr Scand (Suppl)* 1973;234:1–21.
11. Soothill JF. Factors predisposing to food allergy. In: Wilkinson AW, ed. *The immunology of infant feeding.* New York: Plenum Press, 1981:63–9.
12. Granato DA, Piguet PF. A mouse monoclonal IgE antibody anti bovine milk β-lactoglobulin allows studies of allergy in the gastrointestinal tract. *Clin Exp Immunol* 1986;63:703–10.
13. Pahud JJ, Schwarz K. Oral sensitization to food proteins in animal models, a basis for the development of hypoallergenic infant formula. In: *Production, regulation and analysis of infant formula. Proceedings of the Tropical Conference, Virginia Beach, 1985.* Arlington, Va.: Association of Official Analytic Chemists, 1985:264–71.
14. Pahud JJ, Monti JC, Jost R. Allergenicity of whey protein: its modification by tryptic *in-vitro* hydrolysis of the protein. *J Pediatr Gastroenterol Nutr* 1985;4:408–13.
15. Freier S, Eran M, Goldstein R. The effect of immediate type gastrointestinal allergic reactions on brush border enzymes and gut morphology in the rat. *Pediatr Res* 1985;19:456–9.
16. Block KJ, Walker WA. Effect of locally induced intestinal anaphylaxis on the uptake of a bystander antigen. *J Allergy Clin Immunol* 1981;67:312–6.
17. Majno G, Shea SM, Leventhal M. Endothelial contraction induced by histamine-type mediators. An Electron Microscope Study. *J Cell Biol* 1969;42,647–72.
18. Devey ME, Anderson KJ, Coombs RRA, Henschel MJ, Coates ME. The modified anaphylaxis hypothesis for cot death. Anaphylactic sensitization in guinea pigs fed cow's milk. *Clin Exp Immunol* 1976;26:542–8.
19. McLaughlan P, Anderson KJ, Coombs RRA. An oral screening procedure to determine the sensitizing capacity of infant feeding formulae. *Clin Allergy* 1981;11:311–8.
20. Bessler WG, Braun V. Lipoprotein from the outer membrane of *Escherichia coli*: molecular structure and mutagenicity. In: Peeters H, ed. *Protides of biological fluids, 25th colloquium 1977.* New York: Pergamon Press, 1978:33–6.
21. Walker-Smith JA. Cow's milk intolerance as a cause of postenteritis diarrhoea. *J Pediatr Gastroenterol Nutr* 1982;1:163–73.
22. Jarrett EEE. Regulation of IgE antibody responsiveness by ingestion of antigen and by maternal influence. In: Wilkinson AW, ed. *The immunology of infant feeding.* New York: Plenum Press, 1981:71–81.
23. Jarrett EEE. Immunoregulation of IgE responses. The role of the gut in perspective. *Ann Allergy* 1984;53:550–6.
24. Bahna SL. Management of food allergies. *Ann Allergy* 1984;53:678–82.
25. Hamburger RN. Diagnosis of food allergies and intolerances in the study of prophylaxis and control groups in infants. *Ann Allergy* 1984;53:673–7.
26. Gerrard JW. Allergies in breast fed babies to foods ingested by the mother. *Clin Rev Allergy* 1984;2:143–9.
27. Kilshaw PJ, Cant AJ. The passage of maternal dietary proteins into human breast milk. *Int Arch Allergy Appl Immunol* 1984;75:8–15.

28. Coombs RRA, Devey ME, Anderson KJ. Refractoriness to anaphylactic shock after continuous feeding of cow's milk to guinea pigs. *Clin Exp Immunol* 1978;32:263–71.
29. Bullen CL. Infant feeding and the faecal flora. In: Wilkinson AW, ed. *The immunology of infant feeding*. New York: Plenum Press, 1981:41–53.
30. Hanson LA, Johansson BG. Immunological studies of milk. VI. A. The effect of heat on milk proteins. In: McKenzie HA, ed. *Milk proteins: Chemistry and molecular biology, vol. I*. New York: Academic Press, 1970:96–101.
31. McLaughlan P, Anderson KJ, Widdowson EM, Coombs RRA. Effect of heat on the anaphylactic sensitizing capacity of cow's milk, goat's milk, and various infant formulae fed to guinea pigs. *Arch Dis Child* 1981;56:165–71.
32. Heppell LMJ, Cant AJ, Kilshaw PJ. Reduction in the antigenicity of whey proteins by heat treatment: a possible strategy for producing a hypoallergenic infant milk formula. *Br J Nutr* 1984;51:29–36.
33. Aas K. What makes an allergen an allergen? *Allergy* 1978;33:3–14.
34. Haddad ZH, Kalra V, Verma S. IgE antibodies to peptic and peptic-tryptic digest of β-lactoglobulin: significance in food hypersensitivity. *Allergy* 1979;42:368–71.

Food Allergy, edited by Eberhardt Schmidt.
Nestlé Nutrition Workshop Series, Vol. 17.
Nestec Ltd., Vevey/Raven Press, Ltd.,
New York © 1988.

Hypoallergenic Formula: A Feeding Trial in Newborn Infants from Atopic Families

R. Gerke, D. Reinhardt, and E. Schmidt

Department of Pediatrics, University of Düsseldorf, 4000 Düsseldorf 1, Federal Republic of Germany

This report describes a trial with a formula in which the protein fraction in the form of demineralized whey from cow's milk has been subjected to physicochemical treatment, as presented in the chapter by Jost *(this volume)*, and has been tested for hypoallergenicity in an animal model, as described in the chapter by Pahud et al. *(this volume)*. The trial, using a hypoallergenic formula called LHA, was carried out on newborn infants from atopic families born in Düsseldorf between May 1, 1985 and April 30, 1986, each infant being followed up to the age of about 6 to 8 months.

The group of infants for study was selected from the one-year cohort of deliveries in the Department of Obstetrics at the University of Düsseldorf. Only those newborns with a positive family history for atopic disease, whose mothers were determined to breast-feed and consented to the study, were included in the investigation.

The *study design* consisted of three different feeding phases (Fig. 1):

Phase I: Mothers were told that during the first 5 days after delivery, they should always offer the breast first and should afterwards allow the child to take the hypoallergenic formula *ad libitum* to supplement energy intake.

In general, the hypoallergenic formula would be discontinued after day 5, when lactation performance was adequate. During this period, mothers were asked to inform us about the intended date for weaning. During the period of complete lactation, the mother's dietary cow's milk protein intake was not restricted.

Phase II: When the mother was ready to wean her infant from the breast, a second period with hypoallergenic formula, this time fed exclusively, began. The introduction of the first small amounts of hypoallergenic formula was carried out under clinical observation. Infants were then kept on hypoallergenic formula for at least 1 month, until they were at least 6 months of age. Any beikost given during that time was free of cow's milk protein.

Phase III: The transition to feeding cow's-milk-containing formula was carried out under clinical observation for several hours.

Laboratory investigations included an eosinophil count and IgE determination

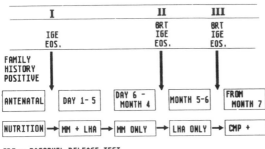

FIG. 1. Study design for the trial of hypoallergenic formula for infants from atopic families (see text).

BRT = BASOPHIL RELEASE TEST

from umbilical cord blood. Samples were taken again at the transition from mother's milk to hypoallergenic formula and again at the beginning of the introduction of cow's milk protein into the feeding regime. In the latter two instances, the basophil release test was added to the eosinophil count and the IgE determination.

PARTICIPATION

It was to be expected that, of the parents whose infants were eligible for study, quite a large number would not give their consent to a study design such as this for various reasons.

Of 909 pregnant women (Fig. 2), 125 (13.8%) presented positive histories in their families. Twelve infants needed intensive care intervention; 33 parents objected, from the outset, to a complicated study design such as this; and 21 mothers left the study because they did not succeed in breast-feeding completely. Other problems were nonallergic diseases of the infant and/or late refusals.

Forty-five infants remained in the study. Clinical observation was possible in all of them. However, not all of the laboratory studies could be carried out because mothers sometimes refused the repeated intravenous puncture.

FIG. 2. A composition of the group of infants studied.

● TOTAL GROUP OF PREGNANT WOMEN	909
● THEREOF: POS. FAMILY HISTORY FOR ATOPY	125 (13.8%)
● DROP-OUTS:	
→ NICU	12
→ OBJECTION TO STUDY	33
→ BREAK-OFF: EARLY WEANING	21
→ OTHER REASONS	14
● NON-ATTENDERS	80
● PARTICIPANTS	45

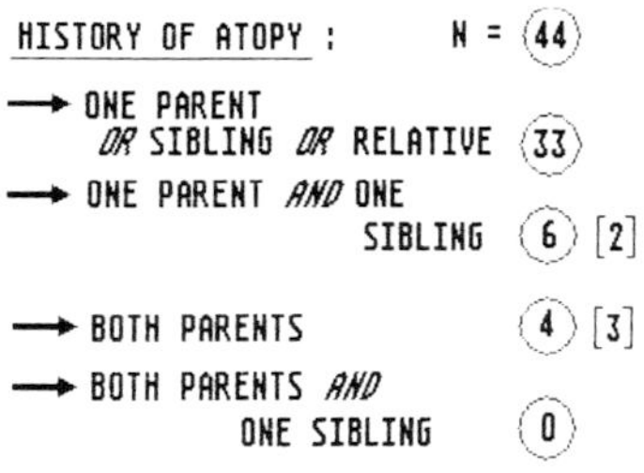

HISTORY OF ATOPY :   N = (44)

⟶ ONE PARENT
    OR SIBLING *OR* RELATIVE (33)

⟶ ONE PARENT *AND* ONE
                SIBLING (6) [2]

⟶ BOTH PARENTS   (4) [3]

⟶ BOTH PARENTS *AND*
              ONE SIBLING   (0)

FIG. 3. Family history for atopic disease in newborns subjected to the trial.

Incidence of Positive Family Histories

Thirty-three infants eligible for this study had one parent or sibling or relative with a positive history of atopic disease; in six infants, one parent and one sibling were involved; in four infants, both parents were involved. Two of the parent-sibling pairs and three of the parent pairs had identical atopic diseases (Fig. 3).

RESULTS

Clinical Observations (Fig. 4)

Phase I: The hypoallergenic formula was well tolerated as a supplement to mother's milk. Comparison with a retrospective control group, using glucose solution as a supplement to mother's milk, revealed a significantly higher weight gain in the study group on day 5.

Phase II: The change from mother's milk to hypoallergenic formula was tolerated without any adverse clinical reaction.

Phase III: Changing from the hypoallergenic formula to the cow's milk-protein-based formula resulted in two infants with a short-term spotty erythematous reaction, starting about 2 hr after first contact with cow's milk protein and lasting for 2 to 5 hr.

FIG. 4. Clinical observations during the trial with hypoallergenic formula in infants from atopic families.

MM + LHA	MM ⟶ LHA	LHA ⟶ CMP
DAY 5: SIGNIF. BETTER WEIGHT GAIN WITH MM + LHA AGAINST CONTROLS WITH MM + GLUCOSE	NO ADVERSE CLINICAL REACTIONS	2 INFANTS: SHORT-TERM ERYTHEMA 1 INFANT: CMP-INTOLE-RANCE, TREATED WITH LHA

One infant developed diarrhea within 24 hr after challenge; the diarrhea disappeared with reintroduction of hypoallergenic formula. The challenge was repeated several days later and took the same course.

Laboratory Findings

It is evident from Fig. 5 that laboratory results are not available in all infants observed for reasons mentioned above. Participation varied between 33% and 80%. Figure 5 shows the number of investigations and also shows the number of pathological reactions at each stage of the investigation for the following three measures: eosinophils, IgE, and basophil release test.

There was little deviation in eosinophils in the three phases. IgE levels gave an increasing number of elevations from Phase I (cord blood) to Phase II (following complete breast-feeding), indicating at least the probability of sensitization processes other than the ingestion of protein. There was, in general, no further elevation of levels between Phase II and Phase III, the latter being at the end of feeding hypoallergenic formula.

In the basophil release test, there was one borderline-positive reaction after Phase II (exclusive breast-feeding) which stayed slightly positive through Phase III. There were two mothers who then refused to go beyond Phase III, which means that they refused to introduce cow's milk. These infants have been continued on breast milk and hypoallergenic formula until this presentation, and they are now 8 months and 9 months old, respectively.

The one infant with a positive basophil release test in Phase II and Phase III tolerated cow's milk challenge without any symptoms. No statement can be made about the two infants who became positive between Phase II and Phase III, i.e., during the phase in which hypoallergenic formula was fed in addition to breast milk. These mothers have, so far, refused the challenge, which is intended to test their breast milk for cow's milk protein constituents.

	EOS.		IgE		BRT	
	NORMAL	PATHOL	NORMAL	PATHOL	NORMAL	PATHOL
PHASE I CORD BLOOD	18 (48%)	0	15 (33%)	2	–	–
PHASE II AFTER MM ONLY	34 (75%)	2	29 (64%)	9	24 (53%)	1
PHASE III AFTER H.A.FORM.	36 (88%)	1	34 (75%)	10	29 (64%)	1[2]

FIG. 5. Laboratory findings in infants from atopic families during the three phrases of the study.

CONCLUSION

This study is based on a relatively small number of cases.

The hypoallergenic formula by itself was well tolerated, as has also been reported elsewhere (1). Furthermore, it did not lead to any adverse clinical reactions following reintroduction at weaning.

Two short-term exanthematous reactions and one manifestation of cow's milk protein intolerance were observed.

Laboratory investigations showed one elevation of the basophil release test during the period of exclusive breast-feeding. Two additional elevations of the basophil release test during long-term breast-feeding in combination with hypoallergenic formula in older infants (8–9 months) were observed, but challenge with cow's milk was refused.

Although hypoallergenic formula has been well-tolerated clinically, it is advisable to continue to change from hypoallergenic formula to cow's milk under clinical observation.

The investigation gives no information about the prophylactic effect of the use of hypoallergenic formula on the prevention of atopic disease in infants.

REFERENCE

1. Zabransky S, Zabransky M. Erste klinische Erfahrungen mit einer hypoallergencn Säuglingsnahrung. *Extracta Paediatr* 1987;11:10–12.

Food Allergy, edited by Eberhardt Schmidt.
Nestlé Nutrition Workshop Series, Vol. 17.
Nestec Ltd., Vevey/Raven Press, Ltd.,
New York © 1988.

Detection of Casein Antigen in Regular and Hypoallergenic Formula Proteins by ELISA: Characterization of Formula Protein Fractions According to Their Molecular Weights

F. Lorenz, M. Seid, R. Tangermann, and V. Wahn

University Children's Hospital, 4000 Düsseldorf 1, Federal Republic of Germany

Together with beta-lactoglobulin, the different types of casein are considered to be responsible for most of the allergenicity of cow's milk proteins (1). Children allergic to either component can only successfully be brought up in the absence of allergens. Replacement of cow's milk proteins by soy bean proteins is often unsuccessful because many children become equally sensitized to soy bean proteins as well (2,3).

Recent progress in the treatment of cow's milk allergy has been made by the introduction of proteolytically digested formula proteins. Digestion procedures were applied based on the experience that peptides with molecular weights below 5,000 are hardly immunogenic.

This report describes our attempt to determine the molecular weights of major protein fractions in three commercial hypoallergenic formula proteins and to answer the question as to whether most of the casein epitopes are removed after proteolysis.

MATERIALS AND METHODS

Protein fractions of cow's milk (pooled from 109 healthy German cows), three different hypoallergenic formulas (LHA, prepared from whey proteins, lot 652CS-FAS, Nestlé, Switzerland; Alfare, prepared from whey proteins, lot 22.203/05DS24, Nestlé; Pregomin, prepared from soy bean and beef collagen, lot 140888, Milupa, Friedrichsdorf, FRG), and two nondigested formulas (Milumil, Pre-Aptamil, both from Milupa) were obtained by brief centrifugation for 15 min at 3,000 rpm and 4°C. The lipid layer on top was carefully removed before soluble proteins were aspirated by a Pasteur pipet.

A rabbit antibody to casein was purchased from Behring (Marburg, FRG). Alkaline-phosphatase-conjugated goat anti-rabbit IgG was obtained from Sigma (Munich, FRG). Normal rabbit serum obtained from a nonimmune rabbit was used to quantitate nonspecific rabbit IgG binding to the microtiter plate.

ELISA PROCEDURE

Protein fractions were diluted to 10^{-1} mg/ml in phosphate-buffered saline (pH 7.4). For coupling to the solid phase of a microtiter plate (Nunc, Copenhagen, Denmark), 200 μl of diluted proteins were added in triplicate to the wells and were incubated at 4°C overnight. Excess antigen was removed by three washings with PBS containing 0.05% Tween 20. Rabbit antiserum was added next, diluted 1:100 in PBS containing 1% gelatin (Serva, Heidelberg, FRG) and 10 mM EDTA. Binding to the solid-phase antigen was allowed for 2 hr at 37°C. Excess antibody was removed as described above, before anti-rabbit-IgG conjugate was added, at a 1:800 dilution, to PBS-Tween. After another incubation period of 2 hr at room temperature, excess conjugate was removed (by washing) before PNPP (Sigma) (diluted to 1 mg/ml in diethanolamine buffer, pH 9.8) was added to quantitate enzyme activity bound to the microtiter plate. The O.D. at 405 nm was read after 10 min at room temperature using an automatic ELISA reader (Flow Laboratories, Bonn, FRG).

Gel Filtration

Isolated protein fractions were separated by HPLC using a Superose 12 column (1.0 × 30.0 cm, Pharmacia, Freiburg, FRG). We applied 100 μl to the column and eluted with PBS at 0.5 ml/min. The O.D. at 280 nm was recorded automatically. The molecular weights of the major protein fractions were calculated from a standard curve using a calibration kit (Sigma, Munich).

SDS-PAGE

Reagents and polymerization procedure of the gels were used as described by the Biorad (Munich) Protein Slab Cell Instruction Manual according to established procedures (4,5). A 5% to 20% polyacrylamide gel was used under nonreducing conditions. A 50-μl sample of each protein fraction was diluted 1:1 with sample buffer, boiled for 10 min, and then applied to the gels for separation; 60 mA was applied until the bromphenol blue marker reached the bottom of the chamber.

RESULTS

Figure 1 shows the six different elution profiles in comparison with the respective external molecular-weight markers. We notice that all three hypoallergenic

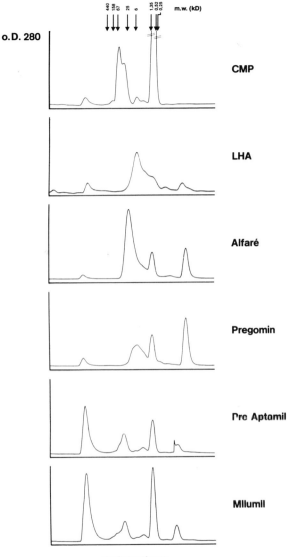

FIG. 1. HPLC elution profiles of protein fractions of cow's milk protein (CMP), three hypoallergenic formula proteins (LHA, Alfare, Pregomin), and two regular formula proteins (Pre-Aptamil, Milumil). Please notice that molecular weight in all hypoallergenic formula proteins is markedly reduced as compared to CMP; in the two regular protein fractions, however, a macromolecular peak occurs, probably representing aggregated material. In all digested preparations, significant amounts of low-molecular-weight peptides appear.

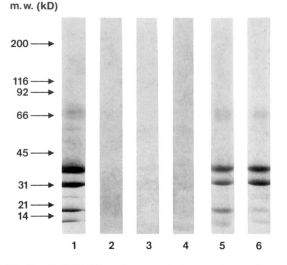

m.w. (kD)

200 →

116 →
92 →

66 →

45 →

31 →

21 →
14 →

1   2   3   4   5   6

1   CMP (10^{-1} mg/ml)
2   LHA (10^{-1} mg/ml)
3   Alfaré (10^{-1} mg/ml)
4   Pregomin (10^{-1} mg/ml)
5   Pre-Aptamil (10^{-1} mg/ml)
6   Milumil (10^{-1} mg/ml)

FIG. 2. SDS-PAGE under nonreducing conditions of cow's milk protein and different formula milk proteins. Although molecular weights of protein bands in regular formula protein are similar to native cow's milk protein, we were unable to demonstrate significant amounts of proteins with molecular weight above 10,000 in any of the digested hypoallergenic materials (lanes 2–4).

formula proteins exhibit markedly reduced molecular weights as compared to cow's milk protein, whereas both regular formula proteins contain a protein fraction with a molecular weight higher than 440,000, probably representing aggregated material.

These observations can be confirmed by SDS-PAGE. In Fig. 2 we notice that cow's milk protein and cow's-milk-derived formula proteins have major bands at similar molecular weights. In contrast, the three hypoallergenic formula proteins are hardly visible despite the fact that comparable amounts of protein had been applied to the gels.

Figure 3 shows that the casein content in all three hypoallergenic formula proteins is markedly reduced as compared to cow's milk protein and regular formula proteins. However, binding of monospecific antibody to casein still clearly exceeds nonspecific binding of normal rabbit IgG, indicating the presence of residual casein epitopes.

DISCUSSION

Based on the experience that peptides with molecular weights below 5,000 are hardly immunogenic, so-called "hypoallergenic" infant formulas have been developed (6). Some of these products contain partially digested proteins, whereas others contain amino acids (Vivonex, Eaton) as the nitrogen source. Proteins used

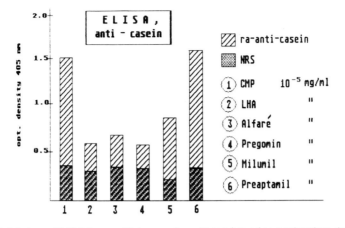

FIG. 3. Solid-phase ELISA to quantitate casein epitopes bound to a microtiter plate. With all protein fractions tested, solid-phase binding of monospecific casein antibody is markedly higher as compared to nonspecific binding of normal rabbit IgG, indicating the presence of residual casein epitopes. However, the digestion procedure in hypoallergenic formula proteins (columns 2–4) has obviously markedly reduced the casein epitope content. From these experiments, however, it cannot be determined whether the antibody is bound to native casein or its digested low-molecular-weight peptides.

for partial proteolysis are either casein [Nutramigen, Pregestimil (Mead-Johnson)], whey proteins [Alfare, LHA (Nestlé), or beef collagen [Pregomin; (Milupa)]. Both pancreatic and tryptic fragmentation of whey proteins in animal experiments completely abolished their capacity to sensitize orally and to trigger systemic or cutaneous anaphylaxis (Pahud et al., *this volume;* see also ref. 7).

Of the different protein constituents of cow's milk, casein and beta-lactoglobulin are most frequently responsible for allergic reactions (8) whereas the other proteins seem to be of minor clinical importance.

Our studies addressed two questions:

1. How effective is partial proteolysis in reduction of molecular weights?
2. Are immunogenic epitopes of a major allergen (casein) reduced or eliminated?

The first question can clearly be answered: By both gel filtration and SDS-PAGE, a significant reduction of molecular weights can be documented for all three hypoallergenic preparations tested. Peptides analyzed by SDS-PAGE are undetectable down to molecular weights of 10,000, indicating effective digestion.

To answer the second question, a solid-phase ELISA was used to detect casein epitopes in a setup that only allows qualitative, not quantitative, results. According to these experiments, the number of casein epitopes recognized by a monospecific antibody is markedly reduced but is still detectable. The question, however, remains to be answered whether these residual epitopes are expressed on traces of undigested casein or low-molecular-weight peptides derived from casein. It also remains to be studied whether these epitopes are able to elicit immune responses *in vivo* following oral administration.

Until these two issues have been sufficiently studied *in vitro* and *in vivo*, we would like to add a note of caution toward abundant and uncontrolled use of this new generation of infant formulas. To date, the possibility cannot be excluded that infants may become sensitized to casein on a "hypoallergenic" diet *in vivo* and will develop allergic reactions as soon as regular cow's milk protein is introduced. Extended clinical studies will show whether this theoretical consideration is of practical importance.

SUMMARY

Several infant formula proteins, including three designated as "hypoallergenic," were analyzed for protein molecular weights and expression of casein epitopes. In all three preparations, major peptides were hardly detectable by SDS-PAGE and were probably markedly smaller than 10,000 molecular weight. Despite this impressive reduction of molecular weight, residual casein epitopes could be detected by a solid-phase ELISA. It remains to be shown whether these epitopes can still elicit immune responses *in vivo* following infant feeding.

COMMENT

On the occasion of the oral presentation of our data (Munich, January 1987) we presented Western blot experiments suggesting that the casein epitopes are expressed on native casein. Unfortunately the putative casein band turned out to be an artifact, so we would like to withdraw these results presented in Munich.

REFERENCES

1. Müller G, Bernsau I, Müller W, Rieger CHL. Cow milk protein antigens and antibodies in serum of premature infants during the first 10 days of life. *J Pediatr* 1986;109:869–73.
2. Halpin TC, Byrne WJ, Ament ME. Colitis, persistent diarrhea, and soy protein intolerance. *J Pediatr* 1977;91:404.
3. May CD, Remigio L, Bock SA. Usefulness of measurement of antibodies in serum in diagnosis of sensitivity to cow milk and soy proteins in early childhood. *Allergy* 1980;35:301–10.
4. Richards EG, Lecanidou R. Electrophoresis and isoelectric focusing in polyacrylamide gels. In: Allen RC, Maurer HR, eds. Berlin: deGruyter, 1974:16–28.
5. Gordon, AH. Electrophoresis of proteins in polyacrylamide and starch gels. In: Work TS, Work E, eds. *Laboratory techniques in biochemistry and molecular biology.* New York: American Elsevier, 1973:123–32.
6. Schmidt E, Reinhardt D, Gerke R. Zum Einsatz hypoallergener Milchnahrungen bei Neugeborenen. *Kinderarzt* 1987;18:627–31.
7. Pahud JJ, Schwarz K. Oral sensitization to food proteins in animal models. A basis for the development of hypoallergenic infant formula. In: *Production, regulation, and analysis of infant formula. Proceedings of the Tropical Conference, Virginia Beach, 1985.* Arlington, Va.: Association of Official Analytical Chemists, 1985:264–71.
8. Wahn U, Ganster G. Kuhmilchproteine als Allergene. In: Wahn U, ed. *Aktuelle Probleme der pädiatrischen Allergologie.* Stuttgart: Gustav Fischer Verlag, 1983:121–6.

DISCUSSION

Comment on Dr. Wahn's Presentation

Dr. Jost: Dr. Wahn has apparently developed a very sensitive test which I think is an interesting tool. I have two comments: First, I have already shown you in my own presentation that, for the antigens we are examining (beta-lactoglobulin, alpha-lactalbumin, serum albumin), the processed protein, which corresponds to the processed protein in LHA preparation, is not devoid of residual antigenicity. I have shown, using solid-phase radioimmunoassay, that we have achieved a reduction in levels of antigenicity of 100-fold or more. This is a point I want to make absolutely clear. It is a realistic industrial objective to reduce the antigenicity of epitopes by this order of magnitude, and only the application of the formula will show whether this is sufficient to meet the needs of the atopic infant. Second, about Dr. Wahn's band which shows specificity to casein: I do not have a definitive answer to this, i.e., to the possibility that our raw material contains casein. We can definitely say that collected whey has a very low casein content indeed, and I think that if you use a very sensitive test you must expect that you may detect some casein breakdown products. Sweet whey contains an important quantity of the κ-casein macropeptide, a glycopeptide of 8,000 molecular weight. Dr. Wahn might have detected reactivity against this fragment, but I am doubtful about this because of the molecular weight at which he observed the reaction. I am also surprised that there is no difference in this particular reactivity between LHA and Alfaré, which has gone through a fractionation process. I am even more surprised to see that the same activity is present in Pregomin, which is apparently not based on milk protein at all.

Dr. Wahn: I think I should add that we did try to quantitate the amount of casein present in comparison with cow's milk protein, but this is difficult because Western blotting is not a quantitative method. However, by trying to dilute the band we found that the content of casein (if it is casein) was of the order of 10^4-fold lower than in raw cow's milk, i.e., about 10,000-fold lower. This still justifies calling it hypoallergenic, although there may be extremely sensitized infants who might still react to this small amount. As to what we have detected, I cannot at the moment say since we do not have monoclonal antibodies to differentiate between α-, β-, and κ-casein, and we shall have to wait until these become available. As regards Pregomin, I was as surprised as you to detect casein epitopes in a product not derived from milk, but this raises the question of cross-reactivity with beef heart protein. We should certainly be asking ourselves whether, if this protein indeed expresses casein epitopes, we are sure that it is not capable of releasing histamine from basophils and causing clinical reactions.

General Discussion

Dr. Strobel: I am impressed about the immunologic testing of these hydrolysates. I should, however, like to add another dimension to the studies. We have heard that IgE is not everything in allergy, and these studies have not addressed cell-mediated immunity at all, although we know that the requirements for the induction of this type of immunity (DTH) are different from antibody immunity. There may be allergens which can induce cell-mediated reactions without causing antibody reactions. I should also like to point out that in these studies the aggregates have been excluded; i.e., the final formula as prepared by the mother has *not* been tested. I think one ought to test this because other substances of potential immunogenicity will be present in the final product apart from the hydroly-sate—for example, starch, which has induced an immune response in hyperimmunized animals.

Dr. Pahud: You are quite right about cell-mediated immunity. This must also be looked at, and we have not yet done so. As regards testing the whole formula, we have been un-able to get any sensitization with oral administration, either with the hydrolysate or with the whole formula. Using parenteral sensitization, we did get a response, mainly against the beta-lactoglobulin.

Dr. Jost: Concerning the SDS gel, we used this method particularly to detect residual protein and not the peptide parts.

Dr. Revillard: You seem to have achieved a very marked reduction in the antigenicity of native whey protein in this study. But I wonder, on the other hand, if the peptides that are present in the preparation are able to block the binding of antibodies to native milk proteins. What is the tolerogenic potency of such small peptides toward the immune re-sponse to native protein, either in terms of antibody production or of cell-mediated re-sponse?

Dr. Pahud: The inhibitory actions of these peptides have been tested in the radioimmu-noassays done in Dr. Jost's group. *In vitro* these peptides do block the probe antibodies, and we are now trying to use the hydrolysate to tolerize animals orally. We have no evi-dence as yet that tolerance is readily achieved by such peptides.

Dr. de Weck: When we look at the antigenicity of these peptides and proteins, we should consider using human antibodies which have been produced against the various milk pro-teins, because the epitopes which can be ''seen'' in milk proteins by the human are not necessarily the same as those seen by a rabbit or guinea pig. Maybe some of the antigens or epitopes which we are concerned about because of their continued presence may not be so relevant, since humans might not be able to recognize them. Have you conducted any studies with human anticasein?

Dr. Wahn: I agree that epitopes recognized by our rabbit antibody might differ from those recognized by human antibodies, but unfortunately the sera we have available from allergic infants contain multispecific antibodies directed not only against casein but also against other proteins. Specific human monoclonal antibodies are not available.

Dr. Von Geiser: We have heard something of the protective effect of breast-feeding and of this LHA preparation. In our hospital, and others too I expect, the nurses sometimes feed infants who are meant to be breast-fed with a cow's milk formula without our knowl-edge. How great do you estimate is the likely effect of small cow's milk feedings in infants who are later fed on breast-milk or hypoallergenic formula?

Dr. Schmidt: Feeding cow's milk during the first days and then breast-feeding is an ex-cellent way of sensitizing an infant against cow's milk. I do not know what would be the effect of substituting hypoallergenic formula for breast-feeding in this situation, but I guess that it would probably not be a very good idea.

Dr. Marini: When you give the hypoallergenic formula to young babies who are nor-mally breast-fed, do they accept it? And what about the case of a mother who wants to continue breast-feeding but has to supplement the feeds because she has not got enough milk?

Dr. Schmidt: Most infants accept the hypoallergenic formula well; a few cases of diffi-culty have occurred, but the change from breast-feeding to formula has always been made at a time when the mothers wanted to wean; so they managed in spite of the difficulty, and the infants took to it after a while. There have been no particular difficulties in mixed breast- and formula-feeding.

Dr. Aas: I am personally very satisfied with what has been presented with regard to this new preparation. I see it as a pragmatic and professional approach to the problem. You will never be able to get a 100% guaranteed nonsensitizing hydrolysate product from cow's milk. But if this preparation has an acceptable taste, which it appears to have, and if it is treated properly by the users, so that they don't create new aggregates with sensitizing epitopes on them, then it is an achievement, and is likely to be better than what we have at present for the majority of infants that we are concerned with.

Food Allergy, edited by Eberhardt Schmidt.
Nestlé Nutrition Workshop Series, Vol. 17.
Nestec Ltd., Vevey/Raven Press, Ltd.,
New York © 1988.

The Dietetic Treatment of Food Allergy

Glenis K. Scadding and Jonathan Brostoff

The Middlesex Hospital, London W1N 8AA, England

The dietetic treatment of food allergy is, in theory, extremely simple, since it only involves (a) the identification of relevant food antigens and (b) the avoidance of relevant food antigens. This can be a most rewarding process because simply by food exclusion, troublesome symptoms can be completely avoided. However, it can also become remarkably complicated, difficult, and fraught with metabolic and psychological problems. Our practice at the Middlesex Hospital consists largely of adults, so my remarks will mainly concern them; however, infants will be mentioned where relevant.

TYPE-I HYPERSENSITIVITY

In immediate-type food hypersensitivities, small quantities of food elicit a reaction in a short period of time, and the identification of the relevant antigens is usually easy and is made on the patient's history. Skin-prick tests or the RAST (radioallergosorbent test) can be used as confirmation if necessary. Avoidance of the specific allergens is safe, effective, cheap, and easy if only one or two food stuffs are involved, but it becomes extremely difficult when the patient is sensitive to a wide range of foods or if there is exquisite sensitivity with anaphylaxis occurring to a minute quantity of the relevant food allergen or even contact with another person who has recently ingested that food: One peanut-sensitive patient developed swelling of mouth and tongue after kissing her boyfriend who had recently eaten them. Similarly, breast-fed children can be sensitized by, and later react to, foodstuffs contained in breast milk, and it may be necessary for the mother herself to avoid highly antigenic substances, such as cow's milk, eggs, wheat, nuts, citrus fruits, shellfish, and fish. (1,2). Professional dietary advice is mandatory (except in cases where one or two unusual antigens are being eliminated) for the following reasons: firstly, to ensure that the substance is really completely removed from the diet, which involves instructions in reading the labels on foodstuffs (Table 1 shows the different forms in which cow's milk can appear on labels in foods); and secondly, to ensure that the long-term diet is nutritionally adequate and that any missing vitamins or minerals are replaced. For babies with cow's milk allergy, various substitutes are available. Hydrolyzed cow's milk protein products are probably the

225

TABLE 1. *Dietetic guidelines from the Department of Nutrition and Dietetics,*
Bloomsbury Health Authority

Milk-Free Diet

Milk and all **milk products** must be excluded from the diet, including all commercially pre-pared foods containing milk derivatives. This diet sheet advises you on how to achieve this; but remember on any restricted diet, it is important to eat a wide variety of permitted foods in order to ensure that you are getting all the nutrients you need in your diet. Milk and milk products are major sources of calcium in our diet, and consideration must be given as to whether a calcium supplement is required. Your doctor or dietitian will advise you.
  It is important to check the labels on manufactured foods for the following ingredients:

  Milk; butter; buttermilk; cream; artificial cream; cheese; skimmed milk powder; marga-rine; yogurt; casein and caseinates; lactalbumin; whey; lactose; nonfat milk solids; hydrolyzed milk protein.

These are all sources of milk protein, milk sugar, or butterfat and must therefore be avoided. **Food manufacturers often change the ingredients of products, so check labels regularly.**

If there is ever any doubt about a product, avoid it.

most popular, though synthetic amino acids together with all necessary vitamins and minerals are now available. Soya derivatives have been used, but sensitization to these is common (3,4). Goat's milk is not recommended because it is deficient in folate and may be contaminated and because there is an 18% incidence of cross-reactivity with cow's milk (5). The tablets and medicines used in replacement ther-apy must also, of course, be free from any offending antigen: Unfortunately, in the United Kingdom there is no necessity for manufacturers to state on the labels the full contents of each of their medicines, and tablets frequently contain sub-stances such as lactose, corn starch, and colorings.
  Rigorous attention to small details is frequently necessary in Type-I sensitivity. Figure 1 illustrates the peak flow chart of an asthma patient with immediate hyper-sensitivity to a variety of foods which produced mouth swelling and later broncho-spasm. She was an inpatient on an elemental diet and spring water only and was not unnaturally getting very bored with this regime. One evening she was allowed out for a drink with her boyfriend on the condition that she had Perrier water and nothing else. Unfortunately, she was given Perrier water with ice and lemon, and the latter resulted in an immediate recurrence of her symptoms. Skin-prick testing with lemon juice subsequently gave a positive wheal, and thus she identified an-other offending allergen. It is also important that the right allergen is avoided. This is illustrated in the case history of another lady who thought she was unable to eat shrimps. Careful analysis of her history showed, in fact, that absolutely fresh shrimps did not usually bother her—the ones that had been treated with preserva-tive proved to be the problem. This was confirmed when we made extracts of both

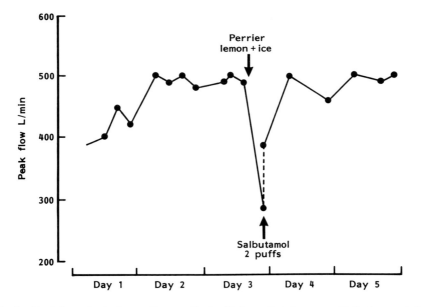

FIG. 1. Peak flow chart of an asthma patient with immediate hypersensitivity to a variety of foods.

kinds and tested her basophil histamine release. Sodium metabisulphite, which is used to preserve shrimps, is also used on a wide variety of other seafoods.

DELAYED REACTIONS TO FOOD

Where the reaction to food is not a Type-I phenomenon but is, instead, delayed and requires large quantities of the food, the diagnosis is much more difficult. It involves a period without any ingestion of that foodstuff during which sensitivity appears to increase, followed by challenge with the food, preferably repeatedly and preferably on a double-blind basis. During the period of dietary exclusion the patient can be maintained on spring water alone if he or she is adult and plump; otherwise, the patient can be maintained on an elemental diet, which contains synthetic amino acids and hydrolyzed maize starch together with all necessary vitamins and minerals. We have had a special version of this diet prepared for our use in which the starch source is rice, since this is less allergenic than maize starch in many patients. One alternative is a highly restricted diet that includes just a few foods such as lamb, rice, cauliflower, pears, and spring water; another alternative is a diet that excludes the major food groups. Our usual choice is a grain-, dairy-, egg-, citrus-additive-, and preservative-free diet. It is our usual practice to exclude also from the diet any food that the patient craves or eats in large quantities.

In a busy clinic it is difficult to undertake double-blind challenges on every patient, so our initial food reintroduction is usually done openly by putting back the relevant food for a week at a time and noting any change in symptomatology. If the food does appear to cause symptoms, it is again withdrawn from the diet, and other food groups are tested.

Before embarking on a prolonged period of restricted eating, it is wise to ensure that the suspect food really is the cause of the patient's symptoms. (This procedure is not recommended outside the hospital, either in infancy or where there have been previous severe reactions.) We have usually performed repeated open challenges. In only a very few of our patients has it proved possible to confirm the results of open challenge by subsequent double-blind challenge. When undertaking this, our dietitian makes lentil puree, which is then put into pots, and the relevant antigen is hidden in some of these pots and is administered in triplicate so that the patient gets a good load of antigen over a period of 2 to 3 days. Plain pots are interspersed in replicate, and the code is held by the dietitian. The order of the pots is thus not known by the patient, nor is it known by the doctor when assessing whether or not the results are positive. This is obviously a time-consuming procedure, and thus far we have found its use only possible in a research setting. However, Nestlé has kindly made available for us coded tins of lentil puree with hidden foods, so we hope to increase the use of such tests.

An alternative type of diet for delayed food sensitivity, where large quantities of food are necessary over a period of several days to elicit a reaction, is a rotation diet. This can also be useful when the offending food items cannot be identified or are multiple. The principle of this is that certain food groups are eaten on one day and are then not eaten again until 3 or 4 days later. In this way the intestine never receives a buildup of one particular food group antigen. A typical rotation diet is shown in Table 2. We have sometimes had success in patients with atopic eczema with multiple RAST sensitivities on this diet. Figure 2 shows such an example. Regular exacerbations of symptoms occurring after a particular day in the rotation suggests that one of the food groups eaten on that day is provoking the patient. This can be further investigated.

Exclusion diets in adults frequently involve the omission of wheat or grains as a whole (6). We have found compliance to be best when patients are given a list not only of what *not* to eat but also of what to eat, with suggested recipes. For this reason we are involved in producing a recipe booklet and a 2-week diet plan.

We have recently reviewed our experience with dietary elimination in 100 adult patients treated at the Middlesex Hospital Allergy Clinic. When those patients who were referred for dietary assessment only are excluded, 93 patients remain. Of these, 41 improved on a diet, meaning that their symptoms either decreased or disappeared entirely. Of the remainder, 21 did not improve, and 31 were either unable to follow the diet or were lost to follow-up. This gives a fairly high failure rate of 56%. However, 44% of patients improved; these patients came from a population which is largely composed of second-stage referrals—that is, patients who have been investigated and treated unsuccessfully at other hospitals for their condition. The majority of them also improved without recourse to any medication other

TABLE 2. Rotation diet

Day	Meat, fish, etc.	Vegetables	Fruits	Beverages	Grains, flour	Nuts	Oils, fats	Sweetener
1	Beef Lamb Cheese	Parsley family: carrot, celery, parsnip, parsley Fungi: mushroom, yeast Spinach	Rose family: strawberry, raspberry Apple family: apple, pear, quince Mango	Milk Tea Apple juice	Oats	Brazil Cashew	Beef drippings Butter	Beet sugar (silver spoon)
2	Fish Shellfish	Sunflower family: lettuce, chicory, endive, artichokes Potato family: tomato, potato, aubergine, peppers	Citrus family: orange, lemon, grapefruit, kumquat, tangerine, lime Avocado Rhubarb	Orange juice Grapefruit juice Camomile tea	Buckwheat Sunflower seeds Ryvita (original) Tapioca	Filbert Hazel	Olive Sunflower oil Safflower oil	100% Maple syrup 100% Maple sugar
3	Poultry Eggs	Mustard family: cabbage, broccoli, cauliflower, kale, turnip, kohlrabi, Brussels sprouts, chinese cabbage, radish, watercress Gourd family: marrow, pumpkin, cucumber, fresh courgette, fresh gherkin	Banana Plantain Melon Pineapple Gooseberry family: gooseberry; red, black, and white currants	Pineapple juice Mint tea	Wheat Corn (maize) Rice (rice cakes) with salt or bran only) Sago	Walnut Hickory Pecan	Corn oil	Cane sugar Molasses
4	Pork	Legume family: pea, beans, lentil, soya, chickpea Sweet potato Lily family: onion, garlic, chive, leek, asparagus	Grape family: grape, raisin, currants, sultanas Plum family: cherry, peach, apricot, plum, prune, sloe Palm family: coconut, date	Grape juice Rosehip tea White wine Soya milk (sugar-free)	Lentil Chickpea Soya Cream of tartar Carob	Peanut Almond	Peanut oil Soya oil Pork lard	

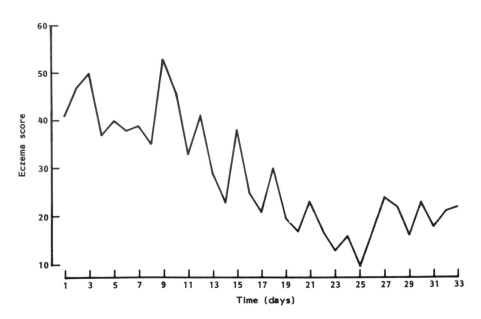

FIG. 2. Effects of a rotation diet on exacerbation of atopic eczema, suggesting that one certain food group provokes the patient. The eczema score was derived by considering the body as being divided into nine parts and alloting a score of 0–10 for each area, depending on the severity and the extent of the eczema there.

than diet, and they now successfully remain on their diet. It would thus seem economically viable to investigate and treat patients from a food sensitivity point of view. The conditions from which these patients suffered are shown in Table 3. It is obvious that many patients were multisymptomatic, as is frequently the case in food sensitivity. The foods implicated are shown in Table 4.

TABLE 3. *Conditions improved by diet in 41 positive responders*

Symptoms	Number of patients
Irritable bowel syndrome	13
Joint pains (including rheumatoid arthritis, lupus erythematosus, systemic and Still's disease)	12
Migraine	8
Lethargy/depression	8
Eczema	5
Urticaria/angioedema	4
Asthma/rhinitis	3
Hyperactivity	3
Pruritus	2
Urinary frequency	2
Crohn's disease	1

TABLE 4. *Foods causing symptoms in positive responders*

Food	Number of patients
Cow's milk	17
Wheat	11
Colorings/preservatives	10
Egg	6
Yeast	4
Rye	4
Tomatoes	3
Nuts	3
Cocoa	3
Banana	3
Cane sugar	2
Citrus	2
Corn	2
Pork	2
Beef	2
Soya	1
Mushrooms	1

REINTRODUCTION OF FOODS

In adults, a 6-month period of food avoidance is usually followed by a trial reintroduction of one food family at a time, usually eaten in small quantities on a rotational basis. If symptoms recur immediately, the food is removed from the diet again for 6 more months. If not, we recommend continued rotational eating, on the basis that this is less likely to cause sensitization. In practice, most patients eat the food every day after a few weeks.

In children with a history of severe reactions, reintroduction is best undertaken in a hospital. Small children (<3 years old) are more likely to lose their allergy quickly (7). The disappearance of food sensitivity varies according to the food: With nuts, peanuts, and fish, the allergic reactions are prolonged (7,8).

There are some more controversial aspects of the dietetic treatment of food allergy which I should like to deal with briefly.

Antifungal Agents

There is a theory which states that chronic candidiasis of the gastrointestinal tract is a major cause of chronic illness from tissue sensitivity to the organism and/or its by-products rather than from direct tissue invasion by the organism itself; the theory also states that chronic candidiasis promotes food allergy by increasing intestinal permeability. We undertook a small survey of 20 food-allergic patients and failed to find any evidence of candida in their stools or of candida antibodies in their blood, nor was there any evidence of abnormal lymphocyte sen-

TABLE 5. *Treatment of chronic candidiasis sensitivity syndrome*

Dietary and nutritional measures

Dietary measures to retard candida growth:
  Low-carbohydrate, yeast-free diet
  Adequate nutrients for optimal immune response, e.g., vitamins (yeast-free B complex, vitamins A, E, C, etc.), minerals (zinc, iron, magnesium, calcium), and fatty acids (evening primrose oil)
  Supplementation to ensure favorable gut flora ecology, e.g., lactobacillus

Pharmacologic measures

Avoidance of drugs promoting chronic candida growth, e.g., antibiotics, steroids, oral contraceptives, etc.
Treatment of candida with antifungal medication, e.g., nystatin, ketoconazole, caprylic acid, etc.

Immunologic measures

Active immunization with *Candida albicans* extracts

Other measures

Treat all inhalant, food, and chemical allergies; e.g., use environmental control, active immunotherapy, and hypoallergenic diets
Rule out associated endocrinopathic conditions, e.g., thyroid, ovarian, adrenal, etc.

---

sitivity to *Candida albicans*. However, there is a trend toward treating patients for this condition, which is called *chronic candidiasis sensitivity syndrome* (9). The basis of treatment is shown in Table 5. This regime has been tried on an *ad hoc* basis in a few patients attending our allergy clinic in whom there was a history of recurrent thrush or of cravings for sugary foods. To date, the results are not overly impressive except in one or two individuals.

Immunotherapy

There is obviously no role for classic desensitization in food allergy. Provocation neutralization techniques have been variously reported as being successful or unsuccessful; at the present time, however, the American Academy of Allergy and Immunology regards the case not proven (10). Two more recent reports support the use of such methods in food allergy following double-blind evaluation. We have performed a double-blind study using this method in perennial rhinitis due to house dust mite (11) and have shown that there is evidence of efficacy. The method has now been extended to a few patients with defined food allergies and has produced benefit in some.

Metabolic Deficiencies

We have recently tested the sulfoxidation capacity of 94 food-sensitive patients and found that the proportion of those who are poor metabolizers by this route is far higher than that in the normal population. It may be that metabolic defects underlie, as well as predispose to, food-allergic reactions.

SUMMARY

The treatment of food allergy is primarily a matter of food intolerance, with the degree of strictness depending on the degree of sensitivity. The diet must be adequate and must not have effects that are worse than those of the disease for which it is being given.

REFERENCES

1. Donnally HH. The question of the elimination of foreign protein in women's milk. *J Immunol* 1930;19:15.
2. Hemmings WA, Kulangara DC. Dietary antigens in breast milk [Letter]. *Lancet* 1978;ii:575.
3. Halpern SR, Sellars WA, Johnson RB, Saperstein S, Reisch JS. Development of childhood allergy in infants fed breast, soy or cow's milk. *J Allergy Clin Immunol* 1973;51:139 51.
4. Dannaeus A, Johansson SGO, Fencard T, Ohman G. Clinical and immunological aspects of food allergy in childhood. *Acta Paediatr Scand* 1977;66:31–7.
5. Hutchins P, Walker-Smith JA. The gastrointestinal system. In: Brostoff J, Challacombe SJ, eds. *Clinics in immunology and allergy, vol. 2, no. 1. Food Allergy.* New York: Saunders, 1982:70–1.
6. Lessoff MH, Wraith DG, Merrett TG, Merrett J, Buisseret PD. Food allergy and intolerance in 100 patients—local and systemic effects. *Quart J Med* 1980;49:259–71.
7. Bock SA. The natural history of food sensitivity. *J Allergy Clin Immunol* 1982;69:173–7.
8. Estebain MM, Pascual C, Madero R, Diaz Pena JM, Odeja JA. Natural history of immediate food allergy in children. In: Businco L, Ruggoeri F, eds. *Proceedings of the 1st Latin Food allergy workshop.* Rome: Fisons SpA, 1985:27–30.
9. Kroker GG. Chronic candidiasis and allergy. In: Brostoff J, Challacombe SJ, eds. *Food Allergy and intolerance.* London: Baillière Tindall, 1986:855–67.
10. American Academy of Allergy. *Adverse reactions to foods.* NIH Publication 1984, no. 84-2442:170.
11. Scadding GK, Brostoff J. Low dose sublingual therapy in patients with allergic rhinitis due to house dust mite. *Clin Allergy* 1986;16:483–91.

Food Allergy, edited by Eberhardt Schmidt.
Nestlé Nutrition Workshop Series, Vol. 17.
Nestec Ltd., Vevey/Raven Press, Ltd.,
New York © 1988.

Prevention of Food Allergy in Infants and Children

Paolo Durand

Istituto Giannina Gaslini, 16147 Genoa, Italy

The presence in a family of an infant or a child with immunologically mediated adverse responses to food causes important feeding problems.

Prevention in at-risk populations and early treatment of food allergy in infants and children include the identification of the mechanisms which are involved in pathogenesis.

At the present time, the prevention of food allergy—frequently mediated by IgE reactions to food and by other mechanisms not involving IgE mediation—might be limited to the following possibilities:

1. Avoidance of potentially allergenic foods during the last trimester of pregnancy and during lactation in infants at risk.
2. Encouragement of breast-feeding, which has the dual benefit of eliminating some of the potential allergenic proteins and providing important immune defenses.
3. Use of pharmacologic agents when food allergic disease is present.

These preventive possibilities will now be discussed in detail (1,2).

AVOIDANCE OF POTENTIALLY ALLERGENIC FOODS

Immunogenicity of potentially allergenic proteins depends on the foreignness, the exposure dose, the frequency of exposure, the age of exposure, the molecular structure, the molecular size and shape, and the multiplicity binding sites (3). Some of the physical properties of the proteins are the heat resistance and the resistance to denaturation and to digestion (4). Very few food-allergenic proteins have been isolated and characterized, but some have been purified. Milk, for instance, is composed of a large number of antigenic components. Most of the 16 antigens found in cow's milk (5), as well as most of the 32 antigens found in bovine whey, are serum proteins; only a few are milk-specific (6).

The major milk proteins—namely, alpha-lactalbumin, beta-lactoglobulin, and casein—have been purified and tested for allergenicity. Denaturation of alpha-lactalbumin, beta-lactoglobulin, and casein modify their properties so that they are less allergenic.

We know that food allergens from the mother's diet can cross the placenta and can be excreted in the breast milk. Casein, and particularly beta-lactoglobulin and ovoalbumin, can be easily demonstrated in the breast milk after ingestion from the mother (7). It is well established that the presence of these substances in breast milk may be responsible for the manifestations of food allergy in some nursing infants. The hypersensitivity phenomena are not dissimilar to the symptoms produced by artificially fed infants.

Therefore, evidence tends to favor the conclusions that the avoidance of highly allergenic food proteins must be considered by the mothers who are in the last trimester of pregnancy and during the period of lactation, to prevent placental or breast milk passage of food antigens from the mother to the infant. However, problems of compliance sometimes occur.

For the infant reacting to cow's milk, there are problems in selecting appropriate feeds without allergenic components. The use of soybean formulas and casein hydrolysate mixtures is indicated in infants and children with symptoms and signs of cow's-milk-protein allergy. However, nearly 25% of the children affected by cow's milk allergy who are fed exclusively with soy formula, as well as nearly 18% who are fed with casein hydrolysate, develop hypersensitivity reactions to these substitutes over weeks or months. Elimination diets are often not easily followed, resulting in lack of compliance. Alternatively, a specialized elemental diet may be useful in selected patients who do not tolerate mother's milk substitutes. Special diets with selected cow's milk substitutes are sometimes refused or are difficult to maintain for a long period of time. Therefore, special care must be taken to avoid suboptimal nutrition and malnutrition.

BREAST-FEEDING

Breast-feeding for the first 4 to 6 months has been claimed as an effective tool in preventing the early development of symptoms of sensitization, especially in high-risk infants.

During the last 50 years, numerous articles have been published addressing the question, Does the exclusion of cow's milk from the infant diet reduce the risk of allergy? In 1983, Burr reviewed 24 articles on this subject (8). In 13 of these 24 studies, allergic diseases were positively associated with cow's milk or mixed feeding, whereas 10 showed no convincing relationship with infant feeding. After Burr's article, there have been seven others published on the subject. Three of them confirm the question under consideration, three do not provide evidence against it, and one presents positive results regarding breast milk (9–13). Some defects are present in many of these studies; very few have been conducted as randomized controlled trials, and sufficient information has not usually been collected regarding early supplementary feeds given to breast-fed infants (Table 1).

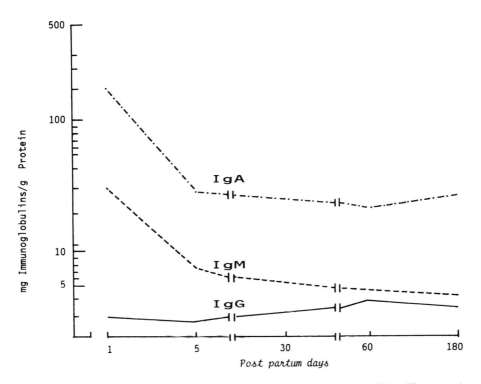

FIG. 1. Immunoglobulin G, A, M distribution in colostrum and in human milk in different periods of lactation.

In conclusion, the results of these studies tend to favor the hypothesis that giving infants cow's milk or the early introduction of solid foods increases the risk of allergic disease.

The promotion of breast-feeding is advised by pediatricians because it seems to offer the dual benefit of eliminating one of the most common sensitizing food antigens while providing important immune defenses. Colostrum and breast milk provide important immune defenses for the infant's gastrointestinal tract, especially during the early neonatal period (14). They contain a number of factors that contribute to its beneficial effect, including nonspecific anti-infective components such as lysozyme, lactoferrin, gastrointestinal mucosal growth factor, and B-cell proliferation factor (15) (Table 2). On the other hand, the transient deficiency or absence of secretory IgA, along with the maturational delay of the gut mucosa during the neonatal period, may predispose the vulnerable infant to macromolecular absorption of intact food protein and absorption of partially degraded food products (13).

According to the previously presented data (Fig. 1; Table 2), there is no doubt about the advantages of breast-feeding. However, in some cases, despite dietary prevention, the symptomatology of food allergy appears.

TABLE 1. *Review of 31 studies that showed epidemiologic evidence for the following: a relationship between allergy and cow's milk feeding (CMF) or mixed feeding; a relationship between allergy and breast-feeding (BF); and the absence of a convincing relationship between allergy and infant feeding*

```
                                         ┌─ 16 positive for CMF or
                                         │   mixed feeding
                                         │
   31 Reported Studies ─────────────────┤    2 positive for BF
                                         │
                                         │
                                         └─ 13 no convincing
                                             relationship
```

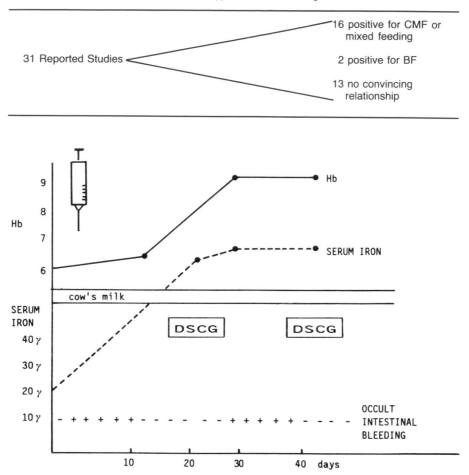

FIG. 2. DSCG effect (100 mg × 4) on the occult blood loss from the intestine in a child with iron-deficiency anemia due to milk intolerance. (From ref. 27.)

TABLE 2. *Immunoglobulins and other factors present in colostrum and human milk*

IgA, IgG, IgM
Lysozyme
Lactoferrin
Growth factor gastrointestinal mucosa
B-cell proliferation factor
T, B cells and macrophages
Lactobacillus bifidum

PHARMACOLOGIC AGENTS

Pharmacologic agents may be useful in the management of specific cases of food allergy (which does not profit by dietary prevention) as well as in treatment of prophylaxis, especially in children when strict avoidance of the offending food cannot be attained. However, the benefit cannot be predicted (16).

The pharmacologic agents are anti-H_1-receptor antihistamines, H_2-receptor antagonists, cinnarizine, pirenzepine, steroids, oral disodium cromoglycate, ketotifen, and inhibitors of prostaglandin synthesis (Table 3).

The mode of action of antihistamines is through competitive inhibition with histamine for receptors on target cells. All antihistamines act best when administered prior to the release of histamine, but the doses of antihistamine needed to control symptoms are large enough to provoke secondary effects such as drowsiness. Only some of the new antihistamines having minimal side effects might be useful in treating food allergy (16).

H_1-receptor antihistamines alone or in association with H_2-receptor antagonists must be given before the exposure to the offending food to prevent symptoms. But despite the good clinical improvement with anti-H_2, several side effects (endocrinologic, hematologic, gastroenteric, and immunologic) have been observed (16).

Food allergens are believed to stimulate mediator release from mast cells in the gastrointestinal tract, thus causing adverse reactions such as, for instance, increased permeability of the gut with absorption of potential allergenic protein into the blood. Sodium cromoglycate acts primarily by inhibiting mediator release at the surface of mast cells. Originally used by inhalation and aerosol to prevent allergenic asthma, oral sodium cromoglycate has been used with favorable results in controlling adverse symptoms in many patients suffering from food allergy not managed by dietary restriction. The drug is effective in preventing gastrointestinal symptoms and amelioration of other symptoms of IgE-mediated food allergy. Oral sodium cromoglycate is a safe drug; however, adverse reactions such as abdominal pain, vomiting, headache, rhinorrhea, and insomnia have been reported (16–21) (Fig. 2).

The medical literature contains some references to the use of oral ketotifen in controlling food allergy. Ketotifen decreases the responsiveness of the autologous mixed lymphocyte reaction *in vitro,* and it seems to be of some utility in the man-

TABLE 3. *Pharmacologic agents in food allergy*

Sodium cromoglycate
Ketotifen

H_1 receptor antagonists
H_2 receptor antagonists
Cinnarizine
Pirenzepine
Prostaglandin inhibitors steroids

agement of patients with food allergy, even if it lacks carry-over effects. Ketotifen seems to be a simple and effective drug, but at present it requires more investigation because an inhibitory effect on lymphocyte proliferation has been reported (22,23).

Steroids for long-term medication should not be used, especially if other drugs can be effective.

Prostaglandins seem to play a role in mediating adverse reactions—especially in the gastrointestinal tract—to certain foods. Inhibitors of prostaglandin synthesis—for example, aspirin and other nonsteroid drugs (indomethacin, ibuprofen)—have prevented symptoms of food intolerance in a group of patients, but there have been some failures (24,25). Pirenzepine, an anticholinergic drug which acts by modulating gastric secretion, seems to be useful in the treatment on gastroenterologic adverse reactions to foods because it defends the intestinal mucosa and controls enteric motility.

NEW APPROACHES TO THE PREVENTION

The prevention of IgE-mediated disorders could be approached by intervention at the lymphokine level to modify IgE production. A search for the "designer gene" to produce lymphokines is in progress.

In summary, the various strategies described above may be useful in the prevention or treatment of the adverse reactions to foods in infants and children.

However, a great deal is still to be learned about the various mechanisms that operate in adverse reactions. Investigations are necessary in order to identify the structure and immunologic properties of food antigens and their relationship to food allergy.

Although pharmacologic agents are of potential value, their effectiveness seems unpredictable. These drugs must be more precisely investigated, not only for their therapeutic benefits but also for adverse reactions and possible side effects.

REFERENCES

1. Bellanti JA. Prevention of food allergy. *Ann Allergy* 1984;53:683–7.
2. Businco L, Marchetti F, Pellegrini G, Cantani A, Perlini R. Prevention of atopic diseases in at risk newborns by prolonged breast-feeding. *Ann Allergy* 1983;51:296–302.
3. Taylor SL, Lemanske RF Jr, Bush RK, Busse WW. Food allergens: structure and immunological properties. Presented at the Third International Symposium on Immunological and Clinical Problems of Food Allergy, Taormina, October 1–4, 1986.
4. Kilshaw PJ, Heppell LM, Ford JE. Effects of heat treatment of cow's milk and whey on nutritional quality and antigenic properties. *Arch Dis Child* 1982;57:842–7.
5. Hanson LA, Mansson I. Immune electrophoretic studies of bovine milk and milk products. *Acta Paediatr* 1961;50:484–90.
6. Lowenstein H, Bjerrum OJ, Wecke E, Wecke B. Characterization of bovine whey proteins by crossed immunoelectrophoresis. *Scand Immunol* 1975;4(suppl 2):155–61.
7. Kilshaw PJ, Cant AJ. The passage of maternal dietary proteins into human breast milk. *Int Arch Allergy Appl Immunol* 1984;14:533–41.

8. Burr ML. Does infant feeding affect the risk of allergy? *Arch Dis Child* 1983;58:561–5.
9. Atherton DJ. Breast feeding and atopic eczema. *Br Med J* 1983;287:775–6.
10. Kajosaari M, Saarinen UM. Prophylaxis of atopic disease by six months' total solid food elimination. *Acta Paediatr Scand* 1983;72:411–4.
11. Kovar MG, Serdula MK, Marks JS, Fraser DW. Review of the epidemiologic evidence for an association between infant feeding and infant health. *Pediatrics* 1984;74:615–38.
12. Van Asperen PP, Kemp AS, Mellis CMA. Prospective study of clinical manifestations of atopic disease in infancy. *Acta Paediatr Scand* 1984;69:89–91.
13. Stahlberg MR. Breast feeding, cow's milk feeding and allergy. *Allergy* 1985;40:612–15.
14. Ogra SS, Ogra PL. Immunologic aspects of human colostrum and milk: I. Distribution characteristics and concentrations of immunoglobulins at different times after the onset of lactation. *J Pediatr* 1978;92:546–9.
15. Juto P. Human milk stimulates B cell function. *Arch Dis Child* 1985;60:610–3.
16. Collins-Williams C. Pharmacologic agents and food allergy. *Ann Allergy* 1986;57:53–60.
17. Freier S, Berger H. Disodium cromoglycate in gastrointestinal protein intolerance. *Lancet* 1973;i:913–5.
18. Kuzemko JA, Simpson KR. Treatment of allergy to cow's milk. *Lancet* 1975;i:337–8.
19. Kingsley PJ. Oral sodium cromoglycate in gastrointestinal allergy. *Lancet* 1974;ii:1011–2.
20. Dannaeus A, Foucard T, Johansson SGO. The effect of orally administered sodium cromoglycate on symptoms of food allergy. *Clin Allergy* 1977;7:109–15.
21. Businco L, Cantani A, Benincori N, Perlini R, Infussi R, De Angelis M, Businco E. Effectiveness of oral sodium cromoglycate (SCG) in preventing food allergy in children. *Ann Allergy* 1983;51:47–50.
22. Zanussi C. Food allergy treatment. *Clin Immunol Allergy* 1982;2:221–6.
23. Dutau G, Sablayrolles B, Rochioli P. Effects protecteurs du ketotifene dans l'allergie alimentaire du nourisson et de l'enfant. In: Michel FB, ed. *Bronches de l'asthmatique*. Paris: Masson, 1982:160–6.
24. Buisseret PD, Youlten LF, Heinzelmann DI, Lessof MH. Prostaglandin-synthesis inhibitors in prophylaxis of food intolerance. *Lancet* 1978;i:906–8.
25. Dodge JA, Hamdi JA, Burns GM, Yamashiro Y. Toddler diarrhoea and prostaglandin. *Arch Dis Child* 1981;56:705–7.
26. Hamburger RN, Heller S, Mellan MH, O'Connor RD, Zeyer RS. Current status of the clinical and immunological consequences of a prototype allergic disease prevention program. *Ann Allergy* (part II) 1983;51:281
27. Panizon X and Ventura Y. *Prospective Pediat* 1980;10:347–58.

DISCUSSION

Dr. Strobel: I am always very impressed when I see your data on the use of disodium cromoglycate (SCG) in the treatment of gastrointestinal food allergy. It is difficult to conceive that SCG could work in this situation since it does not seem to affect the intestinal mast cell, either *in vivo* or *in vitro*, and there is no really sound evidence that it stabilizes mast cells or exerts an anti-IgE effect. There are some conditions where it will reduce antigen uptake, and I suppose it is also possible that it may form complexes with food antigens in the gut, but I have had very variable responses when using SCG under controlled clinical conditions.

Dr. Scadding: I should like to comment on that. We have often failed with SCG as well, but we do find that it is more effective when given after an exclusion diet. Whether this reflects the change in the mast cell population in the gut or some other mechanism, I don't know. We have recently been trying Nedocromil, which is Fison's new drug which is said to have an effect on intestinal mast cells. When used prophylactically in patients with eczema, migraine, and irritable bowel syndrome in a small open trial, there is some evidence of efficacy despite persevering with a full diet.

Dr. Strobel: We have used Nedocromil, and it does not prevent mediator release from rat intestinal mast cells assessed by measuring rat mast-cell protease release (RMCPII). I cannot comment on its effect in children.

Dr. Durand: We use SCG in certain patients who have not been helped by any other treatment. I have no experience about its specific effects on mast cells, but in some cases it has a very good clinical effect, and there may be considerable improvement in the histological appearance of the mucosa.

Food Allergy, edited by Eberhardt Schmidt.
Nestlé Nutrition Workshop Series, Vol. 17.
Nestec Ltd., Vevey/Raven Press, Ltd.,
New York © 1988.

Gut Absorption of Macromolecules: A Short Communication

I. Jakobsson

Malmö General Hospital, Sweden—214 01 Malmö

I should like to tell you about some of our results in studying the absorption of macromolecules. Several methods have been used to do this, with different markers such as bovine serum albumin, ovalbumin, and beta-lactoglobulin. The trouble is that these are all nonhuman food proteins, so you have to consider the possibility of local intestinal and systemic immune responses. We have developed a method using human alpha-lactalbumin, the main whey protein of human milk, as a marker molecule.

We purified human alpha-lactalbumin and developed a competitive radioimmunoassay for the analysis of alpha-lactalbumin concentrations in serum samples. We took blood samples from infants at 30 and 60 min after breast-feeding, and Fig. 1 shows the results of determinations made in full-term healthy infants of various ages. There was absorption of the marker protein, which decreased with age. We also studied 32 very-low-birth-weight infants fed human milk, with gestational ages ranging from 26 to 32 weeks. Serum samples were collected at 2-week intervals until term (Fig. 2). At 30 to 32 weeks of postconceptional age, the serum concentration of alpha-lactalbumin was about 10 times higher than in the full-term infants below 1 month of age. At the postconceptional age of 39 weeks, the values were approximately the same as those found in full-term neonates.

We are also studying absorption in formula-fed infants of varying ages and in infants with different diseases—for instance, cow's-milk-protein intolerance—by giving them a feed of human milk and then taking serum samples. This study is not yet complete, but we have preliminary data to show that there is increased absorption of the marker protein in infants with cow's-milk-protein intolerance as compared to normal infants of the same age. We consider that human alpha-lactalbumin is a good marker for studying macromolecular absorption in infants. We have demonstrated that absorption is inversely related to maturity and that it appears to be increased in infants with acute symptoms of cow's-milk-protein intolerance.

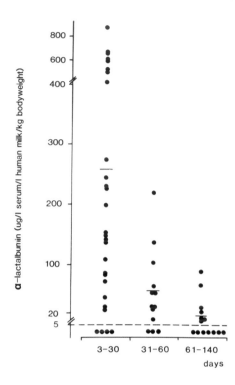

FIG. 1. Alpha-lactalbumin in the blood serum of full-term healthy infants of various ages 30 and 60 min after breast-feeding.

FIG. 2. Alpha-lactalbumin in the blood serum of very-low-birth-weight infants fed human milk, at various postconceptional ages.

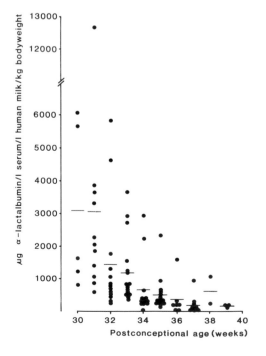

Food Allergy, edited by Eberhardt Schmidt.
Nestlé Nutrition Workshop Series, Vol. 17.
Nestec Ltd., Vevey/Raven Press, Ltd.,
New York © 1988.

Prevention of Allergy Through Nutrition Regimes in Infancy

J. Schmitz and J.L. Bresson

Department of Pediatrics, Hôpital des Enfants Malades, 75015 Paris, France

The increasing use of animal milk for infant feeding during the nineteenth century led to the first reports of allergy to cow's milk at the beginning of this century. The numerous clinical manifestations that cow's milk may trigger in infants are now well known. The following symptoms have been attributed to cow's-milk-protein intolerance: acute digestive symptoms; chronic diarrhea; failure to thrive; urticaria; eczema; recurrent rhinitis or bronchitis; and asthma. Because most of these symptoms are those of atopic diseases, many authors have tried to find whether introducing potentially antigenic proteins as late as possible might delay the appearance of allergic diseases or decrease their incidence, assuming that feeding or avoiding a given antigen might influence the responses to other antigens (1). Fifty years ago in a famous study concerning 20,061 infants followed up during a 9-month period, Grulee and Sanford gave a clear answer to this question; they found that infantile eczema, defined as "any lesions on the face or body," "cradle cap" being excluded, occurred twice as often (1.7%) in partially breast-fed babies as it did in breast-fed babies (0.7%) and seven times more often in the artificially fed group (4.6%) than in the breast-fed one (2). Since that time, however, the possibility of preventing allergic diseases in childhood and later by avoiding antigens in infancy has been hotly debated. We should like first to summarize briefly the main studies conducted during the past two decades on this subject and then to suggest potential reasons that might explain why this question is still open to discussion.

INFANT FEEDING AND THE RISK OF ALLERGY: REVIEW OF AVAILABLE DATA

The numerous studies that have attempted to determine whether or not infant feeding affects the risk of allergy may be grouped according to their design (3). Among retrospective studies, which have the strong disadvantage of relying on a parent's memory, some support, whereas some fail to support, the hypothesis that early contact with antigens is associated with allergy. For example, 22 in a series of 25 infants with symptoms suggestive of cow's-milk-protein allergy had received cow's milk during the first month of life, as compared to 25 of 47 control infants ($p<0.01$), and the patients with cow's-milk-protein intolerance were given formula during their first 7 days in the nursery significantly more often than control infants (4). On the other hand, no association, either positive or negative, could be found between breast-feeding or age at introduction of solid foods and eczema in a retrospective case-control study of 470 subjects aged 1 month to 20 years visiting a dermatology clinic (5).

Prospective studies can be separated into *observational* studies (the most numerous) and *controlled* studies. In the first category, and after the pilot study of Grulee and Sanford (2), a majority of studies involving large series of infants not selected by medical history failed to demonstrate a clear-cut relationship between early feeding and subsequent risk of eczema (6–8), asthma (9), or any other allergic manifestation (10,11). In a large birth cohort of over 1,100 2-year-old children from New Zealand, rates of eczema (6) and of asthma or wheezy bronchitis, as defined by "medical practitioners" (9), were found not to be affected by exclusive breast-feeding during the first 4 months of life. On the contrary, in both cases, parental atopy was highly significantly associated with the occurrence of either eczema or asthma. Interestingly, there was a significant tendency for the risk of eczema to increase with the number, but not the amount nor the age of introduction, of solid foods the child was given during the first 4 months (6). This tendency was not found in the case of early childhood asthma (9). However, in a recent prospective study of 198 infants followed up from birth until $4\frac{1}{2}$ to 5 years of age, in which comparison between those initially breast-fed (regardless of duration) and those fed on cow's milk preparations showed little difference in the incidence of eczema, the latter fell significantly in infants with an immediate family history of atopy when *exclusive* breast-feeding was continued beyond 12 weeks; in the same study, incidence of eczema rose in all breast-fed infants, regardless of family history, when breast-feeding was supplemented with other foods for the same duration (8).

Prospective observational studies concerning infants selected according to familial history of atopy show a clear-cut effect of breast-feeding on the later occurrence of allergic diseases. For example, of 94 infants born to allergic mothers and followed-up for 2 years, 10 of 56 who were bottle-fed and 2 of 28 who were breast-fed, each for a minimum period of 6 weeks, developed asthma ($p<0.06$) (12). However, in a larger group of 250 infants from atopic families, breast-feeding for 3 months or more did not protect against the development of eczema up to the age of 2 years; in fact, 22% of the breast-fed infants, but only 15% of the bottle-fed infants, were affected (13). The fact that breast-feeding may be associated with the development of positive skin tests, suggesting sensitization through mother's milk, was recently confirmed in a group of infants with an immediate family history of atopy followed-up until 20 months of age (14).

Prospective *random controlled or part-intervention studies* are expected to give the most reliable answers to the question raised at the beginning of this chapter. However, since it is ethically controversial to allocate babies randomly to breast milk or to cow's milk, the few available random controlled studies have compared cow's milk to soya preparations, the latter being regarded as nonallergenic. In a carefully controlled study of 292 infants with a family history of allergy, of which 235 could be examined 10 years later, asthma and allergic rhinitis, but not hay fever or eczema (eight cases only), occurred significantly more frequently in controls (in 28, 40, 22 cases, respectively, out of 120) than in soya-fed infants (in 9, 8, 12 cases, respectively, out of 115) (15). Nevertheless, in a smaller, but similarly well-controlled, trial concerning 48 infants with a biparental history of atopy randomized to receive soya or cow's milk from weaning to the age of 9 months and followed-up until 4 years of age, there was no significant difference in the rate of occurrence of atopic diseases between the first (soya, 74%) and second group (cow's milk, 60%), nor was there any difference between these groups in serum immunoglobulins (IgG, A, M, E). In the same study, in which all mothers were encouraged to breast-feed as long as possible, there was no significant difference in the period of complete and or partial breast-feeding between children finally having or not having atopic diseases during the observation period (16). In a part-intervention study of 1,753 unselected infants fed breast milk, soya, or cow's milk, with only a subgroup of these infants being randomly allocated to these regimens, the incidence of allergic diseases was found to be similar in the three groups of infants: 12.5% (45 of 352 breast-fed infants), 14.5% (46 of 317 soya fed infants) and 11.7% (127 of 1,084 cow's-milk-fed infants) after 4 to 7 years of follow-up. Interestingly, the onset of allergy occurred, on average, 6 months later in breast-fed infants than in cow's-milk-fed infants, with the soya-fed children being intermediate (17). However, in a small part-intervention study of 49 infants with a positive family history of allergy, an allergen-avoidance regimen (exclusive breast-feeding for the first 3 months; exclusion of dairy products, fish, and eggs; and avoidance of contact with pets, horse-hair mattresses, feather quilts, etc.) significicantly reduced the incidence of eczema at 6 months (two cases out of 23) and 12 months (three cases out of 23) as compared to control infants (nine cases out of 19 at 6 and 12 months of age, $p<0.01$ and 0.017, respectively) (18).

Finally, more than 30 retrospective, prospective, observational, or controlled studies have been aimed, mainly in the last 10 years, at determining whether breast-feeding and/or antigen avoidance regimens in infants could decrease the risk of allergic diseases later in life. These studies are diverse in their design. Some concern cohorts of thousands of infants prospectively observed; others concern a few dozen randomly allocated newborns. Most of the prospective studies are summarized in Tables 1 and 2, which list all the usually cited literature on the subject. From these tables, it appears that, out of 24 studies, 11 show that breast-feeding decreases the incidence of atopy, whereas 13 show no relationship between infant feeding and allergy, with some of the latter studies even indicating a trend for breast-feeding to be associated with higher rates of atopic diseases (8,13,25).

TABLE 1. *Effect of infant feeding on subsequent risk of allergy: prospective studies concerning infants not selected by medical history*

Authors, year (reference)	Number of infants studied	Duration of follow-up (years/months)	Regimens tested[a]	Atopic disease(s) under study		
				Eczema	Asthma	Others[b]
Observational studies						
Grulee and Sanford, 1936 (2)	20,061	0/9	B/A	+		
Gerrard et al., 1973 (11)	787	1/0–3/0	B/A	0	0	0
Saarinen et al., 1979 (19)	256	3/0	B/C	+ (ns)[c]		+ (ns)
Jakobsson and Lindberg, 1979 (10)	1,079	1/0	B/A	0	0	0
Fergusson et al., 1981 (6)	1,123	2/0	B/A	0		
Hide and Guyer, 1981 (7)	843	1/0	B/A	0	+	
Juto et al., 1982 (20)	70	1/0	B/C	+		
Gruskay, 1982 (21)	908	15/0	B/A	+	+	
Fergusson et al., 1983 (9)	1,110	4/0	B/A		0	
Pratt, 1984 (8)	198	5/0	B/A	0		
Controlled (c) or part intervention (p.i.) studies						
Brown et al., 1969 (c) (22)	379	1/0–2/0	S/C	0	0	0
Halpern et al., 1973 (p.i.) (17)	1,753	5/0–7/0	B/C/S	0	0	0

[a]B, breast milk; A, artificial feeding; C, cow's milk; S, soya preparation.
[b]"Others" denotes gastrointestinal symptoms, recurrent rhinitis, urticaria, etc.
[c]ns, not significant.

WHY IS THE ROLE OF INFANT FEEDING IN THE OCCURRENCE OF ALLERGY SO DIFFICULT TO ASSESS?

The difficulty in proving or disproving the point raised 50 years ago by Grulee and Sanford certainly tells us something about the relationships between infant feeding and atopic disease, and it is thus worth an attempt at clarification.

Methodologic problems may partially invalidate many of the studies (3). For example, one must view with suspicion any observations concerning the type of diet if these observations were collected months or even years after the diet was given to the infant (5,8). Similarly, in part-intervention studies (17,22,29), the regimen was not always randomly chosen by the mothers, who were from families at high genetic risk and were probably choosing to breast-feed in the belief that it

TABLE 2. *Effect of infant feeding on subsequent risk of allergy: prospective studies concerning infants selected by medical history*

Authors, year (reference)	Number of infants selected	Duration of follow-up (years/months)	Regimens tested[a]	Atopic disease(s) under study		
				Eczema	Asthma	Others[b]
Observational studies						
Blair 1977 (23)	244	20/0	B/A		+	
Dannaeus et al., 1978 (24)	36	2/0	B/C	0	0	0
Kaufman and Frick, 1981 (12)	94	2/0	B/A	0	+ ($p < 0.6$)	
Gordon et al., 1982 (13)	250	2/0	B/A	0	0	
Cogswell and Alexander, 1982 (25)	80	3/0	B/A	0		
Van Asperen et al., 1984 (26)		1/8	B/C	0	0	0
Controlled (c) or part intervention (p.i.) studies						
Glaser and Johnstone, 1953 (p.i.) (27)	96	0/7–10/0	S/C	+	+	
Johnstone and Dutton, 1966, (c) (15)	292	10/0	S/C	0	+	+
Matthew et al., 1977 (p.i.) (18)	42	1/0	B/A	+		
Kjellman and Johansson, 1979, (c) (16)	48	4/0	S/C	0	0	0
Chandra 1979 (p.i.) (28)	74	3/0	B/C	+	+	
Moore et al., 1985, (p.i.) (29)	475	1/0	B/S/C	0		

[a]B, breast milk; A, artificial feeding; C, cow's milk; S, soya preparation.
[b]"Others" denotes gastrointestinal symptoms, recurrent rhinitis, urticaria, etc.

would protect their child against allergy (17). Such a tendency may increasingly complicate this type of study and is possibly a partial explanation for the few recent studies in which breast-feeding is negatively or "paradoxically" associated with allergy. Finally, in all studies except two (5,29), clinical assessment of allergic disease was not made blind with regard to the dietary history. Taking into account the emotional load carried by breast-feeding, this limitation may have unintentionally affected the findings.

Since methodologic pitfalls cannot account for all contradictory findings, other reasons for those discrepancies have to be found. Thus it may be that the protective effect of breast-feeding is so difficult to prove because it is small. However, in those studies where breast-feeding is positively correlated with a decrease in allergic diseases, artificial feeding is found to raise the incidence of eczema or asthma two- to threefold (7,15,19,21), or even five- to sevenfold (2,28), as compared to their usual rates, in breast-fed infants. Such a sizable effect is not related to low-population studies of infants, since the clearest protective effect was observed in the biggest population studied (2). Since allergy is a multifactorial condition in which genetic factors play an essential role (6,9,30,31), the contradictory results obtained in these studies could also be explained on the basis that the effect is restricted to a genetic subgroup of infants. Indeed, most of the recent retrospective (31) and prospective studies concerning nonselected infants (6,8,9) found no protective effect of breast-feeding. Although the total number of studies showing such an effect in nonselected infants (5 of 12, Table 1) is only slightly less than that in infants selected for medical history (6 of 12, Table 2), a recent study which found no effect of breast-feeding in the general population was able to show a statistically significant protective effect of breast-feeding in a subgroup of children exclusively breast-fed for 3 months and with a family history of atopy (8). However, some studies have shown, on the contrary, that the protective effect of breast-feeding reached significance only in babies without a family history of atopy (7,21). Thus, the simple presence of atopic diseases in one or both of a child's parents is not sufficient to demonstrate a correlation between breast-feeding and a reduction in childhood atopy, even in a fairly large sample of children (9).

The respective antigenicities of cow's milk and breast milk have to be questioned also. Thus the antigenic properties of cow's milk proteins in recent formulas, which are subjected to longer and higher heat treatment than they were 20 or 30 years ago, are different from those of more traditional preparations. It has been shown in guinea pigs that the anaphylactic sensitizing capacity or the capacity to elicit antibody production of processed cow's milk proteins were considerably reduced by heat treatment, with whey protein being denatured by lower temperatures than casein (32,33). In rabbits, mean hemagglutination titers to casein were identical after repeated parenteral immunization with homogenized cow's milk and a representative commercial formula (Enfamil), whereas hemagglutination titers to alpha-lactalbumin were dramatically reduced after immunization by the commercial formula, probably because of denaturation by the heat treatment used to prepare it (34). Thus the processing of commercial formulas may account for their antigenicity being lower than that of whole cow's milk (35) and may also account for the older studies (2,27) or those with the longer follow-up (15,21,23) being more often associated with allergic diseases.

On the other hand, breast milk is not as antigen-free as is usually thought. Numerous recent reports have demonstrated, by immunoassay, the presence of cow's milk or egg proteins in human breast milk (36–39). Beta-lactoglobulin (BLG) was found in 18% to 53% of single milk samples of lactating women (36,37) as well as in 76% of mothers sampled every 2 weeks until 31 weeks (39). Similarly, oval-bumin was found in breast-milk from 59% of mothers who had ingested a raw egg 4 to 6 hours earlier. Furthermore, ovalbumin in breast milk was of the usual mo-lecular size and was indistinguishable from the native protein in the radioimmuno-assay (37). After a feed of half a pint of cow's milk, concentration of BLG in milk varied from 0.1 to 6 μg/liter in one study; however, in other studies, BLG concentrations were more dispersed and higher, ranging from (a) 5 to 20 μg/liter in single samples from 28 mothers, (b) 5 to 20 μg/liter in single samples from 28 mothers, and (c) 5 to 800 μg/liter in 232 milk samples from 25 mothers (36,39). Variation of BLG concentration was great from one mother to another and from one sample to another in the same woman (13–800 μg/liter) without parallel varia-tion in milk intake (39). The clinical significance for the newborn of these small amounts of antigenic proteins in breast milk remains a matter of debate. On the basis of immediate hypersensitivity reactions on the first known exposures to eggs, milk, and peanut in eight healthy infants exclusively breast-fed, it has been pro-posed that the dose of allergen in breast milk might be sufficient to cause sensitiza-tion but not to cause symptoms (14). However, the presence of diarrhea, vomiting, colic, and exanthema has also been found significantly ($p<0.05$) correlated to high levels of BLG in breast milk (39). Results of recent studies concerned with the effect of maternal dietary exclusion of cow's milk and/or other proteins are similarly inconclusive. The finding that infantile colic in breast-fed infants could be related to the mother's cow's milk consumption (40) was not confirmed by a placebo-controlled double-blind randomized crossover trial including 20 breast-fed infants with persistent colic (41). In this study, rates of colic were not significantly higher on days when cow's milk was given than on days when it was eliminated. Interestingly, rates of colic increased significantly ($p<0.05$) in proportion to the diversity of maternal diet (41). However, in the latter study, cow's milk was re-placed by soya milk. In a subsequent double-blind crossover study concerning breast-fed infants and their mothers, who were challenged with capsules contain-ing powder of either cow's milk whey protein or of potato starch, sequential analy-sis showed a high correlation between infantile colic in breast-fed infants and their mother's consumption of cow's milk (42). In two controlled studies that included 17 and 18 infants and lasted for 12 and 10 weeks, respectively, maternal diet had little influence on eczema, whatever the diet (normal diet, antigen-free diet, or a diet containing cow's milk and eggs or soya as the only known antigens). In both trials it appeared that observed improvement following the antigen exclusion peri-ods was probably spontaneous, since it was not reversed by further test periods (43). It is thus difficult from these studies to assess to what degree cow's milk proteins in breast milk may be responsible for symptoms of allergy in infants; however, since minute amounts of protein may be more allergenic than sizable amounts (44), the presence of these foreign proteins in breast milk may, to a large extent, explain the difficulty faced by researchers in their effort to demonstrate the protective effect of breast-feeding against atopic diseases.

This difficulty—or impossibility—may simply indicate that exclusion of cow's milk proteins in infancy is not sufficient to prevent atopic diseases occurring later in childhood. Indeed, several studies have shown a positive correlation between (a) the number of solid foods given to infants not selected by medical history while they were breast-fed or during the weaning period and (b) the frequency of eczema (6,8). Such a correlation was not found in infants with a family history of atopy (26). It is worth recalling that in the same population in which a correlation could be demonstrated between ingestion of solid foods and eczema, a similar correlation could not be established between solid foods and asthma (6,9). This negative finding would be consistent with the hypothesis that children with eczema are more sensitive to dietary allergens and that children with asthma are more sensitive to inhaled allergens (45). Whatever the degree of validity of this hypothesis, it is important because it stresses that allergic children are simultaneously exposed to allergens by enteric and extraenteric mucosal surfaces. It would therefore be illusory to try to prevent asthma or recurrent rhinitis and, to a lesser degree, eczema by dietary antigen avoidance only, since newborn infants are subjected to many other allergens in their first months of life (46).

REFERENCES

1. Roberts SA, Soothill JF. Provocation of allergic response by supplementary feeds of cow's milk. *Arch Dis Child* 1982;57:127–30.
2. Grulee CG, Sanford HN. The influence of breast and artificial feeding on infantile eczema. *J Pediatr* 1936;9:223–5.
3. Burr ML. Does infant feeding affect the risk of allergy? *Arch Dis Child* 1983;58:561–5.
4. Stintzing G, Zetterström R. Cow's milk allergy, incidence and pathogenetic role of early exposure to cow's milk formula. *Acta Paediatr Scand* 1979;68:383–7.
5. Kramer MS, Moroz B. Do breast-feeding and delayed introduction of solid foods protect against subsequent atopic eczema? *J Pediatr* 1981;98:546–50.
6. Fergusson DM, Horwood LJ, Beautrais AL, Shannon FT, Taylor B. Eczema and infant diet. *Clin Allergy* 1981;11:325–31.
7. Hide DW, Guyer BM. Clinical manifestations of allergy related to breast and cow's milk feeding. *Arch Dis Child* 1981;56:172–5.
8. Pratt HF. Breastfeeding and eczema. *Early Hum Dev* 1984;9:283–90.
9. Fergusson DM, Horwood LJ, Shannon FT. Asthma and infant diet. *Arch Dis Child* 1983;58: 48–51.
10. Jakobsson I, Lindberg T. A prospective study of cow's milk protein intolerance in Swedish infants. *Acta Paediatr Scand* 1979;68:853–9.
11. Gerrard JW, MacKenzie JWA, Goluboff N, Garson JZ, Maningas CS. Cow's milk allergy: prevalence and manifestations in an unselected series of newborns. *Acta Paediatr Scand (suppl)* 1973;234:1–21.
12. Kaufman HS, Frick OL. Prevention of asthma. *Clin Allergy* 1981;11:549–53.
13. Gordon RR, Noble DA, Ward AM, Allen R. Immunoglobulin E and the eczema-asthma syndrome in early childhood. *Lancet* 1982;i:72–4.
14. Van Asperen PP, Kemp AS, Mellis CM. Immediate food hypersensitivity reactions on the first known exposure to the food. *Arch Dis Child* 1983;58:253–6.
15. Johnstone DE, Dutton AM. Dietary prophylaxis of allergic disease in children. *N Engl J Med* 1966;274:715–9.
16. Kjellman NIM, Johansson SGO. Soy versus cow's milk in infants with a biparental history of atopic disease: development of atopic disease and immunoglobulins from birth to 4 years of age. *Clin Allergy* 1979;9:347–58.
17. Halpern SR, Sellars WA, Johnson RB, Anderson DW, Saperstein S, Reisch JS. Development of

childhood allergy in infants fed breast, soy, or cow milk. *J Allergy Clin Immunol* 1973;51:139–51.

18. Matthew DJ, Taylor B, Norman AP, Turner MW, Soothill JF. Prevention of eczema. *Lancet* 1977;i:321–4.
19. Saarinen UM, Kajosaari M, Backman A, Siimes MA. Prolonged breast-feeding as prophylaxis for atopic disease. *Lancet* 1979;ii:163–6.
20. Juto P, Moller C, Enberg S, Bjorksten B. Influence of feeding on lymphocyte function and development of infantile allergy. *Clin Allergy* 1982;12:409–16.
21. Gruskay FL. Comparison of breast, cow, and soy feedings in the prevention of onset of allergic disease. A 15-year prospective study. *Clin Pediatr* 1982;21:486–91.
22. Brown EB, Josephson BM, Levine HS, Rosen M. A prospective study of allergy in a pediatric population. The role of heredity in the incidence of allergies, and experience with milk-free diet in the newborn. *Am J Dis Child* 1969;117:693–8.
23. Blair H. Natural history of childhood asthma. 20-Year follow-up. *Arch Dis Child* 1977;52:613–9.
24. Dannaeus A, Johansson SGO, Foucard T. Clinical and immunological aspects of food allergy in childhood. II. Development of allergic symptoms and humoral immune response to foods in infants of atopic mothers during the first 24 months of life. *Acta Paediatr Scand* 1978;67:497–504.
25. Cogswell JJ, Alexander J. Breast feeding and eczema/asthma. *Lancet* 1982;i:910–1.
26. Van Asperen PP, Kemp AS, Mellis CM. Relationship of diet in the development of atopy in infancy. *Clin Allergy* 1984;14:525–32.
27. Glaser J, Johnstone DE. Prophylaxis of allergic disease in the newborn. *JAMA* 1953;153:620–2.
28. Chandra RK. Prospective studies of the effect of breast feeding on incidence of infection and allergy. *Acta Paediatr Scand* 1979;68:691–4.
29. Moore WJ, Midwinter RE, Morris AF, Colley JRT, Soothill JF. Infant feeding and subsequent risk of atopic eczema. *Arch Dis Child* 1985;60:722–6.
30. Gerrard JW, Ko CG, Vickers P, Gerrard DC. The familial incidence of allergic disease. *Ann Allergy* 1976;36:10–5.
31. Taylor B, Wadsworth J, Golding J, Butler N. Breast feeding, eczema, asthma, and hayfever. *J Epidemiol Community Health* 1983;37:95–9.
32. McLaughlan P, Anderson KJ, Widdowson EM, Coombs RRA. Effect of heat on the anaphylactic-sensitising capacity of cows' milk, goats' milk, and various infant formulae fed to guinea-pigs. *Arch Dis Child* 1981;56:165–71.
33. Heppell LMJ, Cant AJ, Kilshaw PJ. Reduction in the antigenicity of whey proteins by heat treatment: a possible strategy for producing a hypoallergenic infant milk formula. *Br J Nutr* 1984;51:29–36.
34. Eastham EJ, Lichauco T, Pang K, Walker WA. Antigenicity of infant formulas and the induction of systemic immunological tolerance by oral feeding: cow's milk versus soy milk. *J Pediatr Gastroenterol Nutr* 1982;1:23–8.
35. Freier S, Kletter B, Gery I, Lebenthal E, Geifman M. Intolerance to milk protein. *J. Pediatr* 1969;75:623–31.
36. Stuart CA, Twiselton R, Nicholas MK, Hide DW. Passage of cow's milk protein in breast milk. *Clin Allergy* 1984;14:533–5.
37. Kilshaw PJ, Cant AJ. The passage of maternal dietary proteins into human breast milk. *Int Arch Allergy Appl Immunol* 1984;75:8–15.
38. Jakobsson I, Lindberg T, Benediktsson B, Hansson BG. Dietary bovine β-lactoglobulin is transferred to human milk. *Acta Paediatr Scand* 1985;74:342–5.
39. Axelsson I, Jakobsson I, Lindberg T, Benediktsson B. Bovine β-lactoglobulin in the human milk. A longitudinal study during the whole lactation period. *Acta Paediatr Scand* 1986;75:702–7.
40. Jakobsson I, Lindberg T. Cow's milk as a cause of infantile colic in breast-fed infants. *Lancet* 1978;ii:437–9.
41. Evans RW, Fergusson DM, Allardyce RA, Taylor B. Maternal diet and infantile colic in breast-fed infants. *Lancet* 1981;i:1340–2.
42. Jakobsson I, Lindberg T. Cow's milk proteins cause infantile colic in breast-fed infants: a double-blind crossover study. *Pediatrics* 1983;71:268–71.
43. Cant AJ, Bailes JA, Marsden RA, Hewitt D. Effect of maternal dietary exclusion on breast fed infants with eczema: two controlled studies. *Br Med J* 1986;293:231–3.
44. Jarrett EEE. Activation of IgE regulatory mechanisms by transmucosal absorption of antigen.

Lancet 1977;ii:223–5.
45. Hill DJ, Balloch A, Hosking CS. IgE responses to environmental antigens in atopic children. *Clin Allergy* 1981;11:541–7.
46. Kaplan MS, Solli NJ. Immunoglobulin E to cow's-milk protein in breast-fed atopic children. *J Allergy Clin Immunol* 1979;64:122–6.

DISCUSSION

Dr. Wahn: Dr. Schmitz showed that heating cow's milk proteins destroys antigenic determinants in most of them. Is it possible that heating may also introduce new antigenic determinants?

Dr. Schmitz: I know of no studies suggesting that heating milk produces new antigenic determinants. There is some evidence that partial digestion of casein in the stomach may do this, but I do not think heating will.

Dr. Guesry: It is certainly true that boiling whey for 30 min will reduce its allergenicity. It will also drastically reduce its lysine availability and protein efficiency. Thus extreme heat treatment is not feasible as a way of producing a hypoallergenic formula. Lesser degrees of heat treatment must be combined with tryptic hydrolysis or any other process which ruptures the protein chains. Also, I should like to question your negative conclusions. You said that you believed that antigen avoidance should be reserved for the most severely affected patients, but I believe that prevention is better than cure, and since you also showed that you may be able to prevent eczema by strict allergen avoidance, do you really mean what you said about not trying to prevent allergic disease?

Dr. Schmitz: I stand by what I said, that if you examine the relevant literature it does not bring strong arguments for imposing a dietary antigen avoidance regime to unselected infants as an efficient means of preventing allergic disease in the general population.

Dr. Cant: On the whole I would agree with that, but I would like to take issue with you for showing a list of studies for and against an influence of feeding on allergic disease and then trying to make a numerical balance out of it. Let me quote a couple of examples why this cannot work. One widely cited study which purports to show that there is no difference between breast- and bottle-feeding contains the statement ''. . . mothers were deemed to have breast-fed their babies if they gave their babies breast milk exclusively for 1 week and thereafter gave no more than one bottle of cow's milk per day''; so after the second week of life you could be ''breast-fed'' if you had a bottle of cow's milk every day! And several other studies included among their breast-fed groups infants who were given soya milk. It is true that some of the best-designed studies show no difference between breast- and bottle-feeding, but on the whole a critical assessment shows that the balance favors breast-feeding if you want to minimize allergic disease. Also, the question of the effect of weaning is a very important one and has been little studied. Of the 30-odd published studies of the influence of early feeding on the development of allergy, only two to my knowledge have dealt with weaning, and both showed that weaning had a significant effect on the development of allergy. Piglets develop an allergic enteropathy if weaned too early, which is a very important point in husbandry.

Dr. Scadding: When piglets are fed ovalbumin at weaning time it takes a few days for them to mount a cell-mediated response, after which they are tolerant to ovalbumin. However, if you introduce a different antigen during those few days they do not make a cell-mediated response to it and do not become tolerant to it, which suggests that one antigen should be introduced at a time at intervals of several days.

Dr. Kjellman: Whatever the possible effects of diet on the development of allergic disease, we must not make the mistake of promising parents that we can prevent the development of symptoms. In our own randomized studies (and randomization is very important) we see a delay in onset and reduction in severity of symptoms with allergen avoidance. It is possible, however, to calculate an economic effect of the amelioration of symptoms when preventive measures are applied to individuals selected on the basis of screening, using IgE and family history. We have estimated that about $25 (U.S. currency) can be saved for each screened child, which makes screening worthwhile. Now we must concentrate on the search for more selective screening procedures.

Food Allergy, edited by Eberhardt Schmidt.
Nestlé Nutrition Workshop Series, Vol. 17.
Nestec Ltd., Vevey/Raven Press, Ltd.,
New York © 1988.

Influence of Feeding Breast Milk, Adapted Milk Formula, and a New Hypoallergenic Formula on Allergic Manifestations in Infants: A Field Study

Yvan Vandenplas, Michel Deneyer, Liliane Sacre,
and Helmuth Loeb

Academic Children's Hospital, Free University of Brussels, 1090 Brussels, Belgium

Food allergies, particularly cow's milk allergy, often appear to be familial, possibly owing to a genetic tendency to respond with increased IgE production rather than owing to inheritance of sensitivity of specific food allergens. In such persons, milk allergy is common because cow's milk formula is usually the first and most prevalent food in the infant's diet (1). Cow's milk contains more than 25 distinct proteins that may act as antigens in humans. The antigenicity differs from protein to protein and seems to depend on host factors as well as on a combination of genetic, environmental, and adjuvant factors. The most important allergens are found in beta-lactoglobulin (for 60–80% of cow's-milk-allergic patients), casein (60%), lactalbumin (50%), and bovine serum albumin (50%). Measures to reduce the incidence of food allergy are expected to be most rewarding when used in young children. Infants are considered at high risk for food allergy, probably because of the increased intestinal mucosal permeability to incompletely digested macromolecules and the lack of an adequate protection by secretory IgA at the mucosal membrane surface. The risk is especially high in atopic infants, i.e., those from atopic families (2).

Human milk represents a substitute to protect the vulnerable neonate and infant from development of allergies. However, it would appear that mother's milk is not always available for the infant under risk. This provides a situation in which a hypoallergenic milk may come into play. In order to investigate whether a recently developed new hypoallergenic milk formula might contribute to a protection from allergies, 75 infants at risk for an atopy were observed in an open-field study where they received either an adapted formula, breast-feeding, or the new hypoallergenic formula over a total period of 4 months.

MATERIAL AND METHODS

Infants at risk for allergy because of an atopic family history were studied. At least one of the parents or brothers/sisters of the infant had to present clinical symptoms of atopy (Table 1), supported by a positive RAST or a skin-prick test, and symptoms had to disappear if treated. History of allergic manifestations (eczema, urticaria, rhinorrhea, hay fever, chronic bronchitis, asthma, etc.) in the immediate family was available, and consent of the parents was obtained by a questionnaire during the prenatal consultation at 34 weeks of gestation.

Five groups of babies were studied (Table 2). It was decided to include the number of infants necessary to end up with five groups of 15 infants each, because a large number of dropouts in some groups (i.e., breast-fed group) were expected (Table 2).

All babies were followed during a 4-month period. This short period of followup was chosen because of its advantage in permitting a strict separation of breast-fed and formula-fed groups, without adding any other food allergen (e.g., orange juice). All babies stayed at home during the 4-month period.

A screening test for atopy (IgE level) was performed in all infants on the 5th day of life. At 4 months the IgE level was repeated, and a RAST (cow's milk, casein, lactalbumin, lactoglobulin) and a skin-prick test for cow's milk were performed in asymptomatic infants. In symptomatic infants, laboratory investigations

TABLE 1. *Family history: number of atopic persons (father/mother/brother/sister)*

Number of allergic persons	Number of infants
1	40
2	31
3 or more	4
	75

TABLE 2. *Groups of infants studied, including dropouts*

Group 1 ($N = 15$):	HAF exclusively from birth for 4 months. No dropouts.
Group 2 ($N = 15$):	HAF from birth for 2 months; an adapted formula from 2 to 4 months. Four dropouts (parents who refused to change to the adapted formula).
Group 3 ($N = 15$):	Adapted formula from birth for 2 months; HAF from 2 to 4 months. Two dropouts.
Group 4 ($N = 15$):	Exclusively breast-fed for 4 months. Six dropouts.
Group 5 ($N = 15$):	Adapted formula for 4 months. One dropout.

HAF, hypoallergenic formula.

were performed when symptoms were worst, before administration of the hypoallergenic formula.

Cow's milk allergy was suspected if, in the absence of any organic disease such as infantile pyloric stenosis, infectious gastroenteritis, or cystic fibrosis, the infant had symptoms involving the gastrointestinal tract (vomiting, diarrhea, colic, constipation), the respiratory tract (rhinorrhea, bronchitis, asthma), skin (eczema, urticaria), and the central nervous system (irritability, restlessness, drowsiness). Confirmation of the diagnosis was made by demonstrating relief of the symptoms with the avoidance of cow's milk and also by demonstrating the reappearance of symptoms at the reintroduction of cow's milk (3).

The hypoallergenic formula was HAF (Nestlé): The fat consists essentially of vegetable oils (palm, safflower, and coconut oil); the carbohydrates are lactose (70%) and dextrine-maltose (30%); the proteins are derived from a whey protein, hydrolyzed by trypsin under specific conditions. Hypoallergenic tests (radioimmunoassay, immunoallergens, and *in vivo* animal tests) were performed before administration.

RESULTS

Results are shown in Table 3. Zincemia was lower, although still within the normal ranges, in the infants who had received an adapted formula.

TABLE 3. *Evolution of laboratory investigations and symptoms of atopy in all infants*

Parameter	Group 1 (HAF)[a]	Group 2 (HAF/AdFo)[b]	Group 3 (AdFo/HAF)	Group 4 (BF)[c]	Group 5 (AdFo)
IgE > 1.3 U/ml D5 *(N)*	5	6	5	4	6
Range	1.3–2.3	1.7–3.8	1.6–4.0	1.4–3.6	1.4–7.4
At 4 months[d]					
IgE (mean)	2.5	17.2	11.6	7.0	22.3
Range	0.2–6.1	0.2–5.3	0.2–28.4	0.2–19.4	0.2–64.5
RAST+ *(N)*	0	1	1	0	1
Skin-prick test+ *(N)*	0	3	2	0	2
Zn (µg/dl) (mean)	119	83	95	107	80
Range	95–128	66–99	86–112	96–132	45–107
Symptoms of atopy		2–4 months	2–4 months		
N (total)	0	0–6	4–0	1	8
N (with IgE > 1.3)	0	0–3	2–0	0	3
Dermatologic symptoms	0	0–3	3–0	1	4
Gastrointestinal symptoms	0	0–3	2–0	0	4
Respiratory symptoms	0	0–1	0–0	0	1

[a]HAF, hypoallergenic formula.
[b]AdFo, adapted formula.
[c]BF, breast-feeding.
[d]Laboratory investigations were performed either at 4 months or when manifestations were worst.

Group 1

Fifteen infants with a positive family history were fed with HAF exclusively for 4 months. In five of them the IgE level on the 5th day of life was >1.3 U/ml (Table 3). After 4 months, none of these infants had developed symptoms of atopy (Table 3). All infants tolerated HAF very well.

Group 2

Fifteen infants were fed for 2 months with HAF and were then changed to an adapted formula. All infants were free of symptoms at 2 months; however, before 4 months, six infants of this group had developed allergic manifestations which disappeared on HAF and reappeared on the previous cow's milk formula. In four infants there was more than one system involved. In one infant the RAST was positive for beta-lactoglobulin.

Group 3

Fifteen infants received an adapted formula from birth. Four infants had developed allergic manifestations before the age of 2 months. The symptoms diappeared on HAF, but they reappeared with the initial cow's milk formula. Once the diagnosis was established, these infants were changed to HAF, as were the others, and none presented symptoms at 4 months. One infant had a positive RAST for beta-lactoglobulin.

Group 4

One infant in the breast-fed group suffered from eczema before he was 1 month old. The mother appeared to have increased her intake of cow's milk products during lactation. Symptoms vanished when she received a cow's-milk-free diet.

Group 5

Six of the infants with a positive family history and an adapted formula from birth had developed atopic symptoms before the age of 4 months. Symptoms disappeared on HAF, but they reappeared on cow's milk. In five infants, more than one system was involved. One RAST was positive for cow's milk and casein.

DISCUSSION

Atopic disease was confirmed in 18 of 45 (40%) infants with a positive family history who received a cow's milk formula (regardless of the IgE level on the 5th day of life), which was the same as the incidence in our previous retrospective study (2). In the infants with a positive neonatal screening test for allergy [38% ($N = 17$ of 45), as compared to 39% in the retrospective study], atopy was detected in 47% (8 of 17), as compared to 49% in the previous study, performed in a group of 275 infants with a positive family history. So, although the number of infants in each group was small ($N = 15$), the incidence of atopy in the groups' adapted formula (groups 2,3, and 5) was very similar to the incidence we reported before in much larger groups (2).

The frequency of atopic manifestations in our population was low in comparison with the results of other studies, in which the incidence varied from 44.4% to 88.9% (4–8). The large number of infants in whom more than one close relative was atopic ($N = 35$ of 75) increased the risk of atopy for the infant (9). Symptoms coming from the gastrointestinal tract seemed to be most common, which can be explained because the gastrointestinal tract is the first target of the food antigens. Hypersensitivity phenomena in infants are rare in the first month of life. Their peak time of onset is at 4 to 6 weeks in formula-fed infants.

The cornerstone of diagnosis in food allergy is a complete history as well as an unequivocal clinical reaction to elimination of the food and to subsequent challenge under defined conditions (3,10). Laboratory tests may sometimes be useful, but in most cases they are not. A lack of correlation exists between skin tests and oral food provocation. There appears to be a better correlation between family history and food challenge.

The hypozincemia may be related to the atopic condition (11), but low zinc levels in cow's-milk-fed nonallergic infants have been reported (12).

Up to now, discussions on the possibilities of preventing cow's milk allergy have been very theoretical and fundamental, both because of the difficulty in detecting at-risk infants before birth and also because of the lack of acceptable alternative formulas when breast-feeding or human milk from a breast milk bank were not available.

Postnatally, breast-feeding should be the mode of choice, with the mother avoiding overindulgence with any particular food, particularly milk, eggs, and nuts. Supplementation with other foods should be very gradual and should not begin before 6 months of age (13), though this is hard to put into practice in modern Western societies with working mothers. Breast milk can contain foreign proteins which may elicit symptoms of food allergy in the breast-fed infant (14). The fact that only nanogram quantities of foreign antigens are present does not detract from this potential allergenic effect. On the contrary, Jarrett has shown in animals that small doses are more efficacious in producing immediate-type hypersensitivity than are large doses (15). Societal and cultural educational programs about allergy and exposure to food antigens could possibly improve the results obtained with breast-feeding.

When breast-feeding cannot be provided, a number of formulas may be considered. Soy bean formulas have been recommended because of a lower incidence of allergy (16). However, a concern has been expressed regarding a possible increase in the incidence of sensitivity to soy protein with the increase (up to 30%) in its use (17). Other potentially hypoallergenic formulas such as casein hydrolysate, meat-base formula, and heat-treated cow's milk are available, but their usefulness for long-term prophylaxis against food allergy has not been adequately studied, besides other disadvantages (high cost, unpleasant taste, nutritive impairment, etc). Therefore the concept of the new formula we studied is very interesting, both for therapy (in mild cases) and for prevention, though diarrhea may be expected in infants with partial mucosal damage and consequent temporary lactase deficiency.

The effect of exclusive breast-feeding during the first months of life upon prevention of cow's milk allergy appears well established, although there is the possibility of intrauterine sensitization (18). It is justified, however, to strongly suggest exclusive breast-feeding for at least the first 4 months in newborns from a family with an atopic history. If breast-feeding is impossible, a formula like HAF seems an advisable alternative. Whether such a practice may be able to prevent or postpone not only the development of food allergy but also that of allergy in general remains an open question. HAF fed exclusively for 2 months certainly seems only to postpone the appearance of atopy.

REFERENCES

 1. Bahna SL, Furukawa CT. Food allergy: diagnosis and treatment. *Ann Allergy* 1983;51:574–80.
 2. Vandenplas Y, Sacre L. Influences of neonatal serum IgE concentration, family history and diet on the incidence of cow's milk allergy. *Eur J Pediatr* 1986;145:493–5.
 3. Gerrard JW, Shenessa M. Food allergy: two common types as seen in breast and formula fed babies. *Ann Allergy* 1983;50:375–9.
 4. Croner S, Kjellman N-I M, Eriksson B, Roth A. IgE screening in 1701 newborn infants and the development of atopic disease during infancy. *Arch Dis Child* 1982;57:364–8.
 5. Duchateau J, Casimir G. Neonatal serum IgE concentrations as a predictor of atopy. *Lancet* 1983;i:413–4.
 6. Katz DH. New concepts concerning the clinical control of IgE synthesis. *Clin Allergy* 1979;9:609–24.
 7. Michel FB, Bousquet J, Grellier P. Comparison of cord blood immunoglobulin E concentrations and maternal allergy for prediction of atopic diseases in infancy. *J Allergy Clin Immunol* 1980;65:422–30.
 8. Michel FB, Bousquet J, Coulomb V. Prediction of the high allergic risk newborn. In: Johansson SGO, ed. *Diagnosis and treatment of IgE mediated diseases.* Amsterdam: Excerpta Medica, 1981;35–7.
 9. Kjellman N-I M. Development and production of atopic allergy in childhood. In: Bastrom H, Ljungstedt, N, eds. *Skandia International Symposia. Theoretical and clinical aspects of allergic diseases.* Stockholm: Almqvist and Wicksell, 1982;57–73.
10. Stern M, Walker WA. Food allergy and intolerance. *Pediatr Clin North Am* 1985;32:471–92.
11. David TJ, Wells FE, Sharpe TC, Gibbs AC. Low serum zinc in children with atopic eczema. *Br J Dermatol* 1984;111:597–601.
12. Sandstrom B, Cederblad A, Lonnertdal B. Zinc absorption from human milk, cow's milk and infant formulas. *Am J Dis Child* 1983;137:726–9.
13. American Academy of Pediatrics. Committee on nutrition: breast-feeding. *Pediatrics,* 1978; 62:591.
14. Kilshaw PJ, Cant AJ. The passage of maternal dietary proteins into human breast milk. *Arch Allergy Appl Immunol* 1984;75:7–15.
15. Jarrett E. Stimuli for the production and control of IgE in rats. *Immunol Rev* 1978;41:52–76.

16. Johnston DE, Dutton AM. Dietary prophylaxis of allergic diseases in children. *N Engl J Med* 1966;274:717–9.
17. Kjellman N-I M, Johansson SGO. Soy versus cow's milk in infants with a biparental history of atopic disease: development of atopic disease and immunoglobulins from birth to four years of age. *Clin Allergy* 1979;9:347–51.
18. van Asperen PP, Kemp AS, Mellis CM. Immediate food hypersensitivity reactions on the first known exposure to the food. *Arch Dis Child* 1983;58:253–6.

BRIEF PRELIMINARY REPORT OF UNPUBLISHED WORK BY DR. VANDENPLAS

I would like to thank you for giving me the opportunity to present briefly our data concerning a clinical field study we performed in infants at risk of atopy because of a family history of atopy. In a previous retrospective study (1) we demonstrated the increased incidence of cow's milk allergy in infants born to atopic families. We selected 75 infants with a positive family history (in 35 infants, two or more members of the family were atopic) for a prospective study. We studied five groups of 15 infants, as shown in Table 1.

No infants in group 1 developed allergic manifestations. Six infants in group 2 presented with symptoms of atopy after they had been changed to the adapted formula. Infants were considered as allergic to cow's milk when response to an open challenge test was positive. The symptoms improved or disappeared when the infants were returned to the hypoallergic formula but reappeared if the adapted formula was reintroduced. In group 3, four of 15 infants developed manifestations of atopy before 2 months of age, but all infants were asymptomatic during months 3 and 4 (HAF). In the breast-fed group (group 4), one infant developed eczema; this infant's mother had changed her food intake dramatically during lactation, with a much higher intake of milk and milk products than before. The eczema disappeared when we advised the mother to eliminate cow's milk products in her diet. In group 5, eight of 15 infants developed symptoms of atopy, and in each of them the challenge test was interpreted as being positive. Laboratory investigations were performed in the neonatal period as well as at 4 months (or when manifestations were worst) (Table 2).

In conclusion, all infants accepted the hypoallergic formula very well. HAF was effective in the treatment of minor cases and appeared to be effective in the prophylaxis, at least for a short-term prevention. If breast-feeding is impossible for whatever reason, a formula like HAF seems to be a possible alternative worthwhile to study. Of course, before drawing firm conclusions, much more data (double-blind studies, long-term follow-up) are needed.

REFERENCE

1. Vandenplas Y, Sacre L. Influences of neonatal serum IgE concentration, family history and diet on the incidence of cow's milk allergy. *Eur J Pediatr* 1986;45:493–5.

DISCUSSION

Dr. Haschke: I did not understand the study design. You indicated that this was a prospective study and that you had 15 children in each group. How could you be sure that 15 breast-fed infants would remain breast-fed for 4 months? How many infants were involved? What was the dropout rate?

Dr. Vandenplas: It was decided before starting the study to include the number of infants necessary to end up with five groups of 15 infants each, because a large number of dropouts had to be expected (e.g., stopping breast-feeding before 4 months, parents refusing to change to another formula in asymptomatic infants, or parents refusing the reintroduction of the adapted formula if atopic manifestations had disappeared with the hypoallergic formula).

Dr. Wahn: To me it is very surprising that there was such a high rate of atopic symptoms in the formula-fed group. What do you call atopic symptoms?

Dr. Vandenplas: We accepted as atopic manifestations dermatological symptoms such as eczema and urticaria, gastrointestinal symptoms such as colics, diarrhea, and vomiting, and respiratory symptoms such as spastic bronchitis and chronic rhinorrhea. There was certainly an overestimation of allergic manifestations because it was no double-blind study, although the parents had not been informed about the hypoallergic properties of the new formula and a challenge test had to be positive before an infant was considered allergic. One also has to remember that these infants were selected infants and that the data obtained cannot be extrapolated to a general population. The incidence correlates rather well with data from Kjellman (1), who reports an incidence of 53% allergic infants born in families with two atopic persons.

DISCUSSION REFERENCE

1. Kjellman N-I M. *Clin Allergy* 1979;9:347–51.

Food Allergy, edited by Eberhardt Schmidt.
Nestlé Nutrition Workshop Series, Vol. 17.
Nestec Ltd., Vevey/Raven Press, Ltd.,
New York © 1988.

Pathogenic Basis of Food Allergy Treatment

A. Blanco Quiros and E. Sanchez Villares

Hospital Clinico Universitario, Valladolid, Spain 4700

Food allergy is closely linked with children's age, and the condition might be
due to the degree of functional immaturity of the immune system or the digestive
capacity. Guidelines of dietary prophylaxis or treatment must take into account
this pathogenic basis. Another controversial topic in the pathogenesis of food allergy is the role of breast-feeding. It transiently prevents contact with potentially
allergenic foods, but its definitive importance remains uncertain.

We performed a study with 189 cases of food allergy (Fig. 1). Clinical symptoms were detected very early, before 12 months of age in 48% of the children.
This figure was obviously higher (68%) for milk, egg, and cereals (Table 1). The
mean age at onset in children suffering from egg allergy was the lowest (11
months); in children with cow's milk allergy, the age at onset was 13 months. The
high number of patients with fish allergy, coupled with their low age at onset, was
striking (1).

We shall review the pathogenic conditions that could contribute to the development of atopy.

THE IMMATURITY OF THE LOCAL IMMUNE SYSTEM

The intestinal immune system is not completely developed at birth. The immunoglobulin-forming cells (Ig FC) are scarce in the lamina propria, and the intestinal juice is lacking in secretory IgA (sIgA). We found a relative increase of IgM

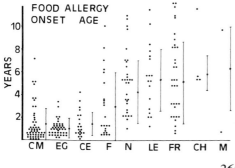

FIG. 1. Onset age of food allergy for 189
children with CM, cow's milk; EG, eggs; CE,
cereals; F, fish; N, nuts; LE, legumes; FR,
fruits; CH, chocolate; M, mother's milk.

TABLE 1. *Food allergy: onset age*[a]

Food	Onset before 12 months of age	Mean age at onset
Eggs	28 of 41 (68%)	11 months
Cow's milk	36 of 51 (70%)	13 months
Cereals	13 of 21 (62%)	15 months
Fish	12 of 23 (52%)	2 years and 9 months
Nuts	1 of 30 (3%)	4 years
Fruits	3 of 35 (8%)	5 years
Legumes	0 of 18 (0%)	5 years and 6 months
Chocolate	0 of 4 (0%)	6 years

[a]From ref. 1.

FC in normal children up to 12 months of age. The ratio IgA/IgM FC was 1.77 ± 0.98 (Fig. 2). Nevertheless, development is faster in secretory immunity than in systemic immunity (2). After this age the ratio increased to 3.00 ± 2.02 (Table 2). Oral immunization of infants with *Escherichia coli* stimulates first the production of secretory IgM antibodies and then later stimulates IgA-type antibodies (3). Maturity of secretory immunity is reached very soon. We could not find significant differences between children 12 to 24 months of age and children who were older.

There is no correlation between the number of Ig FC and the serum immunoglobulin levels because their maturation is independent (4,5). IgE, like the secretory IgA, is produced chiefly in cells lining the respiratory and gastrointestinal tracts. It is present in serum and secretions, although it is not bound to a secretory portion. Contradictory results have been reported with regard to the number of IgE FC in the intestinal lamina propria. Increased numbers have been reported by some (6,7), whereas others have reported normal numbers (8). We found elevated levels

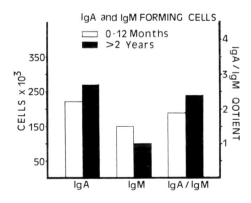

FIG. 2. Density of IgA- and IgM-forming cells in the normal intestinal mucosa according to age. The IgM FC are increased in children below 12 months of age.

TABLE 2. *Density of immunoglobulin-forming cells of intestinal lamina propria in normal children according to age[a]*

Age	N	IgA FC[b]	IgM FC	IgA/IgM FC
0–12 months	5	230 ± 104	152 ± 77[c]	1.77 ± 0.98[c]
12–24 months	10	275 ± 164	103 ± 57	3.00 ± 2.02
> 2 years	9	261 ± 112	119 ± 40	2.37 ± 1.44

[a]From ref. 2.
[b]Cells $\times 10^3$ /μl.
[c]Significant difference with the two other groups $p < 0.05$.

in 23 atopic children as compared with 16 nonatopic patients. This difference increased in older children, with a longer follow-up ($p < 0.02$) (Fig. 3) (4,5).

Nevertheless, we could not find differences between food-allergic patients with or without gastrointestinal symptoms (5). This suggests that the increase of IgE FC is only related to the atopic state, and it is not related to the location of the symptoms or the nature of the allergen. The cause of intestinal, dermatologic, or respiratory siting of clinical disturbances is unknown, but it is not due to the local density of IgE FC. On the contrary, it seems to be a result of the duration of the disease and the progressive allergenic overstimulation (5).

The increased number of IgM FC in the intestinal mucosa was another finding in food-allergic patients, although it was found exclusively in infants up to the age of 9 months (4). These data may reflect an abnormality of local immunoregulation or just a transient deficiency of IgA, as was proposed in infantile atopy by Taylor et al (9). In the IgA-selective immunodeficiency, it is well known that IgM replaces the IgA and can fix the secretory portion. In all our patients the density of

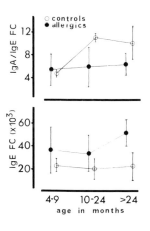

FIG. 3. The density of IgE FC is high in atopic patients, especially in older children. The increase is not related to the location of the symptoms.

intestinal IgA FC was similar to normal controls, but this does not rule out an IgA disturbance.

FOOD ANTIGEN ABSORPTION

It is estimated that 2% of the total ingested proteins are absorbed by the gut in macromolecular form, and therefore this fact might be of considerable importance in the pathogenesis of food allergy (10,11). The permeability is especially increased in preterm infants. Gut closure in humans occurs gradually with fetal maturation; nevertheless, the neonatal intestine may absorb antigenic quantities of ingested protein more readily than the mature adult intestine.

Several factors present within the intestinal lumen and on the intestinal mucosal surface help to control the macromolecular uptake. These systems could be immunologic factors, such as SIgA, or nonimmunologic factors, such as secretions, intestinal flora, peristaltic movement, mucus, etc. On the other hand, there are conditions contributing to pathologic transport of proteins (11). Intestinal helminth infection, acute gastroenteritis, IgA-selective deficiency, and protein malnutrition can increase protein permeability (12). It is debatable whether this increased macromolecular uptake by the neonatal gut could trigger off an allergic response. It has been suggested that during the neonatal period, susceptible infants may become sensitized to specific ingested allergen. With reexposure at a time when much less macromolecular absorption is occurring, minute quantities of allergen may be absorbed and result in allergic symptoms (11). Nevertheless, further studies are needed to ascertain the importance of this intestinal hyperpermeability in food allergy.

BREAST-FEEDING AND FOOD ALLERGY

We could not find significant differences between breast-feeding and bottle-feeding children. The frequency of food allergy was similar in both groups. We found only that breast-feeding postpones the onset date of allergic respiratory symptoms in prematurely born patients. This finding could be due to a higher intestinal hyperpermeability of macromolecules in these children.

In our study, the symptoms occurred at the first known exposure to egg in 24% of egg-sensitized cases, and we observed the same feature in 17% of fish-allergic children. This observation makes us wonder how the sensitization took place. Several authors have proved that intrauterine sensitization is possible. It has also been reported that human milk can contain a small quantity of maternal dietary antigens. It has been shown that there are cases in which allergic symptoms have improved when a specific food has been removed from the maternal diet and recurred when the mother again ingested the food (13). The capacity of sensitization by animal proteins, present in minute amounts in human milk, could be even higher than that of normal artificial feeding.

GASTROINTESTINAL INFECTION AND FOOD ALLERGY

In our study, the onset of allergic symptoms coincided with a gastrointestinal infection in 21.5% (11 of 51) of cow's milk allergy cases. A family history of allergy was also present in seven of these children. Gastroenteritis was less frequent in egg [10% (two of 20)] and cereal [10.5% (four of 38)] hypersensitivity. The mean age of these patients was low: 4 months and 15 days (1).

The relationship between acute gastroenteritis in infants and food allergy is well known. Nevertheless, the exact mechanisms are not clear. The infection causes intestinal damage (14), and it was hypothesized that this injury enhances the absorption of foreign macromolecules and thus leads to secondary sensitization. On the other hand, at present there is increasing evidence suggesting that some viruses can modify the mucosal immunoregulation system. The respiratory syncytial virus infection is associated with an IgE antibody response and a decrease in the number of suppressor T cells, but it is unknown whether these phenomena are postnatally acquired or are inherited. It is likely that the development of food allergy in atopic individuals has less to do with abnormal mucosal permeability than with selective gaps in the immune response (15). Very little is known about the development of the capacity to regulate IgE production and the factors that influence this (15).

REFERENCES

1. Berjon MC, Andion R, Linares P, Fernandez LA, Blanco A. Aportacion clinica y diagnostica de la alergia alimentaria infantil. *An Esp Pediatr* 1987;26:85–90.
2. Blanco A, Linares P, Andion R, Alonso M, Sanchez Villares E. Development of humoral immunity system of the small bowel. *Allergol Immunopathol (Madr)* 1976;4:235–40.
3. Girard JP, Kalbermatten A. Antibody activity in human duodenal fluid. *Eur J Clin Invest* 1970;1:188–96.
4. Linares P, Blanco A, Alonso M, Andion R, Sanchez Villares E. Sistema immunitario intestinal y alergia alimentaria. *An Esp Pediatr* 1977;10:133–40.
5. Blanco A, Linares P, Alonso M, Sanchez Villares E. Pathogenesis of food and gastrointestinal atopy. *Allergol Immunopathol (Madr)* 1977;5:97–100.
6. Shiner M, Ballard J, Smith ME. The small-intestinal mucosa in cow's milk allergy. *Lancet* 1975;i:136–40.
7. Rosenkrans PCM, Meijer CJLM, Cornelisse CJ, Wal AM, Lindeman J. Use of morphometry and immunochemistry of small intestinal biopsy specimens in the diagnosis of food allergy. *J Clin Pathol* 1980;33:125–30.
8. Brandtzaeg P, Baklien K. Inconclusive immunohistochemistry of human IgE in mucosal pathology. *Lancet* 1976;i:1297–8.
9. Taylor B, Normal AP, Orgel HA, Stoken CR. Transient IgA deficiency and pathogenesis of infantile atopy. *Lancet* 1973;ii:111–3.
10. Reinhardt MC. Macromolecular absorption of food antigens in health and disease. *Ann Allergy* 1984;53:597–601.
11. Walker WA. Antigen handling by the gut. *Arch Dis Child* 1978;53:527–31.
12. Reinhardt MC, Paganelli MD, Levinsky RJ. Intestinal antigen handling at mucosal surfaces in health and disease; human and experimental studies. *Ann Allergy* 1983;51:311–8.
13. Shacks SJ, Heiner DC. Allergy to breast milk. *Clin Immunol Allergy* 1982;2:121–36.
14. Hutchins P, Walker-Smith JA. The gastrointestinal system. *Clin Immunol Allergy* 1982;2:43–75.
15. Jarrett EEE. Immunoregulation of IgE responses: the role of the gut in perspective. *Ann Allergy* 1984;53:550–6.

DISCUSSION

Dr. Bellanti: I was interested in the developmental studies that you showed concerning the IgE/IgA ratio in the gut of children. I think the problem of food allergy will be best understood through a study of the development of immune responses and of the gastrointestinal tract. I should like to suggest a mechanism for the development of allergy, particularly with regard to the effects of infection. A few years ago Dr. Frick described how, with the onset of respiratory syncytial virus infection, there is an increased sensitization to other allergens. Similarly you and others have found that acute infection of the gastrointestinal tract can lead to allergy. These studies would suggest that viral infection may cause a disregulation of the T-cell system that regulates IgE. I don't think this is the entire solution, because the effects of acute infectious diseases on disregulation are transient; however, if you consider Epstein-Barr virus, or herpes, or cytomegalovirus, then I think you might see more protracted changes. In his studies in Buffalo, New York, Dr. Ogra has also demonstrated specific IgE antiviral antibodies which, when they react with the antigens, produce a release of mediators which could result in a local increase in permeability to food antigens in the gut or to inhalant antigens in the lung. So the IgE mechanism may enhance the penetration of macromolecules and be the basis for continued sensitization in the atopic patient.

Dr. Blanco Quiros: The mechanism of the relationship between local infection and gastrointestinal allergy must be complex. I agree that two main systems are present. The first is the increase in macromolecular permeability, and the second is the direct action of some virus upon the immunoregulation and the IgE synthesis. I don't think we yet know the exact importance of each mechanism.

Food Allergy, edited by Eberhardt Schmidt.
Nestlé Nutrition Workshop Series, Vol. 17.
Nestec Ltd., Vevey/Raven Press, Ltd.,
New York © 1988.

Dermatologic Diseases Secondary to Food Allergy and Pseudoallergy

Johannes Ring

*Dermatologische Klinik und Poliklinik, Ludwig-Maximilian-Universität,
8000 Munich 2, Federal Republic of Germany*

Adverse reactions to foods and food constituents represent an increasing problem for the practicing allergist (1–4). The spectrum of clinical symptoms ranges from gastroenteritis, urticaria, bronchial asthma, allergic rhinitis, and anaphylactoid reactions to serum-sickness-type reactions with (a) arthralgia and vasculitis or (b) exacerbations of allergic contact dermatitis or (c) atopic eczema.

Many patients complain that headache, tension fatigue, psychological abnormalities, etc. are not clearly defined and are difficult to assess.

CLASSIFICATION OF ADVERSE FOOD REACTIONS

Undesirable reactions to foods can be elicited by a variety of pathomechanisms. In Table 1, a classification of adverse food reactions according to different pathomechanisms is given (5). Clearly, toxic reactions (such as food intoxication) or increased individual sensitivity toward a specific pharmacologic effect of a food or a food additive (intolerance) have to be differentiated from other kinds of hypersensitivity, which can either be immunologically (i.e., allergic) or nonimmunologically (i.e., idiosyncratic) mediated.

When the symptoms observed mimic symptoms of classic allergic diseases, the term "pseudoallergy" is used (3).

In order to define food allergy, the following diagnostic postulates have to be considered:

1. Reproducible elicitation of symptoms by the specific food.
2. Exclusion of other possible causes of incompatibility.
3. Demonstration of immunologic sensitization.

Table 2 gives the definitions of the most important terms used in this context. Here, we will not talk about genuine intoxications by poisoned food or bacterial contamination, nor will we talk about deficiency states (e.g., of vitamins, trace elements, etc.) by which foods can affect health.

TABLE 1. *Classification of adverse food reactions*

Adverse food reaction			
Toxicity		Hypersensitivity	
Intoxication	Pharmacological intolerance	Idiosyncrasy	Allergy
		Nonimmunological mechanisms	IgE, IgG/IgM, IgA (?), cellular
Pharmacological effect, organ toxicity[a]		Unexpected, sometimes "allergy-like" symptoms[a]	Allergic disease

[a]If symptoms mimick allergic diseases, the term "pseudo-allergy" is used.

TABLE 2. *Definition of allergological terms*

Toxicity:	Normal poisonousness
Allergy:	Immunologic hypersensitivity
Intolerance:	Hypersensitivity to normal pharmacologic effect
Idiosyncrasy:	Nonimmunologic hypersensitivity (unrelated to pharmacologic effect)
Pseudoallergy:	Nonimmunologic hypersensitivity with "allergy-like" symptoms

TABLE 3. *Skin lesions possibly provoked by foods*

Erythema	Vesicle
Wheal	Bulla
Purpura	Pustule
Papule	Ulcer
Nodule	Necrosis

There is no specific skin lesion primarily linked to food reactions (6,7), but the whole spectrum of skin lesions can be elicited by allergic food reactions (Table 3). Table 4 gives an overview of dermatologic diseases, which may be evoked by food allergy or pseudoallergy. The most important skin diseases that are possibly evoked by food will be described in detail.

TABLE 4. *Skin diseases possibly evoked by foods*

Pruritus	Panniculitis (?)
Flush	Purpura pigmentosa progressiva
Urticaria	Allergic contact dermatitis
Angioedema	Phototoxic and photoallergic reactions
Atopic eczema	Exanthematous eruption
Swelling of lips and oral mucosa	Melkersson-Rosenthal-syndrome (?)
Stomatitis	Bromoderma
Glossitis (Papillitis linguae)	Acne (?)
Recurrent aphthae	Dermatitis herpetiformis
Immune-complex vasculitis	

URTICARIA AND ANGIOEDEMA

Foods can elicit urticaria (Fig. 1) or angioedema (Fig. 2) by both allergic and pseudoallergic mechanisms (8–10). Various authors have described positive food provocation tests in urticaria (Table 5). Food additives such as preservatives, antioxidants, etc., which are known to elicit or sustain chronic urticaria (3,4,11,14–19), are particularly important (Table 6).

Certain foods contain considerable amounts of vasoactive amines known to provoke urticaria, asthma, or anaphylactoid reactions (1,5,8,20,21) (Table 7).

In this context, special reference has to be made to the syndrome of *contact urticaria* (Fig. 3): Urticaria lesions are provoked by contact with certain sub-

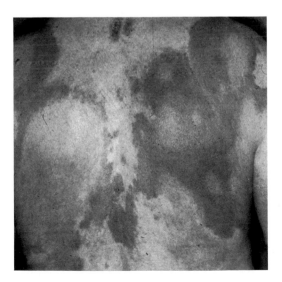

FIG. 1. Urticaria *(Archiv der Dermatologischen Klinik und Poliklinik der Ludwig-Maximilians-Universität München).*

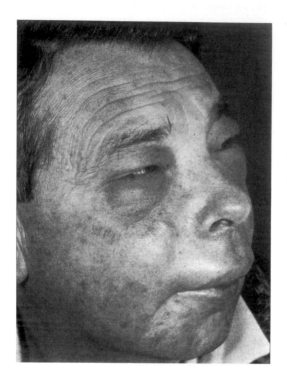

FIG. 2. Angioedema *(Archiv der Dermatologischen Klinik und Poliklinik der Ludwig-Maximilians-Universität München).*

TABLE 5. *Positive provocation tests with foods in chronic urticaria[a]*

Food	1971: Michailoff, Berova (11)	1973: Galant et al. (12)	1975: Wraith et al. (13)	1986: Ring et al. (14)
Milk	24	28	0	2
Fish	22	28	6	12
Meat	19	—	—	4
Egg	18	21	10	5
Vegetables	13	—	—	5
Others	—	28	80	2

[a]Percent positive patients.

stances (22); the diagnosis is done by open patch test (Fig. 4). Many authors have reported food-elicited contact urticaria (1,2,22,23). This syndrome may be mediated by IgE or by nonimmunologic mechanisms.

Most probably, the recently described *protein dermatitis* or gut eczema or butcher's eczema (24), observed in butchers after contact with the animal gut, does not represent a contact urticaria but, instead, represents an atopic eczema provoked by either irritation or allergy to food ingredients (25).

TABLE 6. *Positive provocation tests with food additives in chronic urticaria*[a]

	Warin, Smith (19) (n = 111)	Gibson, Clancy (8) (n = 76)	Juhlin et al. (15) (n = 330)	Hannuksela (7) (n = 137)	Ring et al. (5) (n = 135)
Colors	13	26	18	1	8
Benzoic acid	10	34	11	4	1
Sorbic acid	—	—	9	0	0
Penicillin	15	18	11	0	—
Sulfites	—	—	—	—	2
ASS	41	54	10	18	17

[a]Percent positive provocation.

TABLE 7. *Elicitors of pseudo-allergic food reactions*

Preservatives	Colors	Flavoring	Others
Benzoic acid and derivatives Sorbic acid Nitrites Sulfites Propionate	Azo dyes	Salicylates Glutamate Aspartame	Stabilizers Emulsifiers Guar

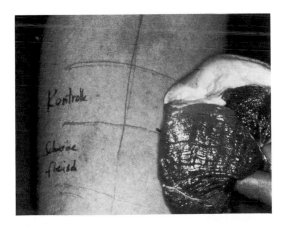

FIG. 3. Contact urticaria to pork meat.

With regard to genuine allergies, certain cross-reactions between foods and pollens have to be mentioned, as in the case of (a) birch and apple or mugwort and (b) certain spices and celery (1,19,23,26,27).

Furthermore, some cases of physical urticaria, especially exercise-induced urticaria or anaphylaxis, may be related or closely connected with food allergy in the

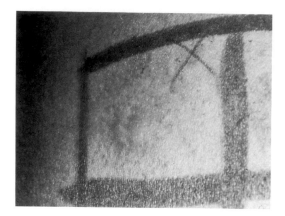

FIG. 4. Positive "open patch test" (after 20 min) in contact urticaria.

sense of a *"summation anaphylaxis"*; these patients seem to only develop symptoms after the combination of physical effort and the intake of the specific food, whereas the food or exercise alone is usually well tolerated (3,23). This makes history-taking in these patients extremely difficult. The time interval between food intake and the physical stimulus may be as long as 48 hr.

ATOPIC ECZEMA

The role of food allergy in the pathophysiology of atopic eczema (Fig. 5) is not well established, although there is abundant literature about this topic (2,28–43). In Table 8, the most important arguments "for" or "against" the pathophysiological role of food allergy in atopic eczema are listed.

There is no doubt that certain foods can provoke atopic eczema in some patients, but this is surely only *one* etiologic factor among many others. There is evidence for IgE-mediated sensitization to many food allergens in patients with atopic eczema (28,37). The relevance of these test results (skin test or RAST), however, has to be proven by elimination or provocation procedures. In the literature, the incidence of positive provocation tests with food-induced atopic eczema are controversial and range between 0% and 84% (quoted in refs. 42 and 44). Only a few controlled studies have been performed, especially by the groups of Atherton's group in London (45,46) and Sampson's group in the United States (47,48). Antigen avoidance by an oligoantigenic diet (strict exclusion of milk and egg intake) led to a considerable improvement in 35% of the children under 8 years of age (45). The most striking finding was that among the children who benefited from this elimination diet, some showed no evidence of sensitization to egg or milk in the skin test or RAST. In another study in adults, an antigen-elimination diet failed to demonstrate clinical effects (46).

The placebo-controlled double-blind study by Sampson and McCaskill reported

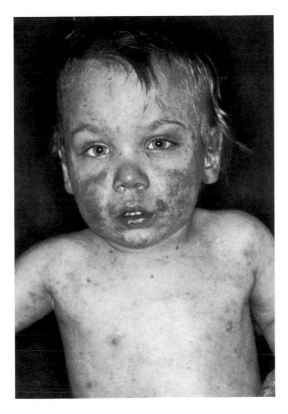

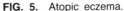

FIG. 5. Atopic eczema.

results of 370 provocations in 113 patients 4 to 24 years old (48). Here, 56% of the patients and 27% of the provocations were positive. Skin symptoms were observed in 84% of cases, beginning within 2 hr as macular erythema and pruritus, sometimes together with wheals; later on, because of the scratch response, excoriations and an exacerbation of eczema were observed.

In 52% of cases, gastrointestinal symptoms were observed; in 32% of cases, respiratory symptoms were observed. The most frequent offending foods were hen's egg (42%) peanut (19%), milk (11%), soy (5%), wheat (5%), chicken (3%), pork (2%), beef (2%), and potato (2%). During positive provocations there was sometimes a rise in plasma histamine levels. It was interesting to note that no child reacted to two different foods from one species. Positive skin-prick tests were more frequent in patients reacting to foods as compared to those who did not react. There was no difference with regard to total serum IgE, history of atopic diseases, or respiratory symptoms. When the identified food was eliminated, significant improvement was observed.

This was a very good study; however, it is still too early to safely state that food allergy plays the decisive role in a rather high percentage of atopic eczema. Another problem that needs to be studied is the influence of pseudoallergic reactions

TABLE 8. *Arguments for and against a role of food allergy in atopic eczema*

FOR
IgE-antibodies against foods more frequent in atopic eczema than in other atopic diseases
Protective effect of breast-feeding
Increased intestinal absorption of potential allergens in atopic eczema
Clinical improvement after allergen avoidance
Positive provocation studies

AGAINST
Only weak correlation between skin test and history of food allergy
Only weak correlation between RAST results and history
Lack of effect of elimination diets planned according to skin test or RAST results
Lack of effect of cow's milk–free nutrition compared to soy in some studies
In adults, provocation tests are often negative

---

in the pathogenesis of atopic eczema. While additives are used in provocation tests in urticaria and angioedema, only limited experience is available with these elicitors of pseudoallergic reactions in atopic eczema (40).

We observed the case of a 38-year-old female patient whose eczema flared dramatically after oral provocation with 500 mg of sodium propionate within 1 day (44).

Another very exciting issue is the question of possibly increased intestinal permeability, which is still controversial (20,33,49,50).

In the practical approach for diagnosing food allergy in atopic eczema, there are several major problems. The relevance of *in vitro* and *in vivo* allergy diagnostics has not been established.

Provocation procedures should always be performed in a blind fashion; however, this may be extremely difficult with certain foods. Furthermore, the exacerbation of the eczematous lesions does not necessarily occur within 1 or 2 hr but may, instead, take as long as several days with successive challenges. At the same time, other factors (psychological influences, other allergens, change of topical or systemic treatment, etc.) may elicit an exacerbation of the disease.

In recent years, special interest has focused on the positive influence of breast-feeding in preventing the manifestation of atopic diseases in childhood (31,32, 41,51–61). As Table 9 shows, there are controversial reports on this topic.

There is some evidence that breast-feeding is indeed able to inhibit, or at least delay, the manifestation of atopic diseases in infants with a high risk of atopy (positive family history in two parents or elevated cord blood IgE). It may well be that breast-feeding not only provides a protective effect by allergen avoidance (e.g., elimination of potential allergens as cow's milk or hen's egg) but also provides a positive protective effect mediated by specific IgG antibodies to food allergens or by other factors contained in breast milk.

Furthermore, the delayed introduction of solid foods seems to be important in the prophylaxis of food allergy in infants (56).

TABLE 9. *Effect of breast-feeding on the manifestation of atopic diseases (literature)*

Studies showing an inhibitory effect	Breast-feeding found to enhance atopic disease	No effect of breast-feeding
Saarinen 1979 (41)	Taylor 1984 (59)	Halpern 1973 (53)
Juto 1982 (55)		Kramer 1981 (58)
Kajosaari 1983 (56)		Gruskay (1982 (52)
Businco 1983 (31)[a]		Van Asperen 1984 (60)
Duchateau 1983 (51)[a]		
Chandra 1985[a] (32)		

[a]Only effective when cord blood-IgE was elevated.

There is no doubt that small amounts of allergens can be detected in breast milk and can elicit allergic reactions in exclusively breast-fed infants. In these cases, a specific avoidance diet has to be recommended to the mother.

On the basis of these findings, only limited therapeutic recommendations regarding food allergy and atopic eczema can be given. The value of oligoantigenic or other very strict general avoidance diets is largely confined to the short period of allergy diagnosis. For long-term therapy, caution is necessary in order not to induce states of deficiency of essential food ingredients or malnutrition. Every dermatologist has seen the sad cases of totally malnourished children as a result of an extreme diet, not at all based on rational allergy diagnosis but rather on ideological considerations.

There are, however, many foods that are easily avoidable (such as spices, fish, etc.). In these cases, specific allergen avoidance represents the simplest and best therapeutic approach.

Oral hyposensitization with ubiquitous foods represents another therapeutic strategy and may work in some patients (62), although there are no prospective controlled studies available.

The use of oral sodium cromoglycate has been recommended by some authors (23,40,63,64), whereas other authors have found it to be ineffective. In an open study over a six-month period in 19 patients with atopic eczema, we found a significant improvement in seven patients with skin-prick test and RAST results suggestive of food allergy (40). The patients were nonselected and had no history of clear-cut food-induced eczematous lesions.

At present, the role of food allergy in atopic eczema remains controversial and certainly represents only one part of the problem for selected individuals. The core of the treatment of atopic eczema remains the careful dermatologic treatment using the right amount of the right corticosteroid in the right vehicle at the right time and the individually tailored emollient during the phases of remission (3,65).

TABLE 10. *Nickel content of various foods[a]*

Food	μg/kg
Lentils	3100
Beans (white)	2850
Peas	2250
Chocolate	2200
Rye (grains)[b]	2700
Peanuts	1600
Milk and milk[b] products	50
Potatoes[b]	250
Raspberry jam	400
Herring	300
Porc	250
Beer	20
Wine (white)	100

[a]Many thanks to Dr. Haeberle from the Department of Dermatology, University of Erlangen, for help in preparing this table.
[b]Influence of acid upon nickel from pots.

CONTACT ECZEMA

Allergic contact dermatitis or contact eczema is elicited by the topical contact of the skin with potential allergens. In rare cases, these allergens may be foods or food constituents. The so-called "protein dermatitis" occurring in butchers or kitchen personnel has been mentioned above (24) (see discussion on contact urticaria). In individuals sensitized to contact allergens, the oral ingestion may provoke a generalized eczematous eruption called "hematogenous," "blood-borne" or "systemic" allergic contact eczema (66).

With regard to food allergy and the frequency of nickel sensitization in the general population, the relevance of nickel contained in certain foods has to be discussed (Table 10). However, before the difficult "nickel-free" diet is recommended (67), the relevance of systemic nickel application has to be proven by oral provocation tests. In some of these patients the characteristic skin lesion consists in a dyshidrosiform eruption of contact dermatitis of the palms and soles (Fig. 6).

PHOTOSENSITIZATION

Photosensitization represents the phenomenon whereby the combination of electromagnetic radiation and the contact with an allergen or another photosensitizing agent provokes skin lesions (68). Among photosensitizing substances are many drugs, but also naturally occurring substances, some of which may be present in foods (Table 11).

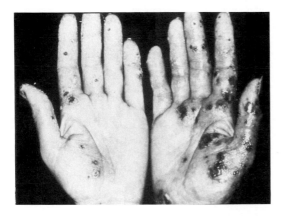

FIG. 6. Dyshidrosiform eczema of palms and soles in nickel-sensitive patients *(Archiv der Dermatologischen Klinik und Poliklinik der Ludwig - Maximilians - Universität München).*

TABLE 11. *Food or food constituents as photosensitizers*

Cyclamate
Dyes

Fig (Ficus)
Lemon (Citrus limon)
Lime (Citrus auranti folia)
Parsley (Anthiscus)
Parsnip (Pastinaca)
St. John's wort (Hypericum)

DERMATITIS HERPETIFORMIS (DUHRING)

Dermatitis herpetiformis presents clinically as an itchy, sometimes burning, eruption of grouped vesicles on an erythematous base; in most patients the vesicles are scratched so that excoriated papules are seen (6) (Fig. 7).

In the pathogenesis of dermatitis herpetiformis as well as gluten-sensitive enteropathy, the role of specific antigliadin antibodies is discussed (69 71). Gliadin represents the alcohol-soluble fraction of gluten. In patients with dermatitis herpetiformis, antigliadin antibodies (of both the IgG class and the IgA class) have been found and seem to correlate with the existence of enteropathy. The same holds true for antireticulin (or antiendomysium) antibodies (71).

One of the hallmarks of diagnosis is that IgA in the direct immunofluorescence in uninvolved skin remains there over long periods, even under strict gluten-free diet (72).

Immunogenetic studies show an association of dermatitis herpetiformis with HLA-B 8 and DR 3 (71).

Iodides, both topical and systemic, will provoke the exacerbation of blisters by a yet unknown mechanism. The efficacy of a gluten-free diet, which it is undoubted in gluten-sensitive enteropathy, is still controversial in the treatment of

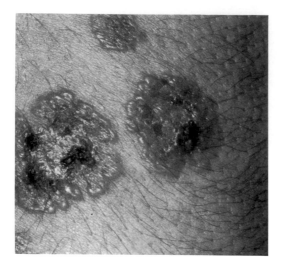

FIG. 7. Dermatitis herpetiformis *(Archiv der Dermatologischen Klinik und Poliklinik der Ludwig-Maximilians-Universität München).*

dermatitis herpetiformis (6,71,72). Sometimes clinical improvement appears only after 6 months of dietary intervention.

ALLERGIC VASCULITIS

Allergic vasculitis (leukocytoclastic vasculitis) represents an immune complex (Type III) reaction leading to perivascular inflammation and extravasation (Fig. 8). Among the common causes of this disease are infectious diseases, drugs, neoplastic conditions, autoimmune diseases, cryoglobulinemia, and others (73).

There are some case reports describing foods as elicitors of allergic vasculitis (74–79) (Table 12). We observed two patients with allergic vasculitis in whom foods were shown to be of clinical relevance by oral provocation tests. Intradermal tests with food allergens had not only produced an immediate wheal-and-flare reaction but also produced marked inflammatory reactions after 8 to 24 hr, which showed histologically and immunopathologically the characteristics of immune-complex vasculitis. The careful avoidance of the most important allergens, together with oral cromoglycate, led to a marked improvement of the condition (75).

Immune complex deposits have also been found in lesions of the oral mucosa in patients with recurrent *aphthae* (80) (Fig. 9).

PRURITUS

Pruritus is a very subjective symptom and is often hard to evaluate. Among the patients with "pruritus sine materia," true cases of food allergy (e.g., against hen's egg) can be found and have to be distinguished from pruritus senilis and pruritus, which are induced by dry skin and exsiccation (3,6,23).

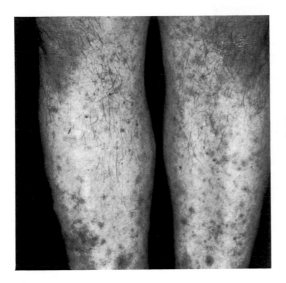

FIG. 8. Food-induced allergic vasculitis on the lower leg.

TABLE 12. *Literature on food-induced allergic vasculitis*

Eliciting agent	Authors	Year
Shellfish	Ancona	1951
Blackberries	Winkelmann	1964
Tartrazine	Kubba, Champion	1975
Tartrazine	Wüthrich	1982
Vitamin B_0	Ruzicka, Ring, Braun-Falco	1984
Foods, spices, vegetables	Eisenmann et al.	1987

OTHER CONDITIONS POSSIBLY EVOKED BY FOODS

In Table 4, many other skin conditions are listed which may possibly be induced by foods in rare instances.

An increasing problem in the office of the practicing allergist concerns patients' subjective complaints related to foods or chemicals in foods. In many of these patients with what we call *clinical ecology syndrome* (81), objective investigations failed to demonstrate any causal relationship between food chemicals and complaints (the crucial test is the placebo provocation) (81–85). Psychological factors such as chemophobia or anxiety and depression seem to represent the major problem of these patients. However, a careful allergological examination has to be done in order to truly rule out food allergy or pseudoallergy.

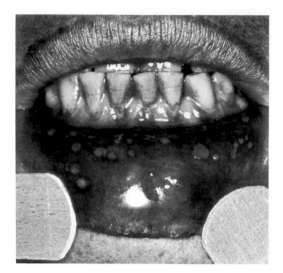

FIG. 9. Aphthae *(Archiv der Dermatologischen Klinik und Poliklinik der Ludwig-Maximilians-Universität München).*

A great deal of research will have to be done to further elucidate the mechanisms and the relevance of these findings. The first step will have to be an improvement in current diagnostic techniques (2,4,13,19,28,40,82,83), possibly by introduction of the intragastral provocation under endoscopic control (IPEC) (86,87).

REFERENCES

1. Lessof MH, ed. *Clinical reactions to food.* New York: Wiley, 1983.
2. May CD, Bock SA. A modern clinical approach to food hypersensitivity. *Allergy* 1978;33:166–88.
3. Ring J. *Angewandte Allergologie.* München: MMW-Verlag Medizin, 1982.
4. Wüthrich B. Allergische und pseudo-allergische Reaktionen der Haut durch Arzneimittel und Lebensmitteladditiva. *Schweiz Rundsch Med Prax* 1983;20:691–9.
5. Ring J. Nahrungsmittelallergie und andere Unverträglichkeitsreaktionen durch Nahrungsmittel. *Klin Wochenschr* 1984;62:795–802.
6. Braun-Falco O, Plewig G, Wolff HH. *Dermatologie und Venerologie,* 3rd ed. Berlin: Springer, 1985.
7. Hannuksela M. Food allergy and skin diseases. *Ann Allergy* 1983;51:269–72.
8. Gibson A, Clancy R. Management of chronic idiopathic urticaria by the identification and exclusion of dietary factors. *Clin Allergy* 1980;10:699–704.
9. Illig L. Pseudo-allergische (anaphylaktoide) Reaktionen der Haut auf Lebensmittelfarbstoffe. *Allergologie* 1982;5:193–8.
10. Juhlin L. Recurrent urticaria. *Br J Dermatol* 1981;104:369–81.
11. Michailov P, Berova N. Gastrointestinal disorders in the pathogenesis of urticaria. *Z Hautkr* 1971;46:609–12.
12. Galant SP, Bullock J, Frick OL. An immunological approach to the diagnosis of food sensitivity. *Clin Allergy* 1973;3:363–72.
13. Wraith DG, Merrett J, Roth A, et al. Recognition of food allergic patients and their allergens by the RAST technique and clinical investigation. *Clin Allergy* 1975;9:25–36.
14. Ring J, Braun-Falco O. Allergie-Diät: Verfahren zur Diagnostik und Therapie von Nahrungsmittel-Allergien und -Pseudo-Allergien. *Hautarzt* 1987;38:198–205.

15. Juhlin L, Michaelsson G, Zetterström O, Urticaria and asthma induced by food and drug additives in patients with aspirin hypersensitivity. *J Allergy Clin Immunol* 1972;50:92–104.
16. Michaelsson G, Juhlin L. Urticaria induced by preservatives and dye additives in food and drugs. *Br J Dermatol* 1973;88:525–32.
17. Schindler H, Bräckle J, Karch B. Kochbuch für Allergiker. München: Ehrenwirth, 1981.
18. Thiel C, Fuchs E. Nahrungsintoleranzen durch Fremdstoffe. *Münch Med Wochenschr* 1983; 125:451–4.
19. Warin RP, Smith RJ. Challenge test battery in chronic urticaria. *Br J Dermatol* 1975;93(suppl 11):19.
20. Boyer J, Depierre F, Tissier M, Jacob I. Intoxications histaminiques collectives par le thon. *Presse Med* 1956;64:1003–4.
21. Moneret-Vautrin DA, Viniaker J, Boissel P, Noel M, Kim K. Effects de l'instillation d'histamine dans l'intestin grêle chez l'homme. I. Variations de l'histaminémie portale et périphérique. *Ann Gastroenterol Hepatol* 1981;17:395–400.
22. Lahti A. Nonimmunologic contact urticaria. *Acta Derm Venereol (Suppl) (Stockh)* 1980;91:1–49.
23. Wüthrich B. Nahrungsmittelallergien. *Internist* 1986;27:362–71.
24. Hjorth N, Roed-Petersen J. Occupational protein contact dermatitis in food handlers. *Contact Dermatitis* 1976;2:28–42.
25. Galosi A, Ring J, Przybilla B. *Kontakturtikaria bei Metzgern. RAST 4.* Freiburg: Berichtsband, Pharmacia, 1984;241–4.
26. Aas K. The diagnosis of hypersensitivity to ingested foods. Reliability of skin prick testing and the radioallergosorbent test with different materials. *Clin Allergy* 1978;8:39–50.
27. Niinimäki A, Hannuksela M. Immediate skin test reactions to spices. *Allergy* 1981;36:487–93.
28. Benton EC, Barnetson RC. Skin reactions to foods in patients with atopic dermatitis. *Acta Dermatol Venereol (Suppl) (Stockh)* 1985;114:129–32.
29. Bierman CW, Pearlman DS. *Allergic diseases of infancy, childhood and adolescence.* Philadelphia: Saunders, 1982.
30. Bjarnason I, Goolamali SK, Levi AJ, Peters TJ. Intestinal permeability in patients with atopic eczema. *Br J Dermatol* 1985;112:291–7.
31. Businco L, Marchetti F, Pellegrini G, Perlini R. Predictive value of cord blood IgE levels in "at-risk" newborn babies and influence of type of feeding. *Clin Allergy* 1983;13:503–8.
32. Chandra RK, Puri S, Cheema PS. Predictive value of cord blood IgE in the development of atopic disease and role of breast-feeding in its prevention. *Clin Allergy* 1983;13:503–8.
33. Fälth-Magnusson K, Kjellman N-IM, Magnusson KE, Sudqvist T. Intestinal permeability in healthy and allergic children before and after sodium-cromoglycate treatment assessed with different-sized polyethylene-glycols (PEG 400 and PEG 1000). *Clin Allergy* 1984,14:277–86.
34. Hanifin JM. Diet, nutrition and allergy in atopic dermatitis. *J Am Acad Dermatol* 1983;8:729–31.
35. Kleinhans D. Zur Immunpathogenese der atopischen Dermatitis (Endogenes Ekzem). *Z Hautkr* 1983;58:925–6.
36. Korting GW. *Zur Pathogenese des endogenen Ekzems.* Stuttgart; Thieme, 1952.
37. von Muyenburg H. Hohe Inzidenz manifester Nahrungsmittelallergie bei Patienten mit Neurodermitis und erhöhten IgE-Spiegeln. *Allergologie* 1984;7:307–15.
38. Rajka G. *Atopic dermatitis.* London: Saunders, 1975.
39. Rajka G. *Atopic dermatitis.* London: Saunders, 1975.
40. Ring J. Nahrungsmittelallergie und atopisches Ekzem *Allergologie* 1984;7:300–6.
41. Saarinen UM, Kajosaari M, Backman A, Siimes MA. Prolonged breast-feeding as prophylaxis for atopic disease. *Lancet* 1979;ii:163–6.
42. Schnyder UM. *Neurodermitis-Asthma-Rhinitis. Eine genetisch-allergologische Studie.* Basel: Karger, 1960.
43. Wüthrich B. Neurodermitis atopica sive constitutionalis. Ein pathogenetisches Modell aus der Sicht des Allergologen. *Akt Dermatol* 1983;9:1–7.
44. Przybilla B, Ruzicka T, Ring J. Die Bedeutung von Nahrungsmittelallergien bei atopischem Ekzem. *Allergologie* 1987 *(in press)*.
45. Atherton DJ, Soothill JF, Dewell M, Wells RS. A double-blind controlled crossover trial of an antigen avoidance diet in atopic eczema. *Lancet* 1978;i:401–3.
46. Atherton DJ. The role of foods in atopic eczema. *Clin Exp Dermatol* 1983;8:227–32.
47. Sampson HA. Role of immediate food hypersensitivity in the pathogenesis of atopic dermatitis. *J Allergy Clin Immunol* 1983;71:473–80.

48. Sampson HA, McCaskill CC. Food hypersensitivity and atopic dermatitis: evaluation of 113 patients. *J Pediatr* 1985;107:669–75.
49. Bloch KJ, Walker WA. Effect of locally induced intestinal anaphylaxis on the uptake of bystander antigen. *J Allergy Clin Immunol* 1981;67:312.
50. MacKie RM. Intestinal permeability and atopic disease. *Lancet* 1981;ii:155.
51. Duchateau J, Casimir G. Neonatal serum IgE concentration as predictor of atopy. *Lancet* 1983;i:413–4.
52. Gruskay FL. Comparison of breast, cow and soy feedings in the prevention of onset of allergic disease. A fifteen-year prospective study. *Clin Pediatr* 1982;21:486–91.
53. Halpern SR, Sellars WA, Johnson RB, Anderson DW, Saperstein S, Reish JS. Development of childhood allergy in infants fed breast, soy or cow milk. *J Allergy Clin Immunol* 1973;51:139–51.
54. Hammar H. Provocation with cow's milk and cereals in atopic dermatitis. *Acta Derm Venenreol* 1977;57:159–63.
55. Juto P, Möller C, Engberg S, Björkstén B. Influence of type of feeding on lymphocyte function and development of infantile allergy. *Clin Allergy* 1982;12:409–16.
56. Kajosaari M, Saarinen UM. Prophylaxis of atopic disease by six months total solid food elimination. *Acta Paediatr Scand* 1983;72:411–4.
57. Kjellman NLM, Johansson SGO. Soy versus cow's milk in infants with biparental history of atopic diseases; development of atopic disease and immunoglobulins from birth to 4 years of age. *Clin Allergy* 1979;9:347–58.
58. Kramer MS, Moroz B. Do breastfeeding and delayed introduction of solid foods protect against subsequent atopic eczema? *J Pediatr* 1981;98:546.
59. Taylor B, Wadsworth M, Wadsworth J, Peckham C. Changes in the reported prevalence of childhood eczema since the 1939–45 war. *Lancet* 1984;ii:1255–7.
60. Van Asperen PP, Kemp AS, Mellis CM. Relationship of diet in the development of atopy in infancy. *Clin Allergy* 1984;14:525–32.
61. Wahn U, Thiemeier M, Ganster G. Kuhmilchallergie bei Säuglingen und Kleinkindern. *Allergologie* 1984;10:361–3.
62. Wüthrich B, Hofer Th. Nahrungsmittelallergien. III. Therapie: Eliminationsdiät, symptomatische medikamentöse Prophylaxe und spezifische Hyposensibilisierung. *Schweiz Med Wochenschr* 1986;116:1401–10.
63. Darlath W. Zur Bedeutung des Mastzellmembranstabilisators Dinatrium cromoglicicum (DNCG) bei der Prophylaxe nutritiver Allergien. *Therapiewoche* 1983;33:3648–52.
64. Molkhou P, Waguet JC. Oral disodium cromoglycate in the treatment of atopic eczema in children. In: Pepys J, Edwards AM, eds. *The mast cell—its role in health and disease.* London: Pitman, 1979;617–8.
65. Braun-Falco O, Ring J. Zur Therapie des atopischen Ekzems. *Hautarzt* 1984;35:447–54.
66. Klaschka F. Hämatogenes Kontaktekzem durch Nahrungsmittel. *Allergologie* 1987 *(in press).*
67. Kaaber K, Veien NK, Tjell JC. Low nickel diet in the treatment of patients with chronic nickel dermatitis. *Br J Dermatol* 1978;58:197.
68. Przybilla B, Ring J, Schwab U, Dorn M. Nichtsteroidale Antirheumatika mit photosensibilisierender Wirkung. *Allergologie* 1986;9:8–15.
69. Doherty M, Barry RE. Gluten-induced mucosal changes in subjects without overt small bowel disease. *Lancet* 1981;i:517.
70. Katz SI, Strober W. The pathogenesis of dermatitis herpetiformis. *J Invest Dermatol* 1978;70:63–75.
71. Leonard J, Fry L. Dermatitis herpetiformis. In: Brostoff J, Challacombe StJ, eds. *Food allergy and intolerance.* London: Baillière Tindall, 1986:618–32.
72. Reunala T, Salo OP. Effects of long term gluten free diet in dermatitis herpetiformis. In: Kukita A, Seiji M, eds. *Proceedings of the XVIth International Congress of Dermatology.* Tokyo: University of Tokyo Press, 1983:411–3.
73. Wolff HH, Scherer R. Allergic vasculitis. In: Ring J, Burg G, eds. *New trends in allergy.* Berlin: Springer, 1981:140.
74. Ancona GR, Ellerhorn MJ, Falconer EH. Purpura due to food sensitivity. *J Allergy* 1951;22:487–93.
75. Eisenmann A, Ring J, von der Helm D, Meurer M, Braun-Falco O. Vasculitis allergica durch Nahrungsmittelallergie. *Hautarzt* 1987 *(in press).*

76. Kubba R, Champion RH. Anaphylactoid purpura caused by tartrazine and benzoate. *Br J Dermatol* 1975;93(suppl 11):61–2.
77. Michaelsson G, Petterson L, Juhlin L. Purpura caused by food and drug additives. *Arch Dermatol* 1974;109:49–52.
78. Ruzicka T, Ring J, Braun-Falco O. Vaskulitis allergica durch Vitamin B6. *Hautarzt* 1984;35:197–9.
79. Winkelmann RK. Food sensitivity and urticaria or vasculitis. In: Brostoff J, Challacombe StJ, eds. *Food allergy and intolerance.* London: Baillière Tindall, 1986:602–17.
80. Lehner T. Immunological aspects of recurrent oral ulceration and Behcet's syndrome. *J Oral Pathol* 1978;7:424–30.
81. Ring J. Das "klinische Okologie-Syndrom": Polysomatische Beschwerden bei subjektiver Nahrungsmittelallergie gegen Umweltschadstoffe. In: Braun-Falco O, Schill WB, eds. *Fortschritt der praktisch Dermatolologische und Venerolologische XI,* Berlin: Springer, 1987:434–6.
82. American Academy of Allergy. Position statement controversial techniques. *J Allergy Clin Immunol* 1981;67:333–8.
83. Breneman JC, Hurst A, Heiner D, Leney FL, Morris D, Josephson BM. Final report of the Food Allergy Committee of the American College of Allergists on the clinical evaluation of sublingual provocative testing method for diagnosis of food allergy. *Ann Allergy* 1984;33:164.
84. Nixon PGF. "Total allergy syndrome" or fluctuating hypocarbia? *Lancet* 1982;i:406.
85. Pearson DJ, Rix KJB, Bentley SJ. Food allergy: How much in the mind? A clinical and psychiatric study of suspected food hypersensitivity. *Lancet* 1983;ii:1259–61.
86. Reimann HJ, Ring J, Wendt P, Lorenz R, Ultsch B, Swoboda K, Blümel G. Der histaminstoffwechsel des Magens bei Patienten mit Nahrungsmittelallergie. *Verh Dtsch Ges Inn Med* 1981;87:823–6.
87. Reimann HJ, Ring J, Ultsch B, Wendt P. Intragastral provocation under endoscopic control (IPEC) in food allergy: mast cell and histamine changes in gastric mucosa. *Clin Allergy* 1985;15:195–202.

DISCUSSION

Dr. Shmerling: When looking for local reactions, is it really necessary to go as far as the stomach? What about the buccal mucosa?

Dr. Ring: There is a lot of controversy about sublingual testing, and the American Academy of Allergy has bluntly stated that this method does not work. I think, however, that you have to differentiate between people whose primary symptoms originate in the mouth, who may be challenged in the mouth, and those with diarrhea or urticaria, in whom you must go to the stomach.

Dr. Guesry: You spoke of reactions to iodine, bromine, and nickel, probably acting through the formation of haptens. Could you enlarge on the mechanism of sensitization by this type of allergen, in contrast to protein allergens? Is there a difference?

Dr. Ring: The mechanism of sensitization is certainly different for these different types of reaction. Iododerma is probably not an allergic response, and there is no obvious immunologic mechanism. Nickel sensitivity is a Type-IV allergic response. It is usually thought, though I do not know on what basis, that nickel is coupled to a protein in the epidermis which acts as carrier protein, transporting it to the Langerhans cells which mediate sensitization to the T-lymphocytes. There are some recent studies which suggest that the nickel molecule coming in contact with the HLA-DR molecule on the surface of the antigen-presenting cell produces a change in the class-II molecule conformation giving the signal for antigen presentation. This is very speculative. What happens when you eat nickel and how it comes to the skin nobody knows.

Dr. Urbanek: We were told by Dr. Frick about increased reactivity in the lungs after food ingestion. Are there any methods for *in vitro* or *in vivo* testing for hyperreactivity of the skin? You said that in some cases there may be a low threshold for reaction to some antigens.

Dr. Ring: This is a matter of current study. It certainly should be possible to test for the postprandial forms of urticaria and anaphylaxis, which show up clearly, using skin-test titrations before and after food challenge. I did not mention urticaria factitia, often thought to have a psychological basis, where striking the skin results in a wheal. Many people with this condition have underlying allergies, suggesting it is not entirely psychological. Perhaps this could form the basis of a test in such patients: dermatographism before and after food challenge!

Dr. Schmitz: You said that eczema might be triggered by itching alone. What, then, provokes the itching in the first place?

Dr. Ring: There are many mediators of itch, including histamine of course, and not all of them are chemical; for example, dry skin per se is a stimulus for itch. In allergy, the release of mediators can be a stimulus.

Dr. Aas: Itch is a very important feature of atopic eczema, and someone once said that eczema is not an eruption with an itch, it is itch with an eruption. It is also a feature of a positive Prausnitz-Küstner test. You can titrate the P-K reaction either with serial dilutions of donor serum or with dilutions of the offending agent and in this way determine, to some extent, the size of the reaction. At the start of any positive reaction you get an itch, up to 5 min before the visible response, though of course the perception of itch is very much determined by the psychological state of the recipient at the time. However, you can also titrate so that you don't get a positive reaction, only an itch. My question touches upon the question of mediators and of whether there are a lot of immunologic and nonimmunologic subthreshold triggers in eczema, among which may be food allergens. It is this: Do you ever try to get an impression of the amount of itch in these patients? I think that the itch is one of the great mysteries in eczema. Some patients with atopic eczema may have a very slight eruption but a tremendous itch, and vice versa.

Dr. Ring: Studies have been done to try to titrate the itch response to different stimuli, and from these it appears that in atopic eczema there is an increased itch response to a particular stimulus, i.e., a reduced itch threshold. However, it is very hard to quantitate itch. We are currently trying out an ''itchometer,'' an itch-watch developed in Newcastle, UK, by Drs. Chadwick and Shuster. This instrument measures the movement of the limbs during the scratch response at night and is at least an attempt at an objective measurement.

Dr. Bellanti: There are observations to suggest that leukocytes in patients with atopic dermatitis have a higher spontaneous release of histamine than normal. We reported a study a few years back in which we injected food antigen into patients and provoked symptoms which were associated with elevated plasma histamine. I have often wondered about this as a possible provocation test. Would it not make sense to bypass the gastrointestinal tract and thus remove one source of variability. One could then titrate a plasma histamine response or a symptom response using carefully selected and quantifiable materials.

Dr. Ring: I agree with you. We also found increased histamine releasability patterns in patients with atopic eczema and sometimes found increased plasma histamine levels. However, one of the big problems we have at the moment is a provocation test for atopic eczema. I was therefore very excited by Mitchell and Platts-Mills' article in which they were able to provoke eczematous lesions on the back by topical contact with extracts of house dust mite (1). Unfortunately we have not yet been able to reproduce this finding, although it is possible that there are technical and galenic difficulties. This problem has certainly not yet been solved.

DISCUSSION REFERENCE

1. Mitchell EB, Crow J, Williams G, and Platts-Mills TA. Increase in skin mast cells following chronic house dust mite exposure. *Br J Dermatol* 1986;114(1):65–73.

Subject Index